The Definitive Yoga User's Manual
For
Yoga Teachers and Students

The
Injury-Free
Yoga
Practice

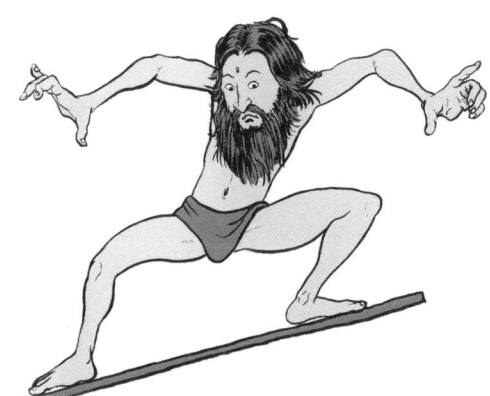

How *NOT* to Get Hurt Doing Yoga!

For purchase, comments, and workshop information, go to:
InjuryFreeYogaPractice.com

© Align by Design Yoga, 2013.

All rights reserved. No part of this publication, The Injury-Free Yoga Practice™, may be reproduced, stored in a retrieval system, or transmitted in any way or by any means electronic, mechanical, photocopying, recording or otherwise, without the prior written permission of the copyright holder, Align By Design Yoga™.

The Injury-Free Yoga Practice™

ISBN: 978-0-9893272-0-6

Published by: Steven Weiss and Align By Design Yoga™
Printed by: Manatee Printers, Inc. Bradenton, FL
Editing Staff:
    Debra Gitterman
    Esther Veltheim
    Ronni Geist, GeistWriters
Design:
    Cliff Berry
    Ronni Geist, Geistwriters
    Carol Weiss
Illustrations:
    Ben Schikowitz
Photography
    Walter Fritz
    Steven Weiss
    Esther Veltheim
    Carol Weiss
Front cover model:
    Jaye Martin

To purchase additional copies of The Injury-Free Yoga Practice™, please visit:

InjuryFreeYogaPractice.com or **AlignByDesignYoga.com**

Dr. Weiss presents the material covered in this book through workshops, seminars, yoga teacher trainings, and chiropractic continuing education. Contact Dr. Weiss through the website, AlignByDesignYoga.com, to inquire about upcoming presentations or to arrange a program. Also, "like" us on FaceBook!

In the unspoken language of the human body,

anatomy is the vocabulary,

alignment is the grammar.

And yoga

becomes poetry.

Steven Weiss

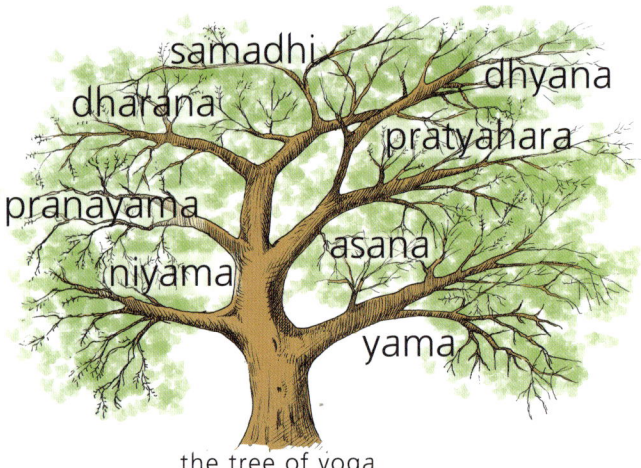

the tree of yoga

As you set up your mat and props for your morning practice, how do you know what the outcome of that practice will be?

- Will your yoga practice finally relieve your persistent back pain or will it make it worse?
- Will some other injury occur in the next hour as you go through your asana routine?

So, how do you know? Can you trust the teacher's instructions to protect you? Are you able to confidently rely on the knowledge you have slowly gathered over years of practice?

This book presents all the principles of yoga alignment necessary for a safe, healthy practice and therapeutic tools to help rehabilitate and restore existing injuries. It explains the underlying anatomy that is the rationale for alignment and how it is applied. You will have all you need to wisely direct and bring self-confidence to your practice.

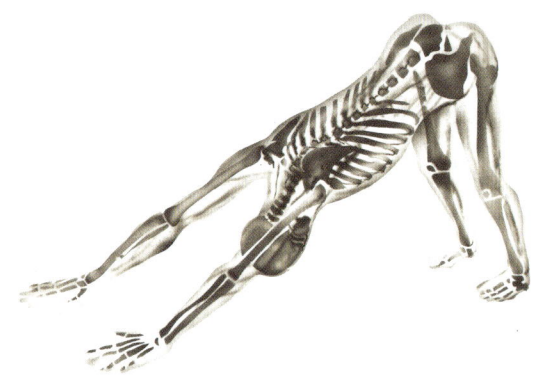

Table of Contents

Preface		1
Introduction		3
Chapter 1	**Yoga and Alignment**	5
	Sthira Sukham Asanam	6
	Hatha	6
	Yoga Asana – an "alignment delivery system"	7
Chapter 2	**Alignment and the Body Systems**	9
	The nervous system	10
	Muscle fibers and myofascia	10
	Body mechanics	10
	Bone density	11
	General Adaptation Syndrome	11
	Wellbeing	11
	Tissue repair and healing	12
	The energetic body	12
Chapter 3	**Raja Principles of Yoga**	13
	Yamas		14
	Ahimsa	Doing no harm	15
	Asteya	Non-stealing	15
	Satya	Truth and wisdom	15
	Brahmacharya	Avoiding unnecessary energy use	15
	Aparigraha	Non-possessiveness	16
	Niyama	Basic life skills and practices	16
	Shaucha	Cleanliness of body and mind	16
	Santosha	Contentment	16
	Tapas	Austerity and endurance	17
	Svadhyaya	Spiritual study and awareness of life	17
	Ishvarapranidhana	Surrendering to universal wisdom	17

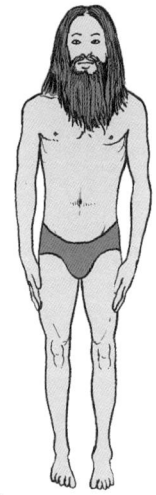
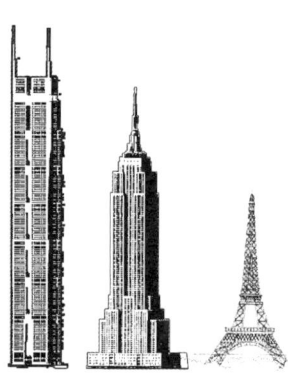

Chapter 4	**Foundations and Orientations of the Hips**	**19**
	Foundations provide freedom	19
	Examples of foundations of the body	20
	Open and closed hips	20
	"There can only be one…"	21
	Engaging open or closed-hip poses	21
	Exceptions to the rule	22
	Linking poses into a flow	22
	Examples of postures in each category of hip orientation	22
Chapter 5	**Integrative Alignment**	**23**
	Hatha's ultimate balance	24
	Interdependence	24
	Human architecture	25
	"First there is a mountain..."	25
	The "baby bear" intention	26
	What is the "just right" effort?	26
	Initiate movement from regions of least mobility	26
	Taking a mobility inventory	27
	The hierarchy of the twist	27
	Hypermobility	28
	Convex vs. concave	28
	The periphery of the body moves faster than at the core	29
	Bones approximate, muscles extend	29
	The center is best	30
	Stretching tips	30
	The quality of Samasthiti	31
	Samasthiti – beyond balance	31
	Moving with Samasthiti	32
	Identifying strengths and weaknesses	33
	Heyam Dukham Anagatam	33

Chapter 6	**Form Follows Function**	**35**
	Stretching	36
	Diaphragms	37
	Aligning diaphragms along the central axis	37
	Follow the curve	38
	Confusion about curves	39
	Using the curves in asana practice	40

Chapter 7	**Anatomy and Physiology – Connective Tissue**	**41**
	Know your medium	41
	Components of connective tissue	42
	Ground substance	43
	Fibers of connective tissue – Collagen	43
	Fibers of connective tissue – Elastin, Reticular	44
	Fascia	44
	Myofascia	45
	Tendons	45
	Tendonitis	45
	Bursas	46

Chapter 8	**Anatomy and Physiology – Ligaments**	**47**
	Micro-pleating action of the ligaments	48
	Wrapping action	48
	How ligament action works	48
	Taking the heat	49
	A little goes a long way	49
	"Two out of three ain't bad!"	50

Chapter 9	**Anatomy and Physiology – Muscle**	**53**
	Anatomy of a muscle	54
	The sarcomere	54
	Stretching is forever	55
	The 10% rule	55
	Speed, time and heat	56
	Scar tissue	57
	Skin deep	57
	Potential for muscle efficiency	57
	The long and short of it	57
	Overstretching	58
	Mixing yoga with athletics...maybe!	58
	The stretch reflex	59
	Deep tendon and stretch reflexes	60
	Habituation	60
	Fast and slow twitch fibers	61
	Muscles and aging	62
	The value of yoga for aging muscles	62

Chapter 10	**Anatomy and Physiology – Cartilage and Bone**	**65**
	Cartilage	66
	Hyaline Cartilage	67
	Bone	67
	Bone Density	68
	Osteoporosis and Osteopenia	69
	Bone's absorptive qualities	69
	Bone re-modeling and the value of good posture	70
Chapter 11	**Align By Design**	**71**
	Need GPS?	72
	The Alignment Grid	72
	Simple triple "S" alignment (skull, scapulae, sacrum)	74
	Lock and Load: Step-by-step stabilization for alignment	74
	The floating ribs	75
	Design and function	75
	Scoop, Scoop, Draw in the Navel, Keeps the low back stable!	75
	Zip it!	76
	Beauty in its simplicity	76
	Just in case…	76
Chapter 12	**Anatomy of the Pelvis and Sacroiliac Joints**	**77**
	The acetabulum	78
	The "sitting" bones	79
	The pelvis rocks!	79
	Sacroiliac joints: the posterior joints of the pelvis	79
	Pubis symphysis: the anterior joint of the pelvis	80
	It's shocking!	80
	Sacroiliac function	81
	Trap door	81
	Open and shut case	81
	Insult and injury	82
	Sacral pump	83
	Something else to chew on	83
	Equator of the body - the sacrum-coccyx juncture	84

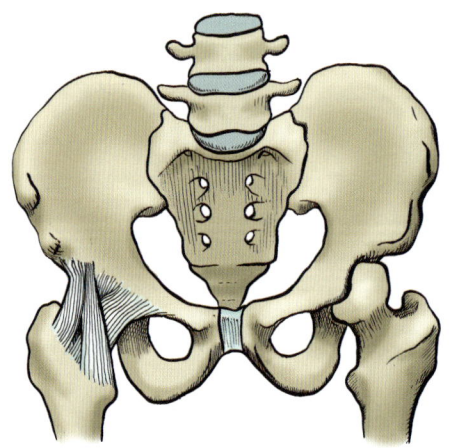

Chapter 13   **Pelvis and Sacroiliac Joints – Alignment Principles**   **85**

    Move from the Mula   86
    Pelvic integrative alignment   87
    Step one - Inward hip release   87
    Step two - Forward tailbone scoop   87
    Baddha Konasana and the bruised sacroiliac joint   88
    Causes of sacroiliac injuries   88
    Evaluating the function of the sacroiliac joints   89
    Marching in place   89
    Observing the sway   90
    Sacroiliac Therapeutics   91
    Therapeutic Supportive Bridge: Setu Bandha   91
    Asana that open fixated sacroiliac joints   92
    Twists when the sacroiliac joints are unstable   93
    Asana and yoga therapy for stabilizing open sacroiliac joints   93

Chapter 14   **Integrative Alignment of the Pelvis**   **95**

    Inward Hip Release   96
    Major anatomical effects of inward hip release   96
    Forward tailbone scoop   97
    Finding the sweet spot   98
    The Human Pez® dispenser   98
    Backward Butt Walking   100

Chapter 15   **The Middle Way**   **101**

    Lower rib cage integration   102
    Method to engage lower rib cage integration   102
    Visualizing lower rib cage integration   102
    Scoop the breastbone, Scoop the tailbone, Draw in the navel   103
    Paired actions   104

Chapter 16   **The Alignment of Sitting**   **105**

Chapter 17   **The Hip Joint**   **107**

    Are you *hip* to this?   107
    How far apart are the feet when spaced hip-width apart?   108
    A snug fit   108
    The swing of things   109
    Hips move in three axes of motion   109
    Mind the gap   109
    Avoid the pinch   110
    Hips in action   110
    In an externally biased world, internal rotation is highly valued   112

Chapter 18	**Hip Extension**	**113**
	Limited range of motion	114
	Experiencing the limits of hip extension	114
	Limited hip extension causes lumbar spine injury	115
	Muscles of hip extension	116
	Quadriceps stretch	116
	Iliopsoas muscle stretch	117
	Extenuating circumstances	117
	Why thigh muscles are massive and tend toward inflexibility	118
	Hip extension and the anterior pelvis	118
Chapter 19	**Alignment of the Legs**	**119**
	General alignment of the legs	120
	The Q-angle	121
	Compensation for a large Q-angle	121
	The specifics of leg alignment	121
	Shins forward-thighs back	122
	Shins in-thighs apart	122
	Lengthwise contraction	123
	Are you pulling my leg?	123
	Roman sandal strapping	123
	Asana Explorations	124
	Reciprocal inhibition	126
	Co-activation	127
	Need a lift?	128
Chapter 20	**The Hamstring Muscles**	**129**
	More ham, less string - muscle to tendon ratio	130
	The function of the hamstring	130
	Basic anatomy of the hamstring muscles	139
	Semimembranosus	130
	Semitendinosus	131
	Biceps femoris, long and short head	131
	Why do tight hamstring muscles cause back pain?	132
	Tips and refinements for the hamstring muscles	132
	Extend the hips, not the knee	133
	Uttanasana - a two-stage strategy	133
	Sitting hamstring stretch	134
	"The poison is the cure"	134
	Rehabilitative stretching of the hamstrings	135
Chapter 21	**Knee Alignment Principles**	**137**
	The muscles of the knees	138
	Extension	139
	Rotation	139
	Knee injury statistics	139
	Vulnerable knee positions	139
	Meniscus- the cartilage of the knee	140
	Roll and glide	140
	Ligaments of the knee - strips and crosses	141

	Hyperextension and the posterior cruciate ligaments	142
	Into the fold	142
	Detailed instructions for knee alignment in asana	143
	The Squat	143
	Meniscus therapy	144
	"X" and "O"	144
	Valgus/varus therapy	145
	Tibial torsion	146
	The patella	147
	Baker's cyst	147
	"Don't it always seem to go…"	148
Chapter 22	**The Ankle**	**149**
	The talus joint	150
	Inverted "T"	150
	Details of ankle alignment while standing	150
	No wrinkles!	151
	The powerful calf muscles	151
	Using accessory muscles to reduce foot sickling	151
	Ankle ligaments	152
	Sprain has sprung	152
	RICE, plus	153
	General guidelines for soft tissue healing response	153
	Ankle support	153
	Collapsed talus joint and foot pronation	154
Chapter 23	**The Feet**	**155**
	No wheelies, please!	156
	Integrative alignment of the foot	156
	Muscles of the arches	156
	How the feet remotely control posture	157
	Additional details on foot mechanics	158
	"Don't stand so close to me"	158
	Eversion and inversion	159
	Plantar fasciitis	159
	Plantar fasciitis rehabilitation	160
	Bunions	160
	Twist walking	162
	The high arch	162

Chapter 24	**Anatomy of the Spine**	**163**
	Architecture of a vertebra	164
	The Disc	165
	Rupture, herniation, bulge	165
	Shear madness	166
	Back pain - mechanical or chemical?	166
	Esoteric qualities can heal disc injuries	166
	Breathless in yogasana	167
	How many movements can the spine make?	168
	Independent facet movement	169
	Hypermobility, clicks and cracks	169
	Yoga - the cause or the cure	169
	The "Dead Zone"	170
	Changes in spinal curves throughout life	170
	Scoliosis - dangerous curves ahead	171
	Scoliosis and mobility	172
	Vital yogic principles for scoliosis	172
	Scoliosis and yoga therapy	173
	Mapping out the spine	173
	Imbalanced spinal mobility	174
Chapter 25	**The Lumbar Spine**	**175**
	Motion of the lumbar spine	176
	The ilio-lumbar ligaments	176
	Happy baby, indeed!	176
	Stiff, or not stiff? That is the question!	177
	Spinal stenosis	177
	When to surrender	178
	Tip of the pelvis, wag of the spine	179
	Don't crush the egg!	180
	The Abdominal Obliques	180
	Keep the spine straight when twisting	181
	The "black hole" of the belly	181
	Spondylolisthesis	182
	Sciatica	183
	Muscle-related back pain	184
	Move gently out of backbends	184
Chapter 26	**Yoga Butt**	**185**
	Springing into action	186
	Pain in the yoga butt	186
	The Righting reflex	187
	Steps to reduce yoga butt posture	188

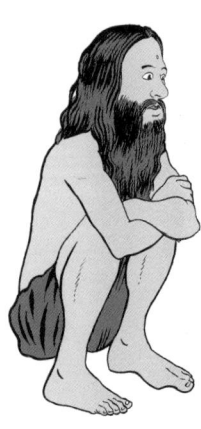

Chapter 27	**The Psoas muscle**	**189**
	Iliopsoas	190
	The elusive psoas	191
	The dual nature of the psoas	191
	Psoas strength in asana	192
	Anterior pelvic tilt, inward hip release and psoas stretching	192
	Hamstring muscles and the psoas	193
	A short, tight psoas muscle	193
	Psoas stretch increases sacroiliac joint mobility	194
	Asana for psoas stretching	194
	The psoas and the abdominal organs	195
	What is the sound of one hip snapping?	195
	Iliopsoas muscle stretch	195
Chapter 28	**The Thoracic Spine**	**197**
	Range of motion in the thoracic spine	198
	The rib cage	198
	The 12th thoracic vertebra	199
	Moving the thoracic spine	199
	Kyphosis - the rounded back	200
	The flat thoracic curve	200
	Chest integration	201
	See-saw rib cage	201
	Rounding the upper back? Not on my watch!	201
	"What is round will roll!"	202
	And, one more thing…	202
Chapter 29	**The Breath and the Bandhas**	**203**
	The diaphragm	204
	The diaphragm during respiration	204
	Diaphragm expiration	205
	Protruding lower ribs	205
	Effective diaphragm engagement	206
	The abdominals	206
	Paradoxical respiration	207
	Nose breathing	207
	Mouth breathing and stress	208
	The heart of the yogi	208
	Blood pressure and yoga	209
	Advanced yogic breathing techniques	209
	Basic three-part breath	210
	Alternate nostril breathing	210
	Holding the breath – Kumbhaka	211
	The Bandhas	211
	Bandhas, from an anatomical point of view	212
	Ujjayi Pranayama - the victorious breath	212
	How loud is the Ujjayi call to victory?	213
	The Valsalva Effect and breath	213
	Back off the bandha!	213

Chapter 30 Shoulder Anatomy 215

Shoulder mobility 216
Mechanical components of the shoulder 216
The gleno-humeral joint 217
Comparing the hip and shoulder "sockets" 217
Biceps tendon 218
Clearance requires external rotation 218
Shoulder dislocation 219
The clavicle and its two joints 219
Not a fashion statement! 219
The acromio-clavicular joint 220
The sterno-clavicular joint 220
The scapulo-thoracic "joint" 221
The scapula - fun facts 221
Where go the palms, so go the shoulder blades 222
Keep your angel wings folded in! 222
Shoulder compensations 223
The serratus anterior 223
Challenges of the serratus anterior 223
The rotator cuff 224
Actions of the rotator cuff 225
Rotator cuff injury 225

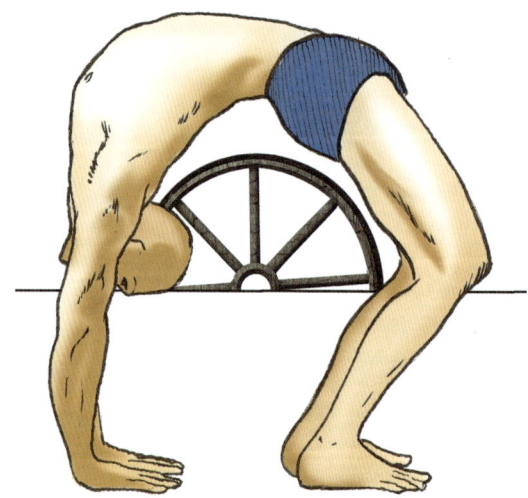

Chapter 31	**Integrative Alignment of the Shoulders**	**227**
	Rules of engagement	228
	Postural pre-requisites for shoulder integrative alignment	228
	Integrative Alignment of the Shoulders	228
	Asana for shoulder alignment exploration	231
Chapter 32	**The Upper Extremities**	**233**
	Out on a limb	233
	Pre-requisites for upper extremity principles	234
	Move from the core, using the shortest levers	234
	Bones draw to the midline, muscles extend out	234
	Triceps muscle rotates toward the midline	234
	Use the triceps muscle to extend the elbow	235
	Samasthiti - equal tension and balance	235
	The elbow	236
	Elbow flexion	236
	Elbow extension	236
	Hyperextension of the elbow	237
	The "eyes" of the elbows	237
	The forearm	237
	Upper extremity alignment	238
	Ventral forearm (palm-side) and wrist move posterior	238
	Middle fingers in line with the seam of pants	238
	Arm counter-rotation provides stability	238
	Arm alignment with the side body ribs	239
	How wide apart are the arms in arm-balancing poses?	239
	Carrying Angle	240
	Carrying on with the carrying angle	240
Chapter 33	**The Wrists and Hands**	**241**
	Wrist and hand relationship	242
	Wrist wrap	243
	Arch of the palm	243
	Weight bearing alignment of the hand	244
	Additional refinements in hand placement	244
	Keep the foundation stable	244
	Spider-fingers	244
	Flexion of the wrist	245
	Wrist extension - less than you think	245
	Carpal Tunnel Syndrome	246
	Sphinx Pose	248
	"Popeye™ arms" therapy	248

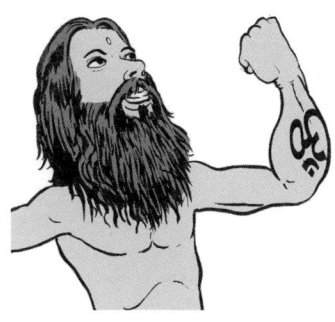

| Chapter 34 | **The Head and Neck** | **249** |

	A balancing act	250
	The cervical spine	250
	Atlas, the first cervical vertebra (C1)	250
	The axis (C2)	250
	The anterior compartment of the neck	251
	Can you see the collarbones?	251
	Foundation for the head and neck	251
	Head and neck posture	251
	Head games	251
	Managing the cervical curve	252
	Cervical spine instability	253
	Hypermobility	253
	Is Headstand safe?	253
	Alignment	254
	Where is the head placed for Sirsasana One?	255
	Considerations for the Headstand	255
	Musculature of the neck	256
	The hyoid bone	256
	Hyoid alignment - the smiling throat of Buddha	257
	How to move the neck	257
	How to align the head	258
	Therapeutic movements of the neck	258
	Easy on the eyes	259
	Using an eye pillow for Savasana	259

Footnotes and References   **261**

Photographic Acknowledgments   **268**

Acknowledgements   **271**

About the author   **272**

About the illustrator   **272**

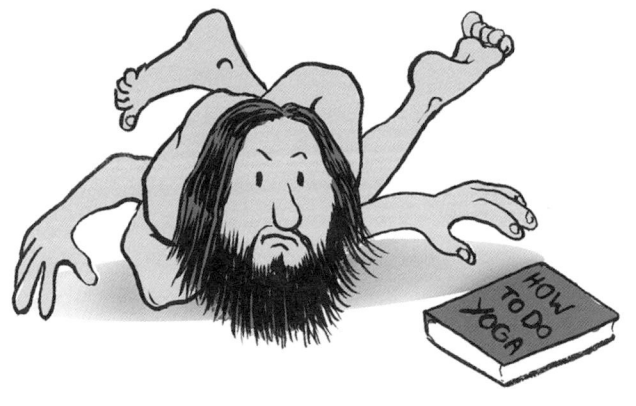

Preface

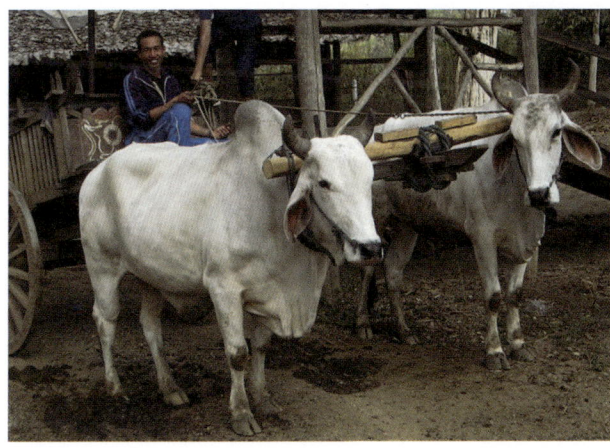

The word *yoga* derives from the Sanskrit term for the yoke that joins the two oxen of an ox cart. In yoga, one ox is the body, the other is the mind. The yoke represents awareness, or consciousness, that binds body and mind in an intimate, dependent relationship. Spirit is the driver, hopefully a compassionate driver who respects the nature of the forces it controls. It is the yoking of body and mind through awareness that produces well-being and safety in action. This allows spirit to achieve serenity and profound satisfaction, in other words, bliss.

Totalism, the theory that to know anything you must know everything, applies to yoga as much as it does to driving a car. When driving an automobile, you cannot know merely how to steer or brake or use turn signals. You must know everything, even if you learn one skill at a time. So it is with yoga asana. There are many steps to creating a yoga posture. It may take many months, perhaps even years, to learn all of the alignment principles and their nuances. This is why yoga is a practice. It requires patience and awareness and, most of all, humility.

Anatomy is another field filled with nuance. To understand anatomy, the subtleties of each structure must be uncovered and each relationship identified and described in the greatest of detail. Anatomy is presented in this book to provide the underlying rationale for the principles of alignment. Many more details could be given for each anatomical topic touched on in this book, but that would detract from my purpose. You, the reader, are encouraged to explore for yourself outside of this text all topics about which you are curious. In this way you will discover specific points of interest and bring additional refinements to your yoga practice.

There are many cross-references and repetitions in this book, particularly where the anatomy and alignment of one section of the body cannot be understood without reviewing its relationship to other parts. Alignment principles often apply to multiple regions of the body and therefore need to be repeated for consistency and clarity.

This book reads more like a novel than a how-to book. I recommend that you start from the beginning and read to the end. Should the sections on anatomy and physiology become challenging, give them a cursory read and return to those chapters another time or as a reference as new material is presented.

What this book is and is not

The system of alignment presented in this book is not a ritualized set of instructions passed down from a specific yoga tradition. The alignment principles are based on the anatomical and mechanical properties of the body. Most anatomically-based alignment concepts for yoga practice evolved from the teachings of Sri B.K.S. Iyengar. Following in his footsteps, Anusara yoga crafted Iyengar's work into a popular, user-friendly system. I have been strongly influenced by the teachings of both of these traditions. But, to be clear, the tenets presented in this book do not contradict the teachings of any school or style of yoga and can be applied to all asana practices without exception. Understanding alignment principles benefits every style of practice and does not interfere with the artful and dynamic flow of any yoga tradition.

Exceptions make the rule

Not all variations and exceptions that exist in the human body can be discussed in this one text. If you sense that a particular recommendation does not apply to you or a particular situation, allow your personal experience to hold merit. Very little in this book, if anything, could be considered unsafe. When in doubt go slow and pay attention!

My hope is that you will begin this journey with a beginner's mind. Allow the slate to be blank, free of attachment to what you expect to find or personal beliefs that you hope to reinforce. If you are willing to let the material in this book unfold like a story from beginning to end, you will get the most benefit from your effort. If the ideas that you read ring true and resonate with your experiences, your yoga practice will powerfully transform.

Recognition of my teachers

Much of the information and many of the terms used in this book are compiled from ideas shared with me by countless yoga teachers, workshop leaders, and mentors. Although much original thought exists throughout these chapters, many of the concepts were developed by other creative and inspiring people. As stated earlier, the material collected from these brilliant teachers is not intended to endorse a specific yoga tradition. For the most part, yoga is an oral tradition, meant to evolve over time and be shared broadly amongst its practitioners. My hope is that this book demonstrates my respect for the original teachers, those known and unknown to me. I also hope I have expanded on their ideas in ways that will be inspiring to you, the reader.

Introduction

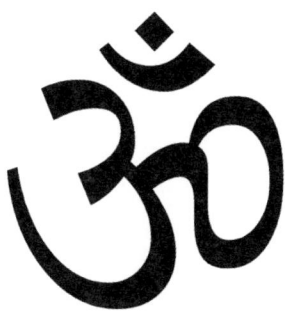

As this book unfolds, it is exciting for me to be on the other side of these printed words, anticipating the journey on which you, the reader, are embarking. In this book I share my observations made in more than thirty years of personal practice, research, and discovery. I explain how subtle shifts in alignment of the human frame can have profound effects on health and vitality. I see no greater privilege than having this opportunity to offer my findings to inquisitive, fellow yogis.

Much of this book is a compilation of the teachings of my mentors. The distinctive contribution I make to the growing body of knowledge about yoga comes from not only my experience as a yoga teacher and diligent practitioner, but also the unique perspective I bring as a holistic chiropractor and anatomy instructor. I have paid careful attention to all that I have viewed and palpated, studied and synthesized. As a chiropractor and yoga therapist, my approach has been to engage therapeutic bodywork with mindfulness and the skillful contact of Sparsa. Sparsa is the Sanskrit term for the place where Prana - life force - and the tissues of the body merge. My observation of countless human forms has impressed upon me not the wide range of our differences, but the remarkable similarities. These commonalities are clues and affirm that there is a single structural design and one set of alignment principles to apply to all asana.

The human body runs the gamut from individuals with rubber-like flexibility at one end to our stiffer brethren. In all of the variations in the human form that I have seen, one thing has been consistent: the powerful influence of structural alignment on the body. Alignment is central to the design of all things mechanical; the human body is no exception. Down to the cellular level, alignment organizes the very essence of what defines a living being.

Yoga has the potential to be one of the most sophisticated and empowering means of creating structural alignment in the body. Clearly alignment should not be an afterthought. Nor should it be considered a facet of advanced asana practice only. Alignment is essential at all levels of practice to ensure that asana are performed safely. In fact, yoga postures need not be overly advanced to be beneficial. The most basic postures are generally the most therapeutic, since they are the easiest ones in which to find precise alignment.

Practicing yoga can be either therapeutic or the cause of trauma. The postures themselves, are not inherently safe or dangerous. The outcome of yoga practice depends on one essential criterion: the successful application of alignment. Applying alignment to the final form of a pose, however, is not what makes asana safe and effective. It is all of the actions engaged from setting the posture's foundation at the start to applying the final tweaks at the end.

Alignment does not happen by simply rolling out the mat or buying the latest clothes. Downloading a soulful chant may open the heart but not the hips. Practicing yoga alignment takes effort. It requires a willingness to apply the principles of alignment with dedicated precision at all times.

Some practitioners mistake alignment for merely a mechanical action. On the contrary, the holistic principles that guide asana alignment originate in yoga philosophy. The ancient yogic teachings offer guidance in not only how to live spiritually, but also how elegance emerges from asana practice through alignment.

This book introduces a system called *Integrative Alignment*. As its name implies, Integrative Alignment organizes the alignment of each part of the body in relation to the whole. Integrative Alignment approaches the mechanical nature of the body, not as something fixed or static, but as a flowing coalescence of vectors of force and internal tensions.

Yoga's greatest teachers

A pilgrimage to the remote reaches of India will not bring us to the feet of our greatest yoga teachers, the ones who guide our daily asana practice. Those teachers are right here, residing within ourselves. *Pain* and *injury* are our greatest teachers. They are the *guru tattwa,* the inner teachers. Rather than something to be cursed, pain and injury are a part of ourselves that can open us to enlightenment and an empowered existence.

Injuries and pain inform alignment. When a posture is correctly aligned, pain abates. Thus, pain is a clear indicator of whether or not a pose is correctly aligned. When an injured area is exercised without producing pain, it heals at an accelerated rate. Without alignment, healing may not occur.

Some yoga traditions view the body as a temple in which the spirit lives. Caring for this exquisite physical form is a tribute to spirit, the humble act of "sweeping the temple floors". The responsibility of all yoga teachers, both our inner teachers and the ones at the front of the class, is to make asana practice a therapeutic and health-enhancing experience. The yogic path to greater awareness and higher consciousness needs to be free of hazards that cause physical injury. This book is offered in service of that intention for all of us who are on this spectacular, life-affirming journey called yoga.

1 Yoga and Alignment

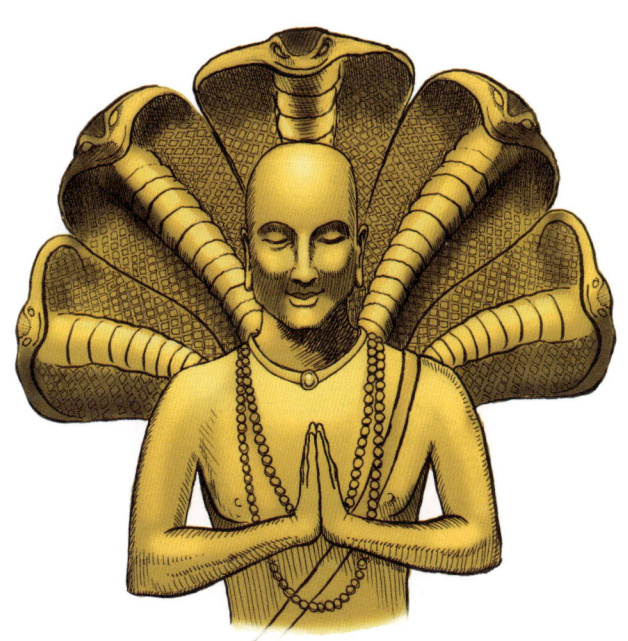

From its origins in South Asia nearly 5,000 years ago, yoga has emerged in the twenty-first century as the fastest growing practice for fitness and well-being in the world.[1,2] Yoga classes are offered alongside Pilates and kickboxing in practically every gym, school, and health club. Many of the principles of yoga, especially those regarding alignment, flexibility, and states of consciousness, are receiving high levels of acceptance and are now attracting researchers in the fields of science, medicine, and psychology.

The yoga studio has become a valuable center for personal growth and human potential. It is a place where students come together and co-create as a conscious community. The ancient philosophies of yoga offer wisdom that can help us navigate the overwhelming demands of modern culture in which we face the dual challenge of a life of material excess and spiritual disconnectedness. Together these two predicaments produce a state of deep and unconscious exhaustion. Yoga's growing popularity is a testament to its ability to remedy the accelerated pace of life, which has become today's norm.

In mainstream media and popular culture, yoga is often categorized as a sport. What makes yoga different from other physical exercise regimens, however, is the intention with which it is practiced. The 2,000-year-old text, the *Yoga Sutras of Patañjali,* provides guidance for the proper intention with which yoga is to be practiced. The "no-pain, no gain" sports mantra is replaced with "no pain, no pain" for the true devotee of yoga.

Of course we want yoga to be magical and filled with ageless wisdom. We expect it to be an all-inclusive, one-stop solution to the totality of life's problems. This desire is unrealistic. The good news, however, is that yoga reliably points a finger in the right direction to follow.[3]

Sthira Sukham Asanam

The physical practice of yoga is called *asana*. Asana comprises poses, or postures and how they are arranged. In Sanskrit, asana means sitting or the seat, referring to the posture or position that is taken. The Yoga Sutra, *Sthira Sukham Asanam*, suggests that the postures and the transitions between them are to be steady (*sthira*) and comfortable (*sukham*).

Hatha

In its most common usage, yoga refers to the practice of *Hatha*. Hatha is a system of yoga formulated nearly 500 years ago by Yogi Swatmarama in the text *Hatha Yoga Pradipika*. Most popular traditions of yoga practiced today have their origins in Hatha. From the Sanskrit terms *ha* meaning sun and *tha* meaning moon, Hatha strives to unify the energy of opposites, particularly those of body and mind.

Asana practice takes the student through a series of increasingly complex movements and forms. From a classical point of view, the purpose of these exercises is to help the yogi develop the ability to sit effortlessly for the long periods of time necessary for the practices of meditation and *Pranayama*.[4]

> Asana practice is an opportunity to discover, establish and maintain alignment as the body moves through increasingly complex movements and forms.

Sri B.K.S. Iyengar states, "Yoga practice is not only the preparation for spiritual awakening; the awakening is inherent in the practice itself."[5]

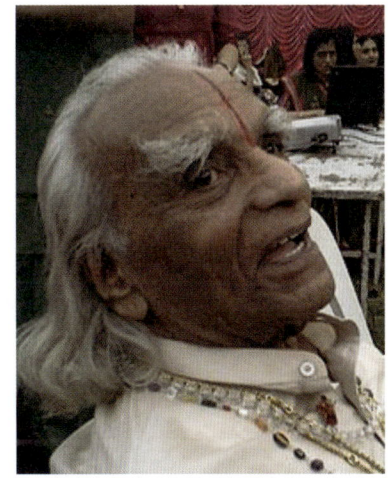

Iyengar regards the individual postures of asana as "archetypal templates." When the student aligns with precision to these forms, a connection to something greater than the posture is achieved. In Iyengar's terms, "Yoga is equanimity. Equanimity is alignment and without alignment there is no equanimity."[6]

Bringing an alignment component into the practice of yoga provides a tool for transforming asana from a simple floor exercise into a powerful mind-body experience.

Yoga Asana – an "alignment delivery system"

The title of this section may provoke a gasp or two from the yoga purist. Yogis often imbue asana practice with the spirituality of Vedic writings and inspirational poetry. Since humankind has yet to engage in a mass jettison of the material form, however, the primary focus of asana remains on developing the physical body.

There is nothing magical or divinely protective about yoga. The alchemy that many yogis experience as a result of their practice does not arise from something supernatural hidden in the form and shape of the poses themselves. Likewise, there is nothing inherently dangerous in the poses. The determinant for the ultimate outcome of asana is alignment and whether or not it has been integrated into the practice. The magic that emanates from asana arises from the power of healing that alignment innately unleashes.

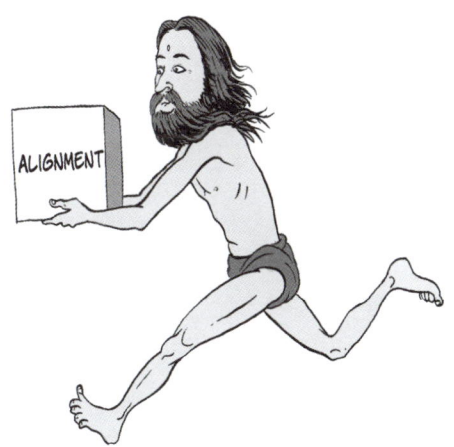

High achievement of human performance, such as being a concert pianist, ballet dancer or professional golfer, requires constant attention to the smallest details and to impeccable form. The appearance of effortlessness that these masters demonstrate results from implacable discipline and hard-earned adroitness.

> When asana is practiced with mindful awareness and with precise alignment, it has Zen-like elegance and refinement.

A mindful yoga practice adheres to the body's anatomical design, which reveals the underlying rationale for proper alignment. In this way, asana provides an elegant and sophisticated "alignment delivery system" for structural health and integration.

Yet yoga is not a panacea. Practicing asana can cause injury just as easily as it can heal. Orthopedists report increasing numbers of injuries directly attributable to the practice of yoga. A recent study by the Consumer Product Safety Commission revealed that common injuries caused by yoga include repetitive strain and soft tissue trauma resulting from overstretching. Joint injuries in the spine and extremities are commonly reported as well. The study also revealed increases in health care costs and a high number of therapeutic services directly attributable to injuries from yoga practice.[7]

Why should so many strains, tears, and compressive injures result from yoga practice? If by its nature yoga is a spiritual and health-restoring experience, it seems contradictory for it to be potentially dangerous. But not every yoga practice is created equal.

Favorable results from yoga depend on a yoga student's dedicated focus on alignment. Poorly aligned postures structurally compromise the body and are the cause of most yoga-related injuries. And yet, when yoga is practiced in coordination with anatomy and proper body mechanics, it is therapeutic and stimulates healing. Increased overall heath and well-being result from an aligned practice.

Still, some yoga practitioners are clearly reluctant to focus on alignment during their practice. They view their time on the mat as a sacred experience, believing that focus on alignment is antithetical to an intuitive and spiritual experience or makes asana practice overly intellectual. If one were to employ a guided-by-spirit, mind-*over*-body approach alone, asana practice would be insufficient and discordant with yoga's basic teachings. Doing so would override the precious and necessary skill of *listening to* the body. Yoga practice should be a seamless, reciprocating interplay between body and mind.

From personal experience, heightened spirituality has emerged as my awareness of alignment has grown. Having more open hips has brought a greater appreciation for life and my sense of wellbeing. My yoga practice became more sacred as my sacrum began to move with greater freedom.

2 Alignment and Body Systems

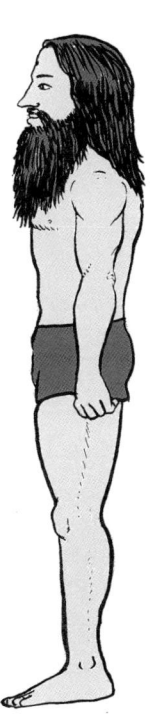

The body "loves" alignment. In addition to giving our yoga postures a more graceful appearance, alignment provides great benefits to our health and wellbeing. Our physiology is more efficient and performs more effectively when the body's many systems are aligned and integrated as a whole. This chapter presents some simple examples of the impact of alignment on a few systems of the body. It is a cursory review and the reader is encouraged to delve deeper into these and all aspects of anatomy whenever the opportunity presents itself.

The nervous system

The nervous system directly or indirectly influences every one of our forty quadrillion living cells. It facilitates communication throughout the body, from the large muscles and vital organs to the smallest capillaries. All of the body's mechanical and organic functions, as well as our sense of balance and spatial awareness, rely on direct feedback from the nervous system. A well-aligned spine is essential. With poor alignment, nerves become irritated or compressed, interfering with their healthy functioning and with the transmission of information from the central nervous system.

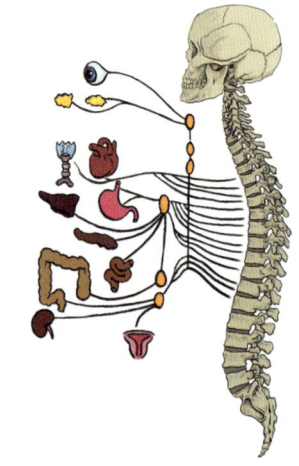

Muscle fibers and myofascia

Muscle contractions produce a force that crosses the joints they affect. Muscles are most efficient when their fibers align obliquely to the direction of that force. Good alignment allows muscles to function most effectively and to develop for optimal performance.

Myofascia, the collagen-rich sleeve of tissue that envelops every muscle fiber, is also sensitive to structural tension. Poor alignment can cause myofascia to torque, over time creating muscular distortions, reducing muscle efficiency, and increasing the potential for injury to muscles, tendons, ligaments, and joints. (See Chapter 9 for more on this topic)

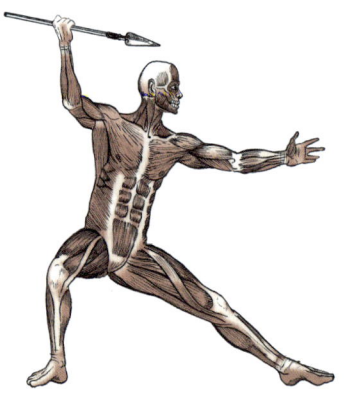

Body mechanics

The wide-ranging array of mechanical operations occurring simultaneously in the body depends on proper alignment in order to be effective. Body mechanics are most efficient when joints remain centered on their axes of rotation. This allows the greatest ease of motion. Proper alignment most effectively positions the body to carry the force and load of gravity.

In yoga, as in any exercise regimen, alignment and a stable foundation should be established before attempting to build strength, flexibility or agility. Developing muscle mass or skill sets upon a frame that is not aligned essentially reinforces the body's operation from a position of stress and creates inefficient habits that are likely to produce injury.

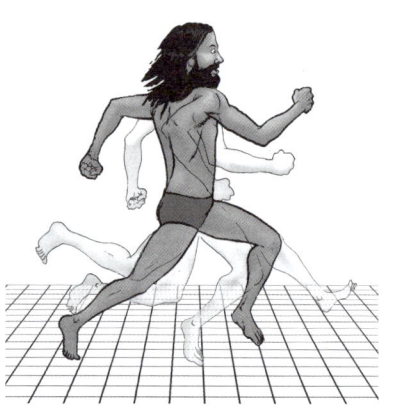

Bone density

The moving body is constantly countering the downward pressure of gravity and the upward force of heel strike. At the same time, bone is being stimulated by contractions of the muscles attached to its surfaces. Additionally, nerves located within the bones are delivering mild electrical stimulation to the many layers of bone tissue. All of these forces have a direct effect on bone density. Alignment attempts to equally distribute the impact of these various forces on bone in order to keep its density uniform.

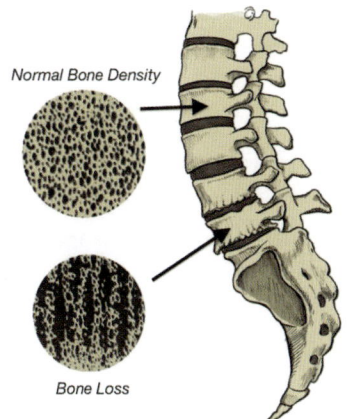

General Adaptation Syndrome

The work of Canadian Nobel Laureate Hans Selye, PhD., has shown that poor alignment is a *stressor* that triggers a bodily response called the *general adaptation syndrome*. In the presence of uncompensated postural imbalances or unchecked muscle tension, stress hormones flood the body. This stress response increases demand on the vascular and hormonal systems. Chronic poor alignment can lead to adrenal exhaustion and a weakened immune system, increasing the potential for disease processes to develop.

The stress response caused by chronic poor alignment is comparable to that of being in a prolonged state of falling backwards out of a chair.

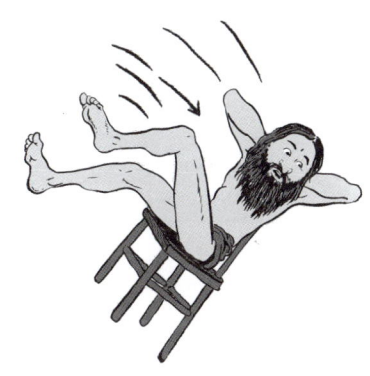

Wellbeing

Studies have shown that yoga increases levels of neurotransmitters such as endorphins that positively affect mood, improve self-confidence and increase life satisfaction.[1] Remarkably, these neurochemicals are present at higher concentrations in locations along the spine that correspond to the vortices (energy centers) of the chakra system.[2] Correct alignment increases the levels of neurotransmitters that produce the positive states of being, while poor posture and improper alignment release stress-triggering chemicals into the body.

Tissue repair and healing

Within the connective tissue of the body, alignment stimulates the repair of microscopic fibers and the formation of new cells. The close contact of cells that proper alignment fosters is essential to the healing process in structures such as skin, muscle, bone, spinal discs and fascia. Effective alignment lessens scar tissue formation, reduces inflammation and prevents degenerative changes.

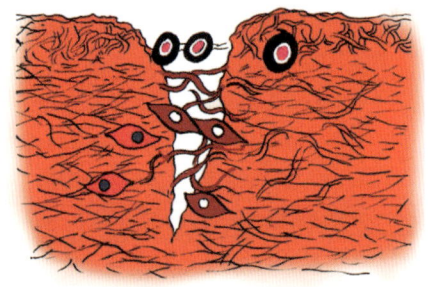

The energetic body

The ancient Sanskrit texts that comprise *The Vedas* (Books of Knowledge), describe a system of 72,000 rivers of energy called *nadis* whose channels run throughout the body transmitting the energy force of life, or *Prana*.

Unimpeded flow of Prana fosters health, vitality and healing. Proper alignment prevents *gunas* or knots from forming along the pranic channels and blocking the pranic flow.

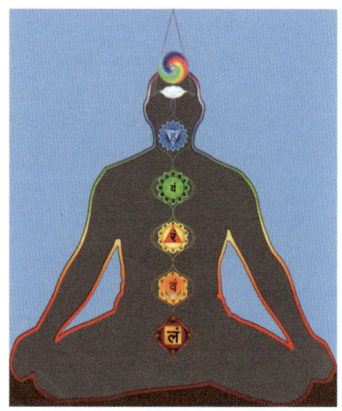

3 Raja Principles of Yoga

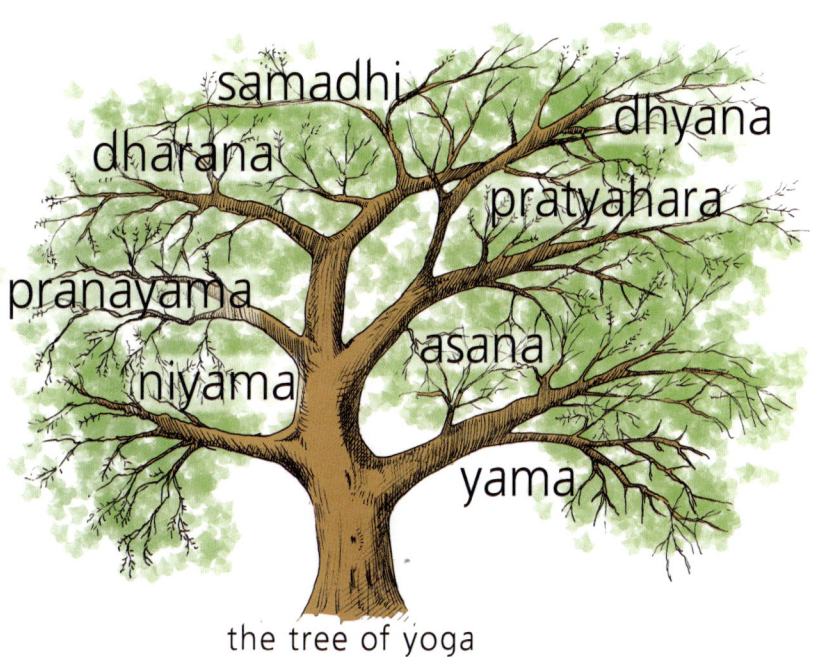

the tree of yoga

In the *Yoga Sutras of Patañjali,* yoga is portrayed as *Astañga,* meaning "eight limbs", in reference to a tree consisting of eight branches. The tree of yoga represents *Raja Yoga,* a "royal union" of practices that challenges the body and mind and puts the practitioner on a regimented path towards spiritual liberation. The yogi "climbs" this framework of ethical, physical and spiritual values, developing mastery in the practices represented by each limb. The ultimate goal is ascension to the top and to reaching *Samadhi,* a meditative state of complete wholeness.

Asana, the third limb from the bottom of the tree is the primary focus of this book. In order to practice asana in the true spirit of yoga, the student relies on the limbs below, *Yama and Niyama*, to serve as a foothold from where asana practice begins.

Yoga teacher Richard Freeman, in his book *Mirror of Yoga* states, "The support built from the first two limbs, the yamas and the niyamas, is an interactive net of kindness and responsiveness to both oneself and to others."[1]

Trauma-yama is not a limb on the tree of yoga!

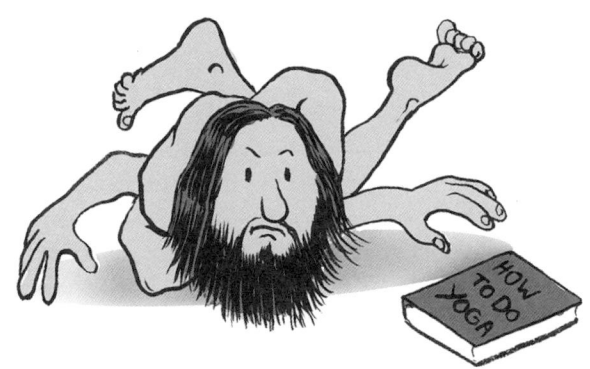

Yamas and Niyamas

Taken from the Sanskrit word for *death*, the first limb of the tree of yoga is *Yama*. The Yamas, according to Patañjali, are comprised of five restraints on behavior. This code of conduct details the "do not" rules for ethical interaction. The second limb, *Niyama*, delineates a set of life skills, observances and practices. The Niyamas establish a set of "to do" rules.

What makes asana practice different from other floor exercise programs is that asana is not merely a physical practice but belongs to a broader system dedicated to spiritual awareness. The principles of Yama and Niyama provide more than a series of ethical guidelines for how the yogi interacts with people and the world around them. Principles of Yama and Niyama are brought directly onto the mat and influence the physical asana postures themselves. Fully integrating Yama and Niyama principles into asana ensures safety and the therapeutic value of yoga practice. Following are the dictates of Yama and Niyama and how they specifically apply to asana practice.

Yamas — Restraints on behavior

- Ahimsa — Non-violence, non-harming
- Asteya — Non-stealing, non-claiming
- Satya — Truth, pureness, and wisdom
- Brahmacharya — Avoiding unnecessary expenditure of energy
- Aparigraha — Non-possessiveness, non-greed, releasing from the grasp of the ego

Ahimsa — Doing no harm, non-violence

Perhaps the most fundamental principle of yoga is to do no harm and remain non-violent. It is easy to understand how this principle applies to the treatment of fellow sentient beings. It is less obvious that it also applies to asana practice. Practicing with ahimsa, not harming oneself, requires knowing what is actually harmful. Many new yoga students, coming from a background of sports and exercise, bring with them a mindset of pushing beyond the limits of steadiness and comfort. It is not uncommon for a new yoga student, numb to the warning signs that they are creating injury, to force a pose.

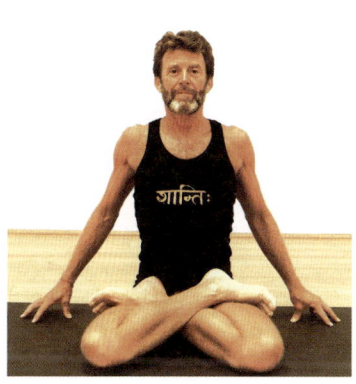

Ahimsa requires students to shift from working hard to "working smart". A smart practice is one that employs alignment and does not force joints beyond their current limits or stretches muscles further than they are capable. That is Ahimsa. Practicing yoga without alignment is dangerous and causes injury. Without exception!

Asteya — Non-stealing, non-claiming

When one region of the body does the work intended for another, it is, in a sense, a form of stealing. For example, a yoga student may have inadequate hip flexibility to correctly perform the Lotus Pose. They may, however, attempt the pose by exploiting the flexibility of the knees or ankles. This dangerously twists and torques the knees and ankles in order to claim completion of the pose.

Satya — Truth, pureness, and wisdom

Forced, poorly aligned asanas have no truth or pureness, nor do they demonstrate the wisdom of our being. They represent a falsity and karmic dishonesty. Satya however can be attained when asana is performed with safety and efficiency.

Brahmacharya — Avoiding unnecessary expenditure of energy

There are many ways to interpret this principle. The term literally means to sit in the chariot of Brahma, the Hindu god of creation. Practicing Brahmacharya is to rise above the machinations of life, taking a dispassionate view of the world and the trivial actions of the self. Applied to asana practice, Brahmacharya is the intention to re-apportion energy so it is not wasted. Practitioners learn to not over-effort and to remain efficient in every movement. The kinesiological term *muscle efficiency* - getting the most power from the least amount of energy - appears throughout this book and is a form of Brahmacharya. Alignment and integration are tools that ensure Brahmacharya in every aspect of asana practice.

Aparigraha   Non-possessiveness, non-greed, releasing the grasp of the ego

It is all too easy to unroll the yoga mat and immediately start comparing ourselves to our classmates. For some students, comparison triggers their competitive nature, and they forcefully go beyond their level of safety. For others, it may elicit the opposite reaction, producing sinking feelings of inadequacy and defeat. Although the ego can be powerfully motivating, it can also lead to actions that limit our potential or increase the likelihood of injury.

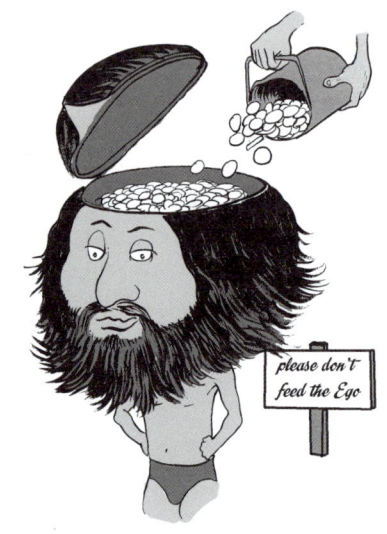

Niyama   Basic life skills and practices

- Shaucha   Cleanliness of body and mind, purity
- Santosha   Contentment in one's place and one's achievements
- Tapas   Austerity, endurance, building up "heat"
- Svadhyaya   Spiritual study and awareness of life
- Ishvarapranidhana   Love, respect and surrendering to the wisdom of the universe

Shaucha   Cleanliness of body and mind, purity

Shaucha can mean literally keeping the mat, props and practice space clean and orderly. This Zen-like discipline frees the mind of distractions. Those who have spent years folding blankets in Iyengar classes know well this form of Shaucha. Another example of Shaucha is the early morning practice of *Kriya* yoga, a ritual of cleansing and hygiene.

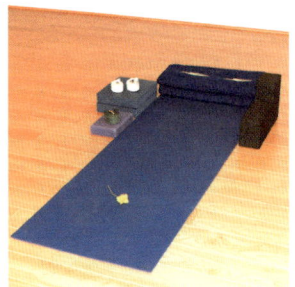

Santosha   Contentment in one's place and one's achievements

Santosha is finding peace and contentment during every practice, in every posture and in each moment. Santosha occurs when the yoga student acknowledges gratitude for what they are able to accomplish and for the privilege of having a life that provides the opportunity to include yoga practice.

Tapas   Austerity, endurance, building up "heat"

The quality of Tapas in asana practice is expressed by maintaining focus, passion and intensity.

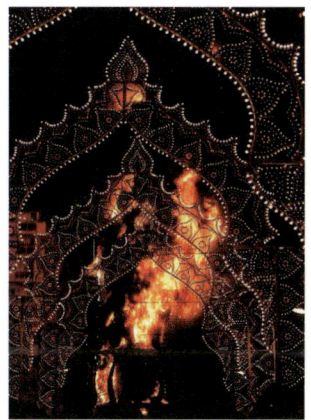

Svadhyaya   Spiritual study and awareness of life

Knowledge acquired from spiritual study can be applied to asana practice. The act of implementing Yama and Niyama principles in asana practice is the practice of Svadhyaya. Another form of Svadhyaya is developing the awareness and meaning of sensations the body emits during practice, from weakness and pain to power and pleasure.

Ishvarapranidhana   Love, respect and surrender to the universe's wisdom

To practice with deep respect and to surrender to both the endless challenges and the opportunities that asana offers demonstrates Ishvarapranidhana.

The yogi cultivates patience with and acceptance of the concept of *practice*, which, by its nature, is *never complete*, perhaps infinite. A further example of Ishvarapranidhana is establishing unyielding trust in the inner healing power of the body and the ability of asana to unleash it.

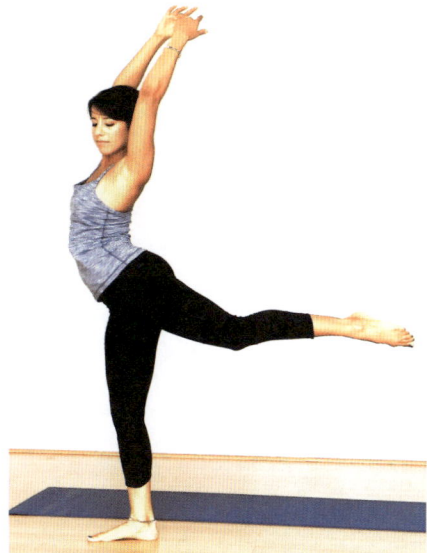

4 Foundations and Orientations of the Hips

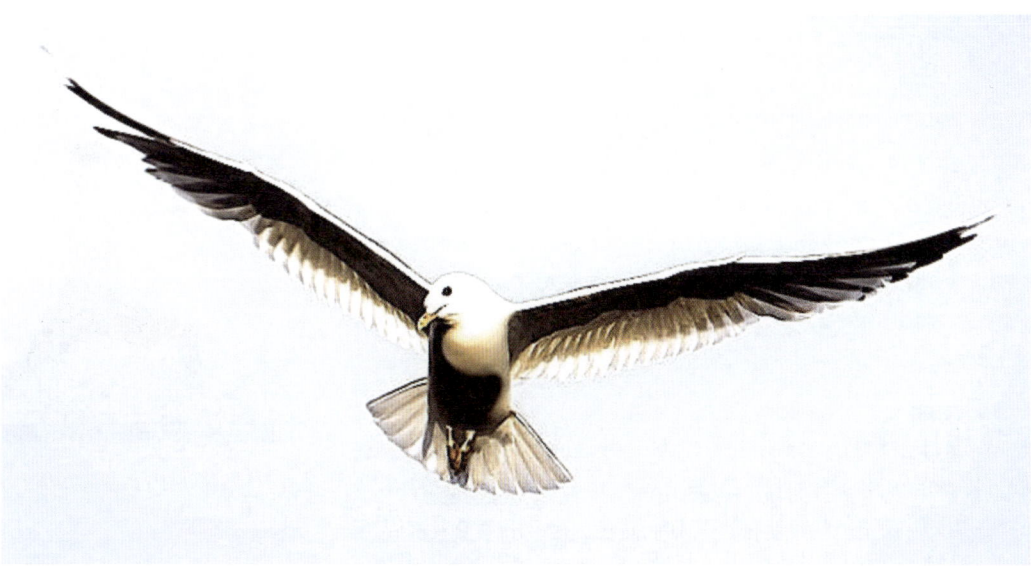

Foundations provide freedom

Many people are drawn to yoga for the sense of liberation it offers. Yoga can release the practitioner from rigidity in body, mind, and spirit. And yet, every asana requires a stable foundation. Asana, like the human spirit, flourishes when it remains grounded. Even birds use thermal pressures in the air as a foundation from which to soar.

Not always obvious in its outward appearance, every structure requires a stable foundation that holds firm and supports all that resides within. The architecture of the body contains multiple foundations. Beyond establishing the precise alignment of each foundation, it is important to integrate each foundation with all others and with the body as a whole. In the upcoming chapters of this book, specific instructions for establishing foundations will be presented in detail.

Examples of foundations of the body

- The feet set the foundation for the legs.
- The legs create the foundation for the pelvis.
- The pelvis forms the foundation for the lumbar spine.
- The shoulders and upper back provide the foundation for the neck.

Each yoga posture aligns one foundation over another to establish a stable, integrated structure. Should the yoga student become fatigued while holding a posture, it is best to come out of the pose before the foundations fail. This honors the body and helps avoid injury.

Open and closed hips

With very few exceptions, every yoga pose is founded on one of two hip orientations. All postures - standing, sitting or inverted - employ either an *open-hip* or *closed-hip* position. The hip orientation determines not only the position of the hips but also the relationship between the hips and the legs and feet.

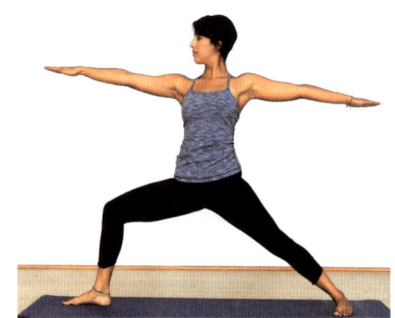

In the open-hip position, it is useful to visualize open-hip poses as if they are performed between two panes of glass, moving only in the two dimensions of horizontal and vertical. In establishing an open-hip pose, the legs open out to the sides along the *frontal plane* that passes through the body's center from side to side. Students square their hips to face the long side of their mat.

Open Hip – Warrior two

In open-hip poses, the legs widen and the feet separate to the approximate distance where the ankles align vertically with the wrists of their outstretched arms. The rear foot in open-hip standing poses is parallel to the back of the mat.

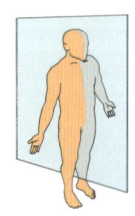
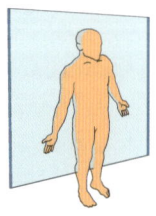

Sagittal plane   *Frontal (Coronal) plane*

The closed-hip position orients along the *sagittal plane* that passes through the center of the body from front to back. The legs move either forward or back from the hips without shifting the pelvis as it faces forward on the mat. In most postures, the distance between the legs in closed-hip postures is two-thirds to three-quarters the width utilized in the open-hip position. The hip joint of the rear leg rotates inward to help square both hips to the front of the mat. The rear leg and foot also turn inward to remain in line with the center of the hip. If the placement of the rear foot is not adequately facing forward, the integrity of alignment between the hip, knee and leg is compromised, resulting in considerable strain and possible injury to the knee.

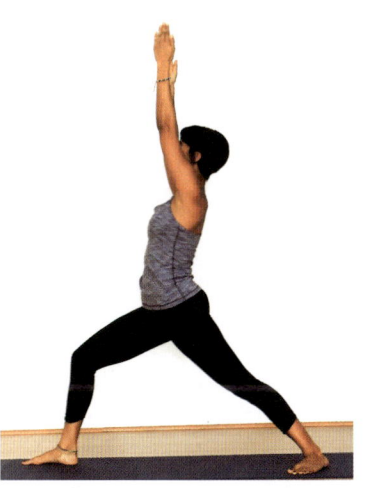

Closed hip - Warrior One

"There can only be one..." [1]

The two orientations of the hips are clear-cut positions and we can think of every yoga posture as falling into one of these two categories. Students find themselves in trouble when, at the initiation of an asana, they do not establish a foundation based on the correct hip orientation.

Despite similarities in name of some yoga postures, they do not often have the same hip orientation. For example, Warrior One is a closed-hip pose, and Warrior Two is open-hipped. Although similar in name, they fall into different hip-position categories and require completely different foundations. The same is true for Triangle, which is open-hipped, and Revolved Triangle, a closed-hip posture. Transitioning from one posture to the other without completely adjusting the alignment of the feet, legs and hips will cause significant strain and trauma. This is a common error that occurs in asana practice and a frequent cause of yoga-induced injury.

Engaging open or closed-hip poses

Each asana begins with the feet and legs placed according to the hip orientation of the pose: open or closed. In some circumstances, a student might not have adequate flexibility to start a posture with the hips square to the required orientation of the pose. In other instances, a student may lose the alignment of their hips when moving deeper into the pose. In either situation, the student should attempt to go as far as they can in the direction of correct hip orientation but not force the action, always staying steady and within comfortable limits. As long as the student has a clear intention and energetically attempts the correct form, the asana is safe and therapeutic. Warrior One is the best example of a situation where the hips may not fully attain their open or closed orientation. In Warrior One, only the most flexible students can bring the rear hip fully around and completely square to the front.

Exceptions to the rule

In some yoga traditions, the position of the hips in **Janu Sirsasana** (Knee Head Pose) is set diagonally between the open and closed orientations. There may be other examples of exceptions to the only-one hip orientation rule, but they are rare and would be unique to a particular style of yoga. Often in these cases, one hip orientation is still predominant and students should energetically favor that position. In Janu Sirsasana, the closed-hip position is favored.

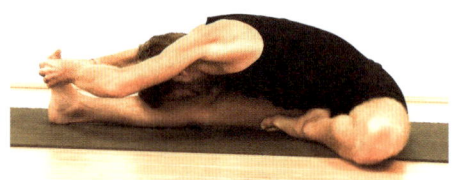

Linking poses into a flow

There are traditional groupings, or *vinyasas* of yoga postures. **Surya Namaskar**, the Sun Salutation, is the most common. Advanced yogis can link together virtually any group of postures and create a flowing vinyasa practice while correctly shifting their hip orientation and alignment. This is not the case, however, for less experienced students. Less experienced students become disorientated, unable to negotiate abrupt changes in foot position, leg width and hip orientation required by the poses. If yoga teachers choose to create complex asana sequences, it is the teacher's responsibility to guide their students with the critical instructions necessary to allow them to orient their poses safely.

Examples of postures in each category of hip orientation

Open-hip postures
- Triangle
- Warrior 2
- Extended side angle
- Warrior 3
- Wide-angle forward fold

Closed-hip postures
- Revolved Triangle
- Warrior 1
- Pyramid pose (Parsvotannasana)
- Half moon
- Lunge

> It is the actions taken to create a posture, not its final position or appearance that makes asana safe and therapeutic.

5 Integrative Alignment

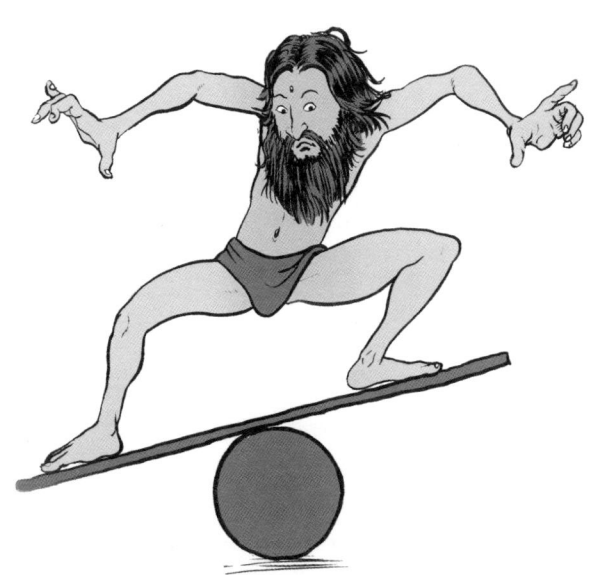

When yoga students decide to bring alignment into their practice, how should they go about it? Is imitating pictures in the many yoga books and journals enough? Can they scan their memory banks for the instructions once heard in a yoga class or workshop? Is there a set of principles relevant to a student's skill level and physical condition that can be trusted? A reliable alignment system is one that allows students to become stronger and more flexible as they advance, injury-free in their yoga practice. Such a system must be consistent at all times with the anatomical and mechanical design of the body.

Although it may seem daunting, learning proper alignment and how to engage it during yoga practice is not overly complex. Despite wide variety in human form and shape, color and size, all human bodies share the same "owner's manual". The way each region of the body integrates with all other regions remains virtually the same in every pose. Of course modifications are necessary to allow for a yogi's unique body structure, but these are adaptations, not new or contradictory rules.

This chapter introduces a number of alignment principles that allow yoga practice to be therapeutic and advance safely. Collectively called *Integrative Alignment*, this system combines many of the principles developed by yoga's most inspiring teachers with fundamentals of anatomy, physiology, and structural biomechanics. Integrative Alignment brings a new level of precision and cohesiveness to asana. It can transform a beginners practice to one that demonstrates advanced alignment and grace. Integrative alignment is comprehensive and its principles do not change from asana to asana. Importantly, integrative alignment is appropriate and consistent with all styles and all traditions of yoga.

> **Alignment** establishes the ideal position of individual parts. It forms the relationships that groups or forces adopt with each other.
>
> **Integration** is the act of coordinating individual parts into a unified, singularly functioning whole.

Hatha's ultimate balance

Yoga asana is in a perpetual balancing act between *movement* and *stability*. *Flexibility* is required to achieve movement and *strength* provides stability. Integrative alignment brings these two opposing forces into balance.

Interdependence

In the flow of a yoga practice, each part of the body moves independently while maintaining a relationship with all other parts. All parts align with each other to function harmoniously as a fully integrated system. This is called *interdependence*. These interdependent relationships are not static nor are they forced to rigidly perform a pre-determined set of movements. Rather, interdependence is dynamic, fluid and responsive to the ever-changing positions of the body. It is a sophisticated system of organic cogs and wheels, pulleys and levers, influencing not only the large joints and muscles but also structures on the cellular level. Some examples of interdependence are obvious: movement of the shoulder contributes to rotation of the wrist. Some examples are subtler: when the throat is drawn back, the jaw muscles relax.

Lack of interdependence is also observable: drawing back the lower ribs may cause the chest to drop and the shoulders to roll forward. Yoga practice can identify habitual patterns in our movements and posture and provides a method to align the body with interdependence.

Human architecture

Like all structures, the human frame has an underlying design, a blueprint of sorts. By adhering to this blueprint in asana practice, the yoga student can establish a stable foundation that provides support, load-bearing, resiliency, and longevity. Along with a solid foundation, the blueprint directs the student's overall alignment and integration for maximum benefit from each posture.

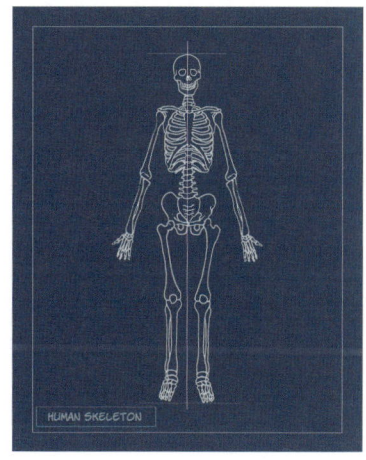

Basic asana most easily express the body's structural blueprint. In simpler postures, students are able to establish alignment without the additional challenge of performing advanced feats of acrobatics. For this reason, yoga therapy relies on basic yoga postures to provide effective rehabilitation.

"First there is a mountain, then there is no mountain, then there is."
Donovan

The alignment principles employed in **Tadasana**, the Mountain Pose, are followed in every other asana. Tadasana, yoga's most basic posture provides the clearest view of the universal blueprint and expresses the body's design in its simplest form.[1] It can be argued that there is only one pose in yoga, Mountain Pose, and that all other poses are merely advanced manifestations of the one. This basic alignment is also referred to as *neutral* posture.

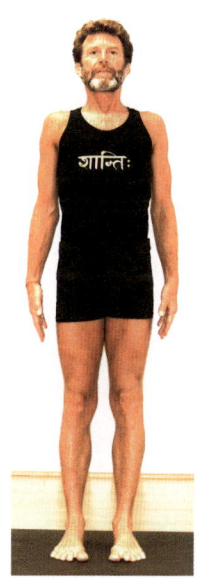

Asana becomes more complex as a student's practice advances and following the blueprint of Mountain Pose more challenging. As the blueprint becomes more obscured by the complexity of the postures, the art of yoga becomes one of discovery – a constant search for alignment and structural integrity.

> Most students of yoga consider B.K.S. Iyengar the pioneer of yoga alignment principles. Our present-day understanding of alignment and many of the concepts presented in this book would be severely limited if not for Mr. Iyengar's knowledge and dedication. Others, including John Friend, founder of Anusara yoga, expanded the groundwork done by Mr. Iyengar. Friend amassed and refined innumerable yoga alignment cues and introduced a single set of instructions applicable to every asana.[2] This book is strongly influenced by study of and direct instruction in Iyengar and Anusara yoga.

The "baby bear" intention

In Astronomy there is a concept called the Goldilocks[3] Zone which demarcates regions in the universe that meet criteria for life to exist on another planet or moon, the "just right" conditions. Yoga practice has its own baby bear, "just right" standard. Yoga students face the predicament of needing to know how deeply to move into an asana in order for it to be challenging and yet remain safe.

Yoga teacher Suzie Hurley of Tacoma Park, MD tells her students, "It's not how far you go; it's how you go far!"[4]

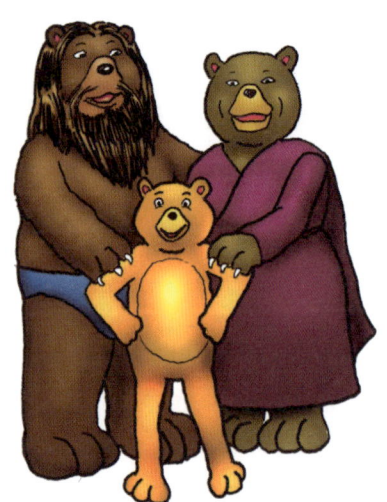

Kofi Busia is a Sanskrit scholar and one of B.K.S. Iyengar's first students. His Santa Cruz, CA, yoga classes are well known for long-held poses. While challenged with a ten-minute headstand, the class may be prodded by Busia with these stirring questions, "If you have already come out of the pose, why have you come out? But if you are still in the pose, why are you still in it?" This perplexing inquiry fills the minds of the students who are hoping to find the peaceful middle ground between over effort and giving up. As in the children's story *The Three Bears,* the journey of asana begs the questions, *What is too much? What is too little? What is just right?* The art of yoga practice resides in mastering the "just right" degree of effort.

What is the "just right" effort?

Yoga postures are safest and most therapeutic when they do not exceed the ability of the yoga practitioner to maintain a steady and stable foundation. The yogi must retain alignment in the most challenged regions of the body and keep the overall posture fully integrated. Asana practice that does not satisfy these basic guidelines is, unfortunately, a trauma-inducing experience.

Initiate movement from regions of least mobility

This principle is instrumental in preventing yoga injuries. Significant differences exist in the mobility of different regions of the body and in individual joints. Yoga practice begins by identifying the least mobile place involved in a particular pose and movement initiates directly from that place. For example, the upper back is less mobile in extension than the lower back due to its anatomical design. When moving into a "backbend" the asana should initiate from the upper, not the lower back. Also, the neck, which is especially mobile in extension, refrains from movement until the upper back has adequately opened.

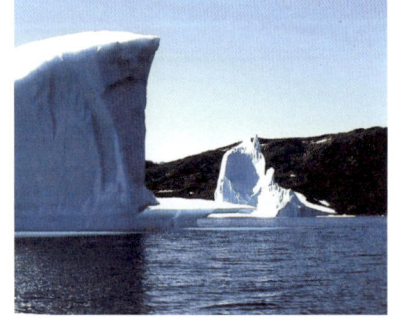

Taking a mobility inventory

Moving into asana by initiating from the least mobile place is a step-by-step process. The first action when undertaking a yoga posture is to *establish a stable foundation*. In standing poses the foundation usually resides in the feet, while in sitting poses, it is the pelvis. Once the pose is stable, an assessment is made of mobility in the body, taking an inventory of sorts. Joint mobility and muscle flexibility are evaluated and "ranked" from the most limited to the most freely moving. Movement into the asana then begins, starting with the least mobile region first. Each region moves as fully as possible without creating strain or compromising alignment anywhere in the body. The process continues step-by-step through the ranking order from lesser to greater mobility until, at last, the most freely mobile region participates in the asana as well.

This approach may at first seem remedial and quite tedious. It is, however, more akin to a self-guided meditation, bringing focus and awareness to the subtleties of the body. Personal assessment and step-by-step procedures are used with any endeavor worth mastering. The seasoned airline pilot runs through a checklist before each flight. A world-class concert pianist warms up with scales before each performance. With practice, the mental effort quickly drops behind the scenes and the process becomes almost unconscious.

The hierarchy of the twist

The seated twist is an excellent pose for exploring the principle of initiating movement from the least mobile region.

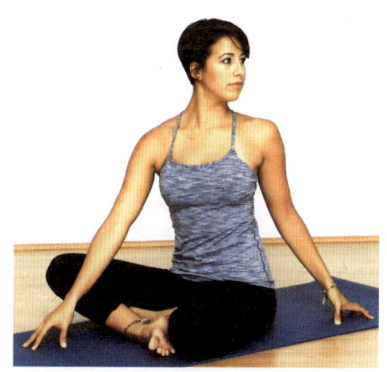

In a typical, non-injured spine, the pelvis remains stable and forms the foundation of the pose. The spine lengthens in its entirety to create joint space and increase ease of motion. The least mobile region involved in the twist is almost always the upper thoracic spine; therefore, movement begins from here. The lower thoracic spine moves next, then the lumbar spine, followed by the mid-cervical region, then the upper cervical vertebrae. Being the most mobile, the eyes perform the final movements.

Often students begin this pose by looking into the direction of the twist. In fact, it is common for teachers to instruct students to look first and then twist. Unless this instruction is part of a deliberate neuromuscular exploration, such as that used in the Feldenkrais Method®, it is not appropriate or safe.

Hypermobility

When a joint moves too much, meaning beyond its natural range of motion, it is called *hypermobile*. If a joint moves too little, it is *hypomobile*. When movement is within the limits of normal motion it is "just right".

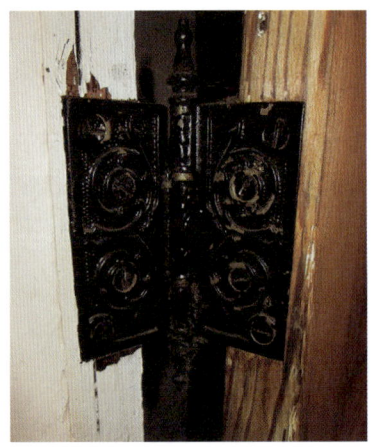

Hypermobility is not a normal state. It can result from an injury or from habitual, repetitive movements that cause instability. Hypermobility may also be of genetic origin. At first, hypermobile joints do not necessarily misalign. Instead, they move farther than their design permits. Over time, hypermobility will overstretch and weaken the soft tissues of a joint. As in the illustration of a door with a loose hinge, the unstable hinge creates aberrant movements and, in time, will likely lead to misalignment and significant damage.

In the body, hypermobile joints become inflamed and eventually suffer degenerative changes. Arthritis is a predictable result of long-term hypermobility. Yoga can be an excellent therapeutic modality for arthritis. Asana should always be modified to be appropriate for the severity of the condition.

For yoga to be effective and not a source of additional aggravation, however, students must clearly identify hypermobile joints and attempt to stabilize them in order to limit their movements. When ranking the hierarchy of movement, hypermobile joints should be engaged last when possible. Hypermobile joints are kept well aligned and engaged with the least amount of force and effort possible.

Convex vs. concave

According to principles of geometry, points on the convexity of a curve move faster and farther apart compared to similar points on the concave side. In keeping with the principle of initiating movement from the least mobile area first, the spine should move by first lengthening the concave side of the curve (the direction the pose is being bent toward). The concave side would otherwise become compressed when laterally flexed if space is not increased. This can result in nerve or disc damage.

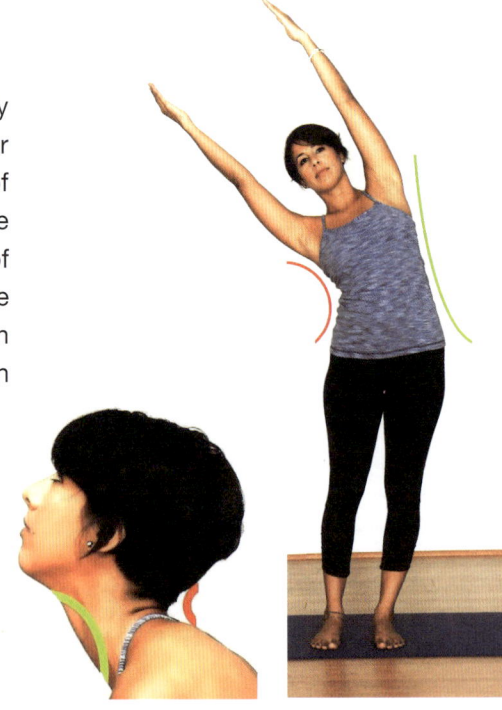

> Lengthen into an asana from the side of flexion to prevent compression.

The periphery of the body moves faster than at the core [5]

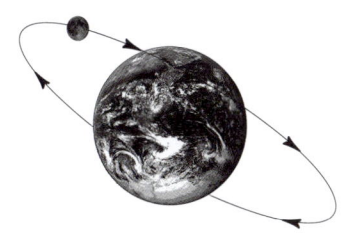

The regions closest to the midline of the body move less and more slowly and than the regions farther from its center. When initiating a yoga posture, therefore, start movement from the central core or midline of the body. Continue to align and move the rest of the body following an outward progression. If the greater relative mobility of the outer body regions is not compensated for, injury is likely to occur. Put another way, to prevent injuries during practice, maintain focus on core alignment and let the posture build from there.

> Move from the core and reach from the core.
> And for teachers, teach from the core.

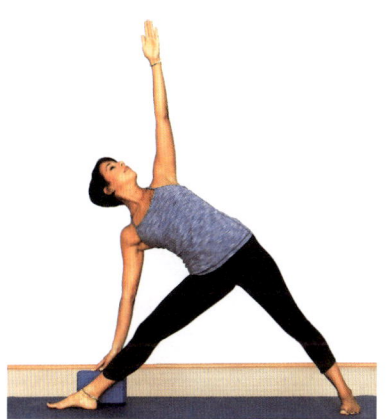

In the example of **Utthita Trikonasana** (Triangle Pose), enthusiastic students often raise their arms overhead immediately as they bend into the pose. Triangle Pose properly begins by first engaging the spine, then rotating the chest and shoulder. Finally, the arm and hand are extended straight out from the shoulder. *The arm should never move beyond the shoulder.* Moving the arm farther than the shoulder is a common cause of shoulder injury.

Bones approximate, muscles extend [6]

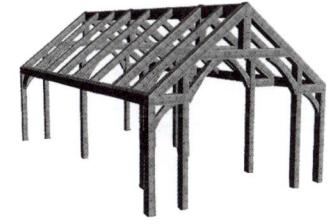

"Reach, stretch, lengthen, extend!" These are popular prompts yoga teachers use to encourage students to deepen their postures. On the surface, these instructions seem straightforward and make sense. Upon closer inspection, however, they prove to be contrary to safe body mechanics. The skeleton is analogous to the framework of a house. It provides support and stability. The soft tissues - ligaments, tendons, muscles and fascia - are not designed to carry significant weight. That would be like attempting to support a house by the sheetrock panels used for its walls.

When a yoga student reaches and extends outward in a pose, the joints separate, shifting more of the weight-bearing responsibilities onto the soft tissues around the joint. Extending the joints places strain on the tendons and ligaments that are designed to anchor and stabilize and not be overly stretched. Once overstretched, tendons and ligaments are no longer able to provide adequate stability for the joints, which initiates the process of joint degeneration.

Consistent with anatomical principles, B.K.S. Iyengar instructs his students to energetically draw the bones in toward the midline of the body. Once a posture is secure and centered on the skeleton, the muscular tension that was used to draw the bones inward softens and releases outward to the periphery. Stretching in yoga postures takes place in the muscles, not in the bones, tendons, or ligaments.

The rehabilitation of inflamed tendons (tendonitis) responds well to drawing the bones into their joints by reducing strain on the tendon attachments. It also protects the tendons from tearing during resistance training or any heavy lifting activities.

The center is best

Joints are designed to function most safely and enjoy their fullest range of motion when they are centered and aligned along a common central axis. With the bones centered in this way, joints are most stable and best able to handle the demands of weight bearing.

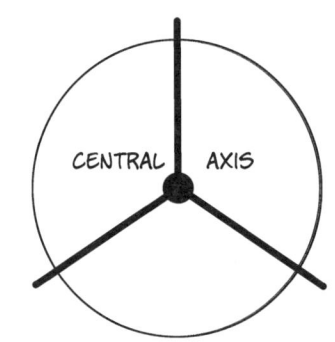

Stretching tips

Shorter muscles have more strength and are more efficient than longer muscles. At the same time, they are tighter and less flexible than their longer counterparts. For example, the masseter muscle of the jaw is one of the shortest and yet most powerful in the body.

An injured, aged or weakened muscle shortens to gain more power and in the process becomes tighter and less flexible. From a survival point of view, it is worth the tradeoff. (See Chapter 9 for more details on muscle physiology)

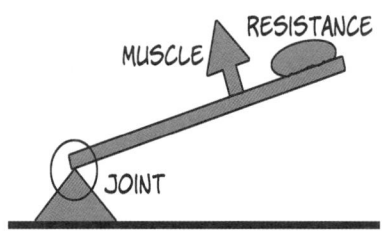

For maximum flexibility, initiate stretches from the thick, fleshy center of the muscle, commonly referred to as the *muscle belly*. Continue the stretch by extending from the muscle belly outward toward the tendons.

Likewise, when engaging a muscle for strength, contract the muscle belly first. The tendons naturally draw inward, toward the muscle belly. The force of contraction, if initiated at the tendon, will easily tear the tendon where it attaches to the bone.

> Bones draw firmly into the center of the joints and hug toward the body's central core, creating a stable frame.
>
> Stretching initiates from the muscle belly and lengthens outward.

The quality of Samasthiti

Equal standing, Balanced stillness

From the Sanskrit:
>Sama: same, upright, straight
>Sthiti: stillness, steadiness, standing

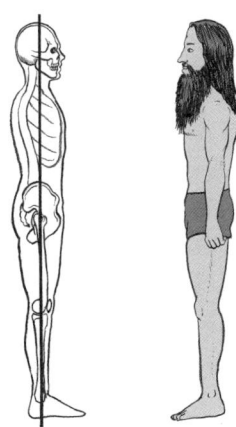

In some yoga traditions, the term *Samasthiti* is used interchangeably with **Tadasana** (Mountain pose). Samasthiti is better applied to yoga practice when it describes the "quality" of an asana where tension throughout the musculature has been made equal and balanced and, on an energetic level, a sense of equilibrium has been achieved. Samasthiti brings centering and balance to yoga postures. Equal length, tension and balance of weight are established along every body surface that the yogi can access. Tension in every muscle and tissue is balanced and equal in all directions, right down to each side of every nail bed. The quality of Samasthiti is especially important for an asana practice intended to address scoliosis, the abnormal lateral curvature of the spine. (See Chapter 24 for more details about this subject)

Samasthiti – beyond balance

Although we like to imagine the human structure as a balanced structure, its asymmetry and disproportions are numerous. Applying Samasthiti wherever these imbalances can be found will greatly improve the safety and performance of asana.

A few examples will make the point clear:

The muscles of the chest and front of the shoulders are approximately 30% stronger than the muscles of the upper back and rear shoulders. Additionally, the shoulders have almost 30% more flexibility in their movements toward the front of the body as compared to movements toward the back. And importantly, our lifestyle activities are predominatly forward-facing. To create Samasthiti, place greater focus on extension of the thoracic spine and shoulders and developing strength in the upper back muscles.

The calf muscles are nearly 30% stronger than the thin musculature of the front shin. Pointing the toes strengthens the calf while pressing through the heel more effectively strengthens the front shin muscles. Pressing through the heels to engage "neutral feet" brings Samasthiti to asana, including postures that are non-weight-bearing.

In a gym, a knowledgeable weightlifter does not do sets of biceps curls without balancing his routine with triceps extension exercises. This too, is Samasthiti.

Moving with Samasthiti

When engaging a region of the body, attempt to activate and control the movement from every possible surface in a balanced and integrated fashion. Movement of each joint should be as precise and performed with as much conscious awareness as if carrying a full pot of boiling water safely across a room.

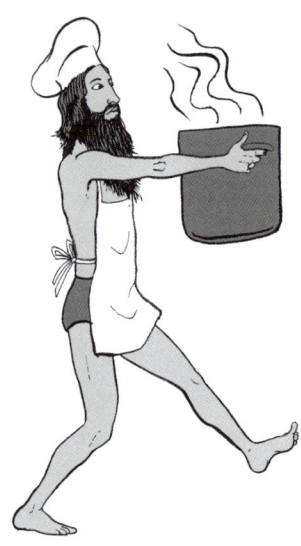

Here is one example: When the shoulder is quickly pulled back, the tendency is for the outer shoulder to move faster than the inner shoulder, causing the joint to externally rotate. Instead, draw the shoulder back equally from the inner armpit and the outer surface. This produces a purer, cleaner movement of the shoulder to the posterior.

Examples of imbalanced efforts:

A limber yogini may exploit her flexibility to go deep into a pose without focusing on establishing stability.

A yogi kicks up into handstand from his more comfortable and stronger leg and never practices the pose using his weaker side.

A flexible yogini can open her hips in flexion and extension, as in **Hanumanasana** (Full Closed Hip Split), but cannot externally rotate the hips to stack the knee over the ankle, as in **Agnistambhasana** (Fire Logs Pose). Will she focus her practice on her specific areas of limitation or always avoid the challenging postures?

A yogi transitions easily from pose to pose in a vinyasa but is challenged when holding asanas for long periods. Will he adapt his practice and hold poses longer to build strength or continue to practice only a fast-flowing style of yoga?

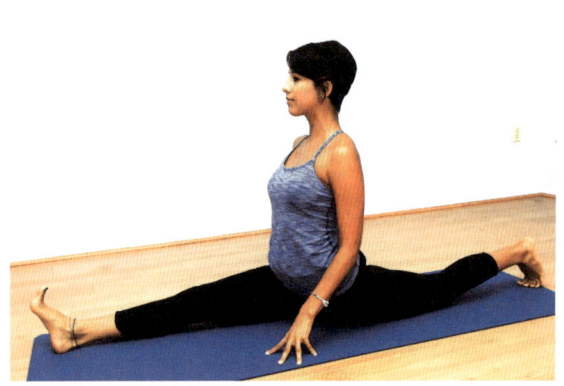

Hanumanasana

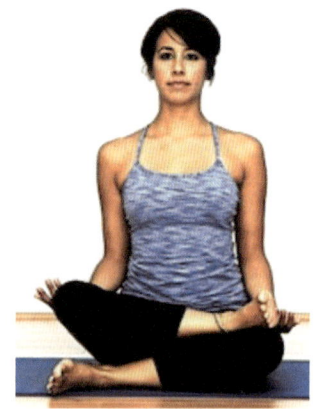

Agnistambhasana

Identifying strengths and weaknesses

Yoga is a transparent practice. It strips away all facades, displaying our personal strengths and revealing our hidden weaknesses.

"Always put your best foot forward!" This is an exclamation familiar to most yoga students and a proclamation rarely questioned. Most of us have become accustomed to taking advantage of our personal strengths to be successful. This way of thinking, however, should be reconsidered when stepping onto the mat. In fact, this initial misstep may be at the heart of many injuries in both yoga and sports. It is often the reason for lower levels of performance. From a yogic point of view, exploiting our strengths does not encourage balance and integration. Instead, it calls on existing skills and achievements and does not allow our less developed abilities to emerge and improve.

Yoga asana is best practiced by first humbly identifying the nature of our weaknesses, limitations and challenges. With a non-judgmental intention, asana initiates from those more recalcitrant areas, allowing them to be expressed at their present level of capability. As the less developed aspects of our practice improve, a strong and safe practice can evolve and the yogi can manifest his true potential.

When we can identify the causes of our limitations and focus on their resolution, our journey becomes one of grace.

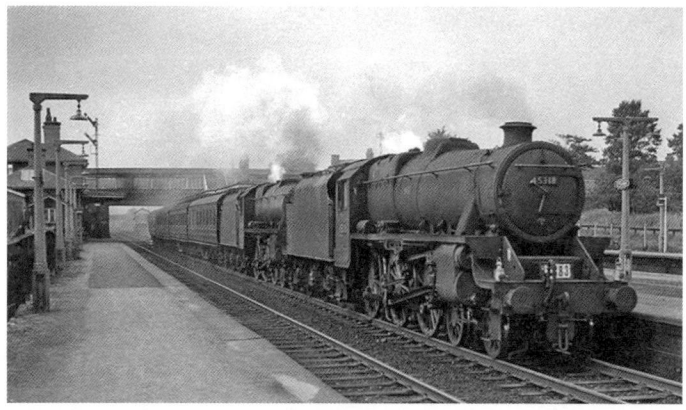

As with a traveling train, it is not the fastest car but the slowest that determines the quality and pace of the trip. Increasing the power of the engine cannot overcome the restrictions caused by a rear car with a rusted axle or stuck brake.

Heyam Dukham Anagatam

The pains that are yet to come can be, and are to be, prevented.

This Sanskrit phrase was recited in the *Yoga Sutras by Patañjali* more than two millennia ago. It is one of the underlying precepts of yoga practice. It reminds the yogi that asana practice should not cause trauma but instead have protective and therapeutic value. This edict and the guiding principles of Yama and Niyama (described in Chapter 3) set the ground rules for a safe and integrated practice of yoga.

6 Form Follows Function

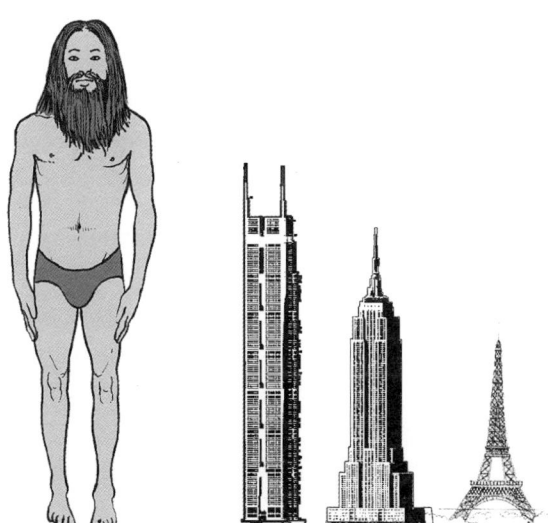

In the fields of biology, architecture and technology, the 19th Century adage, "form follows function," holds true.[1] Things *look* the way they do because of *what* they do. The form that the human body takes is the adaptive expression of the inherent drive of all living things to be as efficient and effective as possible.

This principle applies to asana practice. The form of a posture is the overt expression of the body's underlying function. The appearance of a well functioning body demonstrates good alignment. Poor alignment distorts the body's natural design, producing an unappealing form that implies dysfunction. Vitality and our innate healing processes become something clearly visible and embedded in our posture when we live in alignment.

Finely tuned by evolution, the structures of our body function in specific, predetermined ways. The tissues that stretch should do the stretching while those designed for support should do exactly that. One goal in asana practice is to not force any aspect of the body to function contrary to its design, which inevitably causes injury.

The structural tissues of the body are comprised of a class of organic material called *connective tissue*. Connective tissue anatomy and physiology will be reviewed in detail in Chapter 6. Connective tissue takes many forms, each designed to accomplish a specific set of functions. One form of connective tissue is bone. It is rigid and firm and provides a stable framework upon which the human body is organized. For this rigid frame to achieve movement, joints and specialized forms of connective tissue have evolved.

> Use the structures of the body according to their design.

Structures are most vulnerable to injury when the body transitions between motion and stillness.

Stretching

Stretching is commonly thought to be a capacity of muscle tissue alone. This is not exactly true. There are additional structural tissues involved, and these generally limit stretching. By understanding the capabilities of these different components, yoga students can stretch carefully and effectively and thereby avoid injury. Some important stretching concepts are presented below, followed by an extensive exploration of stretching physiology in Chapter 7.

As the following chart[2] illustrates, muscle tissue stretches the most easily. Muscle tissue is surrounded by myofascia, a collagen-rich sleeve of connective tissue that envelops every strand of muscle from the largest fiber to the smallest fibril. Myofascia can safely stretch only 10% of its resting length. This is considerably less than muscle tissue's ability to stretch to nearly 200%. Myofascia is the limiting factor in stretching. Most injuries resulting from overstretching that are assumed to be the result of muscle trauma are more likely myofascial trauma.

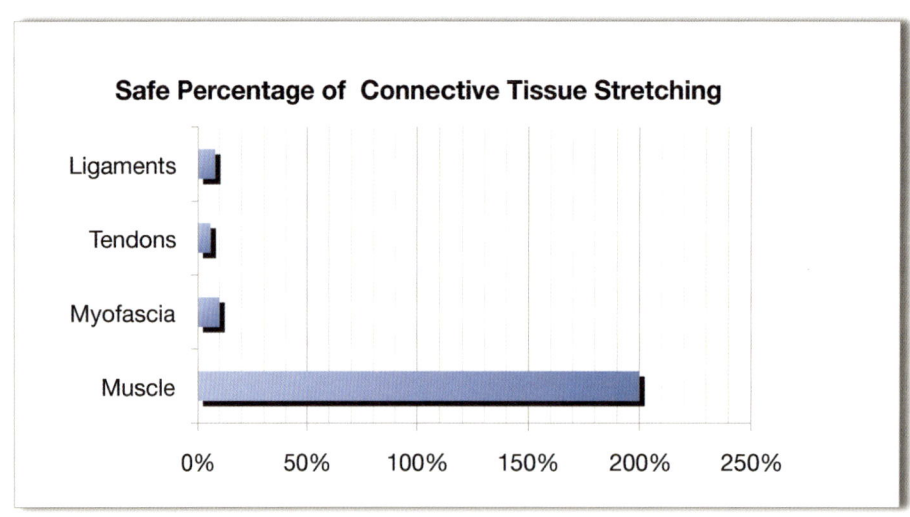

Like myofascia, muscle tendons are not designed for stretching. The tendon's job is to anchor muscle to bone. Tendons, comprised mostly of collagen, are thick and inflexible cables that transfer the power of muscle contractions across joints. A stretched tendon is a common yoga injury and results in tendonitis.

Ligaments are also not intended for stretching. Ligaments stabilize joints by binding bone to bone. They keep joints aligned and prevent aberrant movement while allowing a normal range of motion. Additional discussion on ligament tissue physiology is found in Chapter 8.

Diaphragms

Composed of muscle and connective tissue, diaphragms are structures suspended to create cavities above or below them. A structure is considered diaphragm-like when it does not maintain complete contact with its underlying structures. Most well known is the thoracic diaphragm, the primary muscle of respiration that separates the thoracic and abdominal cavities. Other tissues that are diaphragm-like are the plantar fascia, perineum, diaphragm, soft palate, the fascia of the palm of hands, as well as the eardrums. When the body is fully aligned and its parts integrated, these diaphragm-like structures do not bear weight and are free of tension. In yoga practice, the core diaphragms can be engaged through an energy locking system known as the *bandhas*. More details on the bandhas will be presented in Chapters 12 and 28.

In some esoteric traditions, it is believed that pranic energy transmits through the diaphragms, vibrating like the auditory membrane of a stereo speaker. The palms of the hands and soles of the feet, also having diaphragm-like qualities, are considered to be sites at which prana enters and exits the body.

Aligning diaphragms along the central axis

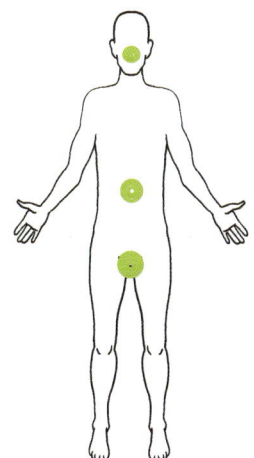

When a diaphragm is muscularly engaged, it lifts from its center, forming a dome-like shape. The pelvic floor, the thoracic diaphragm and the soft palate lift and align in a vertical line that exits the posterior fontanel of the skull. Lifting these core diaphragmatic structures aligns the pelvis and torso on its central axis. This lifting action occurs by engaging the bandhas. Yogis who can engage the bandhas of the palms of the hands and the souls of the feet may also experience the integrating effects of alignment there. Chapter 28 explains in detail how to engage the bandhas.

Follow the curve

The spinal curves formed while in a simple standing posture demonstrate the spine in its *neutral* position. The depth of the spinal curves may be deep or flattened. The degree of curve in the neutral position is a result of gravity, genetics and attempts to balance the countless stresses that occur during a life of habits and injuries. Spinal curves constantly shift, adapting moment by moment to the changing movements and positions of the body. Changes in the shape of the curves directly influence the mobility and stability of the spine.

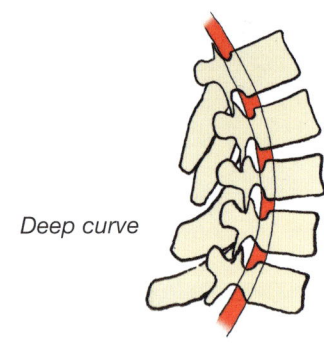

Deep curve

In the case of a whiplash injury, the curve of the neck flattens and may even reverse. A straight or reversed curve creates excessive spinal hypermobility and offers minimal stability. If not for the severe muscle spasms that accompany whiplash injuries, the injured neck would have little integrity and become incapable of supporting the head. Hypermobility of the neck resulting from a straight or reversed spine creates risk of debilitating damage to the spinal discs and nerves.

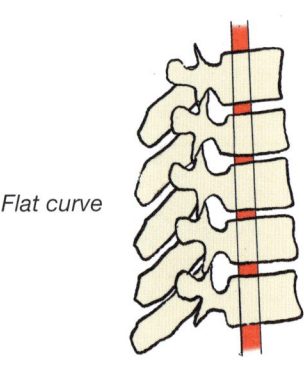

Flat curve

When comparing spinal curves, slight differences may be observed between individuals. Some yoga students, by nature, have straighter spines than their classmates, often merely a natural genetic occurrence. A healthy, straight spine usually makes a person more flexible, overall. To compensate for hypermobility and the instability that may accompany a reduced curve, an opposing curve may deepen to provide the needed stability. For example, hypermobility from a flattened, upper thoracic curve may be offset by a deepened lumbar curve. A flexible yoga student may unwittingly exploit this compensation when performing backbend poses, causing compression injuries to the lumbar discs. Integrative alignment principles help yoga students control their spinal curves and find a neutral, balanced position that offers safety and stability.

Another example of this depth-of-curve imbalance occurs when a flat, poorly formed lumbar curve actuates the thoracic spine to round as an attempt to establish stability.

Despite the complaints by yoga students of stiff and rounded lower backs, most have the ability to deepen their lower back curvature in the classic Cat-Cow sequence. In fact, many stiff-backed yoga students are actually not stiff but instead, hypermobile in their lower spine. For them, muscle shortening and tightness is the limiting factor and not the actual curve of the spine or the movement of the vertebrae themselves.

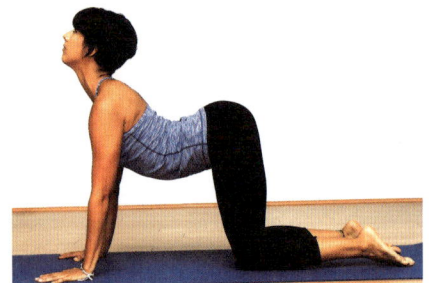

> A deep curve is less mobile but more stable. Flatter curves have greater mobility but are less stable and provide less support.

Confusion about curves

When a fishing pole bends, the distant end comes into closer reach. At first glance, the pole seems to be more flexible when rounded. What actually happens, however, is that as the pole bends, it stiffens as a result of a build up of kinetic energy. The pole is more stable while bent and better able to resist the pull of fish. When the pole is straight, its flexibility is obvious as it wobbles, free of stored energy.

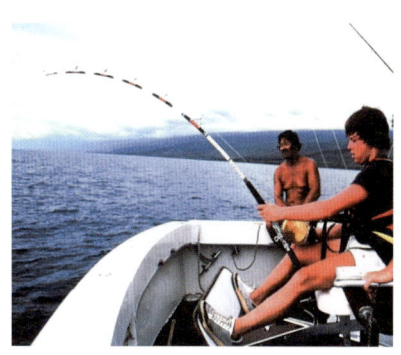

Similar confusion about curves arises in our understanding of the spine. In forward bending yoga postures, a rounded upper back might allow students to reach their toes more readily, however, roundedness deepens the thoracic curve and limits movement rather than increasing it. If the lower back is rounded, the lumbar curve flattens, causing its supporting ligaments to become overstretched. The result is lumbar hypermobility and an unstable lower back.

Aging can also deepen spinal curves. After many years of life, some people appear to shrink. This indicates that curves in the spine are deepening, often accompanying the unfortunate collapse and fracture of vertebrae. Increased curvature is the body's counteraction to a weak and deteriorating bone structure, it being the body's attempt to stabilize its frame. Deepening curves reduces spinal mobility, a trade-off to protect the joints. Some forms of arthritis and other conditions of aging can cause the spine to become rigid and immobile, leaving it straight instead of deeply curved. In these cases, students will benefit from a slow and aligned practice that carefully moves into poses that deepen their curves. Cat-Cow and **Astangasana** (Knees-Chest-Chin Pose) are two examples of poses that carefully deepen the spinal curves. More details on the spinal aging process are available in Chapter 24 and 25.

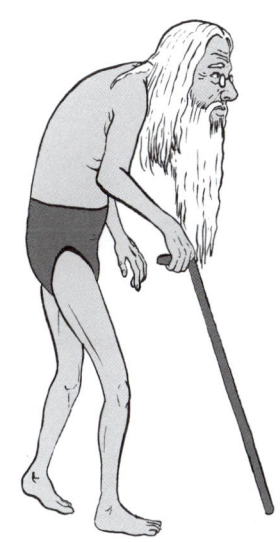

Using the curves in asana practice

With most human activity dominated by the front of the body, the spine and shoulders are predisposed to rounding forward. Yoga practice should not encourage spinal rounding. Every asana is instead, the opportunity to lengthen the spine and square the shoulders.

A yogi moves into a posture by first lengthening the spine. The longitudinal stretch of the spine flattens the curves and increases the space between the joints, creating greater potential for mobility. Once the desired position of the posture has been reached, the yogi slightly releases the lengthening stretch to allow the curves to again deepen. The restoration of a deeper curve brings stability to the posture.

In contrast, when the student is preparing to load the spine in a weight-bearing position, the curves deepen for spinal stability. Lifting with a lengthened, flat spine would easily result in injury. More details on spinal mechanics and safety in movement are presented in Chapter 24, 25, and 28.

If the thoracic spine rounds in forward bending postures, the shoulders also round forward, limiting upper back mobility. The chest collapses and breathing becomes impaired. The head and neck lose their foundation and the bandhas and diaphragms are unable to align along the central axis of the body. Good alignment in Janu Sirsasana keeps the chest forward of the shoulders until the yogi has completed all movement and releases into the final posture.

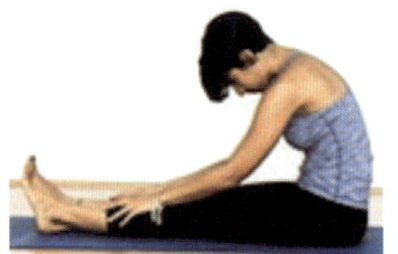

Paschimottanasana   Sitting Forward Fold

In all forward bending asana, the primary movement is forward flexion of the hips. Initially, the torso holds the **Tadasana** (Mountain Pose) alignment as the spine actively lengthens. A small egg-sized curve is maintained in the lower back. The upper back lifts and flattens, the chest moves forward, and the shoulders shift further onto the back. When the hips reach their full capacity to flex forward, the torso begins to release toward the legs, still leading the movement from the chest. Once the student reaches his maximum forward movement with a flat upper back and a curved lumbar spine, he can release all tension in the back and surrender the position of the curves. Limited flexibility of the hamstring muscles is common. Tight hamstrings interfere with full actualization of the posture by preventing the pelvis from fully flexing and the lumbar spine from maintaining its curve.

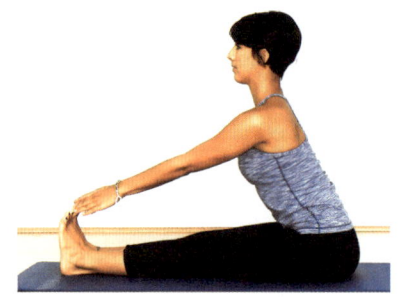

7 Anatomy and Physiology Connective Tissue

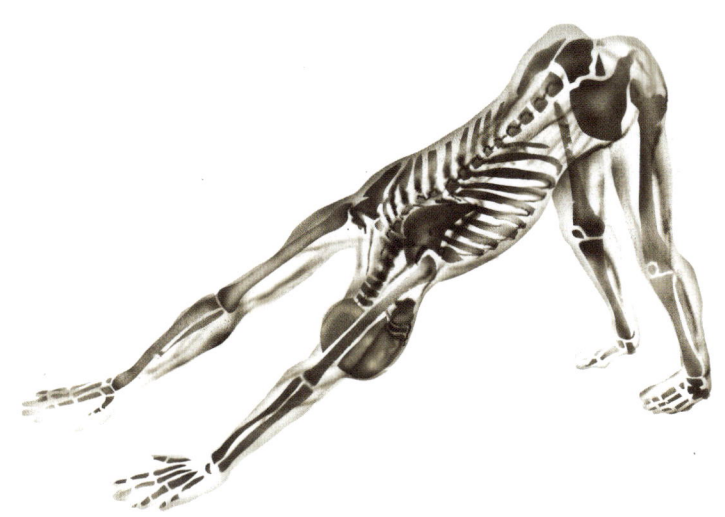

Know your medium

Every artisan and designer involved in the creative process compiles extensive knowledge of the materials and instruments used in their work. Material tolerances and compatibilities must be well understood to change the formless into expressions of organic beauty. This is true in the art of yoga. How well yoga students understand the anatomy and physiology of the body directly impacts on their ability to create a masterful asana practice. Knowledge brings wisdom to asana practice that allows it to flow with the intelligence of the body, not against it.

The primary component of structural anatomy is connective tissue. Like a creature in a science fiction movie that materializes from the primordial soup of a dark lagoon, human structures emerge from a formless aggregate of embryonic connective tissue.

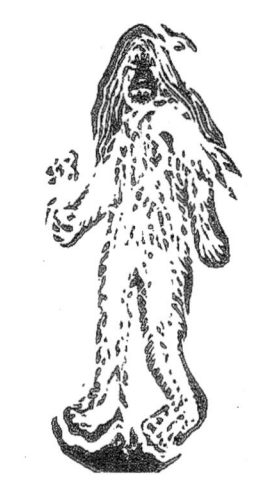

In the adult, fascial connective tissue forms a contiguous envelope that covers every layer of bone and muscle and runs over every blood vessel and organ, forming a head-to-toe cocoon. Connective tissue interweaves muscle with bone so completely that a severe muscle contraction generally will fracture the bone before it pulls the tendon free.

Ligaments, tendons, bone, cartilage, myofascia, fascia, and skin are all forms of connective tissue. Muscle, considered a separate class of tissue, has connective tissue components woven into its structure. [1]

Components of connective tissue

Connective tissue is the primary material of the mechanical and structural components of the body. Three primary elements comprise all connective tissue - ground substance, fibers and cells. The ratio of these three elements determines the type of tissue and how it functions.

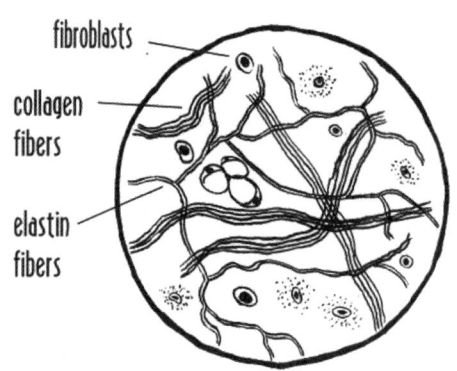

Additionally, minerals infiltrate into some types of connective tissue, such as bone and cartilage, changing their structure and how they function.

Ground substance
- Water
- Sugars
- Proteins

Cells
- Fibroblasts
- Immune cells
- Fat cells

Fibers
Collagen fibers [2]
- Type 1   Tendons
- Type 2   Cartilage
- Type 3   Bone
- Type 4   Muscle lamina/ cell membrane

Elastin fibers
Reticular fibers

Ground substance

Ground substance is a watery, glue-like gel that makes up the base structure of all connective tissue. It creates diffuse, sticky web material that holds together the other connective tissue components. Ground substance is a viscous suspension made up of mostly water and protein-sugar compounds called proteoglycans and glycosaminoglycans. Water makes up 85% of ground substances in infants, decreasing to 70% and lower in adults.

The higher the quantity of ground substance in a type of connective tissue, the more flexible it becomes. The myofascial sheathings surrounding muscle tissue, which are made of connective tissue, are abundantly coated on their inner surfaces with ground substance to provide lubrication for the moving muscle.

Ground substance also facilitates electrochemical communication and nutrient transport throughout the tissues of the body.[3] Connective tissue, having limited blood supply depends on the watery, viscous nature of ground substance to serve as its primitive circulatory and nervous system.

Fibers of connective tissue

Collagen

Collagen is the most abundant protein in the body. It exists in very high concentrations in skin, bone, cartilage, ligaments, tendons, and fascia.

Collagen is made up of the amino acids proline and glycine, which string together to form long chains that wrap into a triple helix shape. Collagen proteins form rough fibers that are designed to *resist stretching*. They contain small, unfettered strands with hook-like projections that reach out to surrounding fibers and cross-link with them to inhibit motion. This starkly contrasts with the cross-linking mechanism of muscle fibers that is designed with smoother strains that propel the fibers to promote motion, not limit it.

To be powerful, cable-like and tensile (resistant to stretching), the average collagen fiber can stretch only 10% beyond its resting length before it tears and ruptures. Collagen also becomes damaged if repetitively compressed, crimped, or bent. Once stretched, changes in collagen length are permanent. Wrinkling of our skin is an example of permanent collagen stretching. There is a need, however, for some degree of functional flexibility in tissues high in collagen, such as ligaments, which must be flexible to allow joints to flex. To accomplish this, ligaments strategically wrap around joints and *micro-pleat,* a process of folding and unfolding at predesigned locations. These design modifications create a "pseudo-stretching" action at the joints to provide mobility. More details on ligament physiology are presented in Chapter 8.

There are at least sixteen types of collagen fibers. Almost all are Types 1-4 that at best can stretch 10% of their resting length. One of the obscure types of collagen is significantly more elastic than the others. If a person inherits a high percentage of this type of collagen fiber, they will have more flexibility than the norm, perhaps able to exhibit contortionist-type abilities.[4]

Elastin

Elastin fibers are smooth and configured into a double helix structure. They have the ability to deform and return to their original size and shape. Elastin can stretch 200% of its resting length before rupturing. Muscle fibers are composed mostly of elastin.[5]

Reticular fibers

Reticular fibers are thin, delicately woven strands that form the soft meshwork that supports lymph tissue and bone marrow. They are sometimes categorized as collagen Type 3 fibers.

Fascia

Fascia is the rudimentary, underlying structural system for the body, forming delineated borders around body structures. Derived from the Latin term for *band* or *bandage*, fascia is a tough membrane made of densely packed collagen fibers. The collagen composition of fascia limits its ability to stretch beyond 10% of its resting length. Fascia encases every structure of the body, from the smallest vessels to the larger organs and bones. Fascia's enveloping design allows it to transmit and distribute nerve impulses and circulate vital nutrients to local tissues.

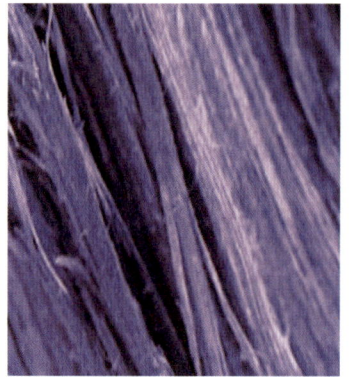

The collagen fibers of fascia generally organize in a longitudinal direction, running parallel to the structures they cover. In this layout, they can provide structural support to the tissues they surround. In some locations, however, fascia runs either horizontal or perpendicular to surrounding structures, such as in the respiratory diaphragm, the pelvic floor, the soft palate, the palms and the soles of the feet. In these locations, fascia is a more independent structure.

Fascia can provide a modest degree of support but a fraction of what bone or cartilage can deliver, being too flexible to be significantly weight bearing.[6]

For example, the plantar fascia supports the vaulting of the foot as it forms its arches. If the joints of the foot spread apart or if the intrinsic musculature of the foot weakens, the fascia becomes overstretched and the arches collapse. When the fascia is forced to provide an excessive amount of structural support, it can become swollen, inflamed or torn, what is called *plantar fasciitis*.

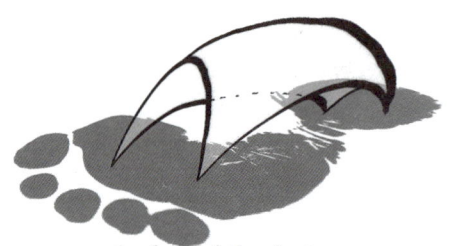

Arches of the foot

Myofascia

The fascia specifically associated with muscle tissue is called *myofascia*. Thirty percent of overall muscle mass is composed of myofascia. From the smallest muscle filaments, called *fasciculi,* to the largest bundles, muscle is enveloped in myofascia. The function of myofascia is to bind together muscle fibers and spread their impulses of contraction. Myofascia also reduces the friction that can occur between muscle fibers.

In the center of the muscle, the muscle belly, myofascial fibers are loose and randomly arranged. They become progressively denser at the ends of the muscle where the fibers are more tightly packed and more parallel in their alignment. The tapered ends of muscles compress their multi-layered sheaths of myofascia to form a seamless tendon.

When a muscle stretches, the limiting factor to how far the muscle can lengthen is the high collagen content of the myofascia. Collagen creates more than 40% of the overall resistance to lengthening that muscle confronts.[7]

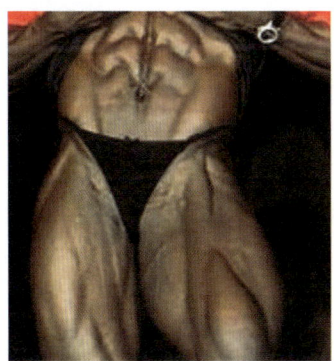

In weight lifting and other resistance training programs, when muscle fibers enlarge, they become compressed against the myofascial sheaths and flexibility reduces. To rectify the "muscle bound" phenomenon, a dedicated stretching program is a necessary tool for the athlete.

Tendons

As muscle and myofascia taper at the bone to where they attach, the individual myofascial sheaths that cover each muscle fiber bind together to form a common cord, or tendon. Tendons are thick, fibrous and cable-like. They are designed to anchor muscle to bone and to transfer its power of contraction across the joint. The high percentage of collagen fibers in tendons provides great tensile strength, or resistance to stretching. The limited elasticity of tendons enables them to efficiently convert muscular energy into mechanical action on the joint. The limited ability of tendons to stretch ranges from 8% where the tendon emerges from the muscle to only 4% at its attachment to the bone.

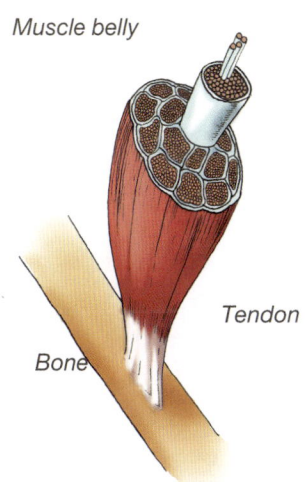

Muscle belly

Tendon

Bone

Tendonitis

Tendons are not designed to stretch beyond their limited tolerance. However, small numbers of muscle fibers migrate into the tapered ends of tendons. These fibers have enough contractile tissue to allow a minimal degree of stretching but stretching can quickly result in tendon strain. If forced to overstretch, the myofascial sleeves covering the tendon become inflamed.

Normally, the muscle fibers that taper into the tendon sheathing move freely, similar to a plastic straw encased loosely inside a paper wrapping. If tendon sheathings that are inflamed are forced to slide, they can tear, like the paper wrapping on a straw after it has become wet and matted. Prolonged inflammation or extensive tearing causes tendon tissue to become permanently overstretched and lax. This results in permanent loss of efficiency and power in the muscle-joint system. Unfortunately, with a minor injury, a healed tendonitis never fully returns to its pre-injury effectiveness. Many baseball pitchers develop tendon laxity in the shoulder of their throwing arm. Some may receive a surgical procedure that shortens the tendon as a method of restoring its tensile strength.

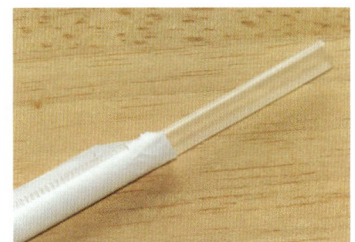

As a yoga therapy for tendonitis, a splint can be placed across the injured tendon, using a strap to reduce the mechanical pull and tension on the inflamed or torn tissue.

Cryotherapy (icing) reduces inflammation and is a first step in protecting the tendon from damage. Icing tendons reduces swelling that results from inflammation. Because micro tears tend to recur during rehabilitation, ice therapy can continue throughout the recovery stage.

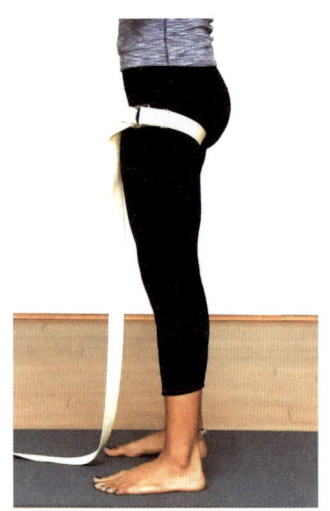

Bursas

Muscle tendons cross over joints in close relation to each other, exerting powerful forces moving in multiple directions. Creating space between the individual tendons reduces friction that can build up between the bones and close-lying tendons. To reduce the strain on these tissues, bursas are positioned at approximately 150 high-friction, mechanically stressed locations throughout the body. Bursas are formed from an out-pocketing of myofascia that is filled with serum-like fluid. Excessive strain created by the tendons can cause inflammation of the bursa. Bursitis is an extremely painful condition that becomes exacerbated by movement of the involved joint.

Bursitis responds well to ice therapy, which reduces inflammation. When joints are precisely aligned and the musculature is balanced across the strained area, the irritated bursa will be calmed and can eventually recover.

The principles of *integrative alignment* presented in this book are excellent tools for the yoga student suffering from bursitis, making asana a valuable tool for healing. Often, introducing slight adjustments to the alignment of an inflamed joint will reduce pain and increase its ranges of motion. As with all yoga therapy, paying careful attention to pain and the actions that reduce it provides the best guidance when using asana as a therapeutic modality.

8 Anatomy and Physiology Ligaments

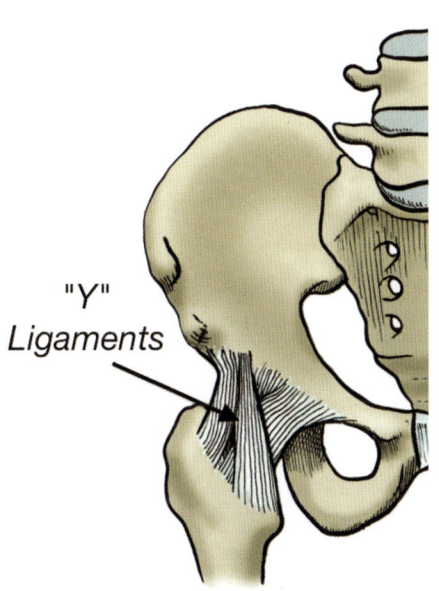

"Y" Ligaments

Contrary to animated images of a barebones skeleton, by itself our underlying frame would appear as a random pile of bones. When assembled, joints form where the bones meet. Without the joints, the human frame would be strong and stable. But of course, our skeleton must also be mobile, so movable joints are necessary. To accommodate both flexibility and stability in the joints, a complex ligament system evolved which allows joints to rapidly and easily change their function.

The structural ligaments of the body are thick fibrous straps that bridge bone-to-bone across the joints. They are positioned to maintain an alignment of the joints that is ideal for full and safe range of motion. The tissues of the average ligament stretch to approximately 8% of their resting length.

Micro-pleating action of the ligaments

Ligaments are made up of mostly collagen fibers. As described in Chapter 7, collagen provides ligaments with excellent resistance to stretching but it is quite unforgiving when crimped or bent. To create flexibility without damaging the non-elastic collagen-rich ligament tissue, a system of extremely small folds, or *micro-pleat*s are built into each ligament. These micro-pleats enable ligaments to shorten and lengthen safely by folding or unfolding at designated locations. The design is similar to an accordion-type window blind.

Wrapping action

Along with micro-pleating, an additional characteristic of ligaments is that they wrap around the joint, winding and unwinding around the joints in concurrence with the micro-folding action. This wrapping action produces torque on the ligaments to produce stability and can tighten or loosen the joints as needed.

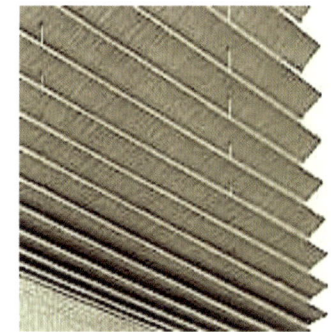

How ligament action works

When ligaments micro-pleat, they loosen and unwrap from the joints, increasing the joints' freedom of movement.

Ligaments loosen when a joint moves in any of these three directions: *internal rotation, flexion or adduction.* In asana that require joint flexibility, moving in these directions will release the ligaments and allow greater and safer mobility.

When ligaments un-pleat and wrap farther around their joints, they become stretched, tight and taut. This produces stability. Ligament un-pleating and wrapping occurs when joints move in the directions of *external rotation, extension and abduction.* Movement in any combination of all three actions stabilizes the joints. In some situations, these actions are performed as actual movements. Other times, the actions are "energetic" or isometric muscle contractions.

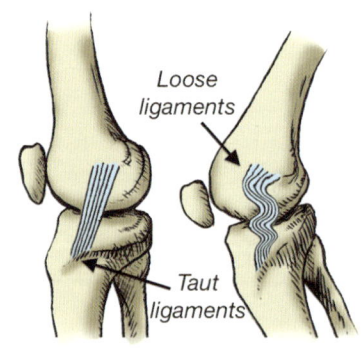

Ligaments Loosen	Ligaments Tighten
•Flexion	•Extension
•Internal rotation	•External rotation
•Adduction	•Abduction

Taking the heat

Friction in ligaments created by the pleating and un-pleating of its collagen fibers produces a sizable amount of heat. Heat is beneficial to muscle tissue and in low amounts helps mobilize joints. Heat, however, causes inflammation, which can damage the cartilaginous surfaces of the joints. The more collagen fiber content in a ligament, the more heat that is produced. Elastin fibers, on the other hand, produce considerably less heat than collagen fibers. To reduce the heat around joints, ligaments have a greater concentration of elastin fibers than is found in tendons. Conversely, the higher collagen content in tendons produces higher amounts of heat, which is beneficial for muscle function and blood circulation.

A little goes a long way

A small increase in the elastin content of a ligament produces significant increases in flexibility. The proportions of collagen and elastin in a ligament have evolved to correspond with the mechanical demands on the ligament. Examples of ligaments with high elasticity are the cervical sections of the *ligamenta flavum* and *ligamenta nuchae*, located along the spine in the neck and upper back. The high elastin content of these ligaments increases their ability to stretch to as much as 25% of their resting length, which is significantly greater than the 8% stretching capacity ligaments typically display. In animals such as cows and dogs, these two ligaments are large and well developed in order to support the weight of their heads in a suspended position while providing wide ranges of motion.

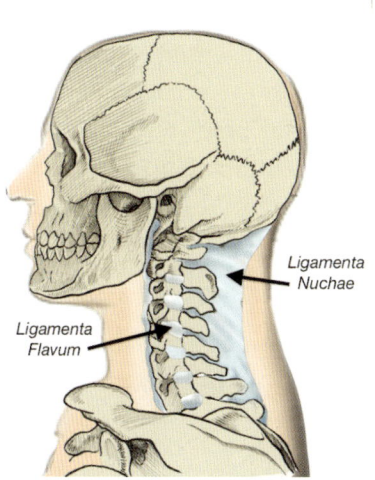

In contrast, the collateral ligaments of the knee have very little elasticity, and their movement relies almost exclusively on wrapping and micro-folding actions. If knees are habitually hyperextended, their ligaments can become overstretched and weak. Overstretching the ligaments of the knee results in permanent laxity and instability. Prolonged episodes of swollen knees also permanently weaken the ligaments.

Genetic predisposition also determines the ratio of elastin to collagen fibers present in ligament tissue. These differences, though slight, significantly affect flexibility and are one of the reasons for observed differences in flexibility among individuals.

"Two out of three ain't bad!"

In the full expression of **Virabhadrasana Two** (Warrior Two), the front leg is meant to flex to 90° angles at both the knee and hip. Many students find this aspect of Warrior Two difficult, causing the muscles in their thigh muscles to burn and their front leg to quickly fatigue. When the front hip and knee flex, the ligaments of these joints loosen, making the front leg less stable and forcing the quadriceps muscles to overwork. Flexion of the hip and knee are part of the pose's design and cannot be changed, however, the actions of abduction and external rotation are available to tighten the ligaments and stabilize the joints. To engage these actions in the front leg, the student aligns the outer thigh in a forward (*sagittal*) line that tracks from the outer buttock, through the outer knee, to the outer edge of the foot. This position produces abduction in the joints of the front leg. External rotation can be added with a firm, isometric contraction of the knee and hip in an outward rotating direction.

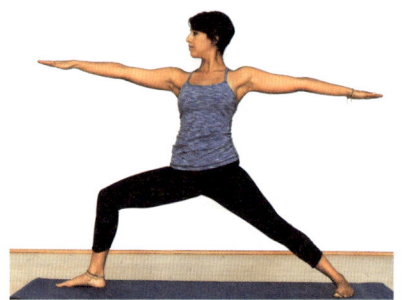

Badda Konasana   Bound Angle Pose

Sometimes the final position of an asana is contrary to the functional design of the ligaments. In Bound Angle Pose, the goal is to open the hips and release the knees toward the floor. The posture is challenging because the hip movements used in this pose - external rotation and abduction - tighten the ligaments and actually limit movement. To compensate for the ligament tightening caused by these movements, the yoga student initiates the pose by first lifting the thighs and bringing them toward the midline, engaging flexion and adduction. As the thighs are released into the final position of the pose, the hips firmly counter-engage (eccentric contraction) with internal rotation, thereby keeping the ligaments loose. By first moving in a direction that releases the joints, the final pose can be both deeper and safer.

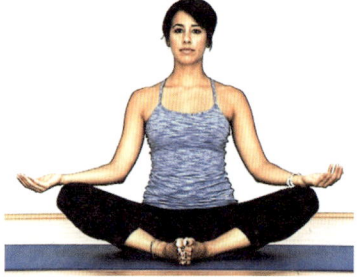

Virabhadrasana One   Warrior One

In Warrior One, one of the major challenges is getting the rear hip square to the front of the mat. Another challenge is keeping the rear foot on the floor and pressed evenly through its four corners. Warrior One positions the rear hip into extension, a direction of movement that tightens and restricts the hip ligaments. To accommodate this limitation of the hip ligaments, the rear hip internally rotates and the thigh is firmly lifted. The rear leg also isometrically draws toward the midline (adduction). Internal rotation and adduction of the rear hip are joint movements that make squaring the hips easier.

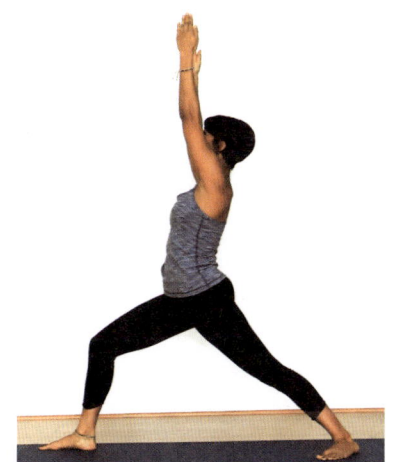

> To enable the hips to square toward the front of the mat, the hip of the rear leg internally rotates to release and loosen its ligaments.
>
> The ligaments of the front hip and knee externally rotate to make the ligaments taut and provide stability.

Vrkasana   Tree Pose

In balancing postures, the weight-bearing leg must be stable. This requires ligament stability at the hip, knee and ankle. To accomplish this, the yogi isometrically contracts the joints using external rotation, extension, and abduction.

The final position of the lifted, bent knee of Tree pose is in a position of abduction and external rotation, two ligament-tightening directions. To bring more flexibility to the hip of the lifted knee, first lift the knee toward the midline so that flexion and adduction are engaged. This loosens the ligaments before the pose continues toward its final configuration. Once the leg is in place, abduction and external rotation are engaged, helping to hold the foot stable against the inner thigh of the standing leg.

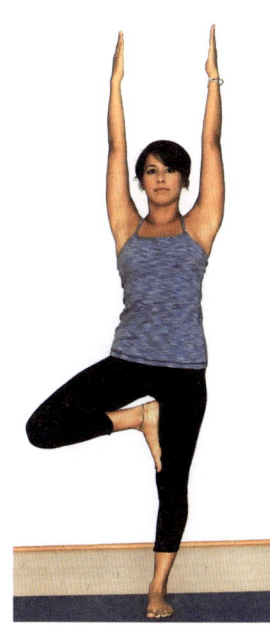

9 Anatomy and Physiology Muscle

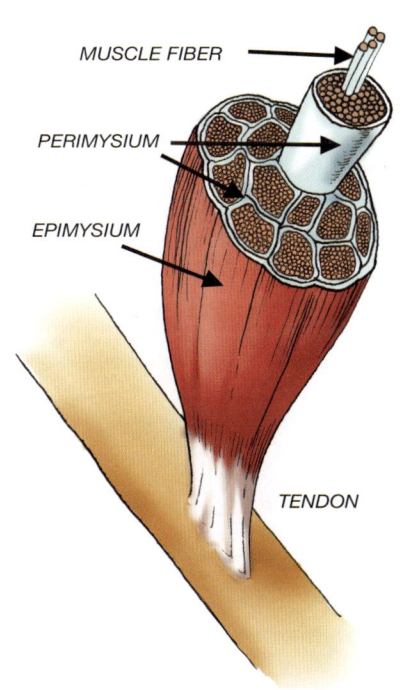

The part of the body that draws the most attention from yogis tends to be their muscles. In asana practice, muscles stretch to increase flexibility and contract to provide strength. Although muscle is not usually categorized as connective tissue, it cannot function without its intimate partner, a specialized type of connective tissue called *myofascia*.

Anatomy of a muscle

A thick telephone cable sliced through its diameter would reveal an internal appearance similar to that of muscle. Muscle consists of strands (of muscle), each surrounded by a sheathing of myofascia. The smallest filaments of muscle are arranged into bundles of varying lengths and sizes called *fasciculi*. Bundles of fasciculi form fibers. Muscles are formed from bundles of fibers. The larger and stronger the muscle is, the greater number of fibers that are bundled together. Some small muscles, such as those of the hand that provide delicate and precise movements, contain fewer fibers per bundle. Myofascia, as described in Chapter 7, encapsulates every strand and every bundle, creating an elaborate relationship between muscle tissue and myofascia. The myofascia that surrounds the outermost muscle fibers is called *epimysium*. The bundles closer to the bone are covered by *perimysium*.[1]

The sarcomere

Muscle fibers consist of unique cells called *sarcomeres*, a term derived from the Greek word for *fleshy part*. A sarcomere has two parts: myoplasm, the contractile portion of the cell, and sarcoplasm, the cell's gel-like center. Sarcomeres vary in size and contain high amounts of elastin. Although the long parallel fibers of muscles differ greatly in size, from 10μm up to 30cm in length, the design and function of sarcomeres remain the same. Individual muscle fibers rarely run the entire length of a muscle. Instead, they collectively form an overlapping, almost haphazard network that spans the bones. As mentioned previously, fibers usually align obliquely to the lines of force that the muscle exerts on the joints, and this orientation provides the greatest strength and efficiency.

Each sarcomere contains millions of bands of myofilaments, which are made up of two proteins. The protein *myosin*, seen under a microscope, forms the thick, dark "A" bands that lay end-to-end between the two "Z" lines. *Actin*, the other protein, makes up the thinner filament "I" bands.

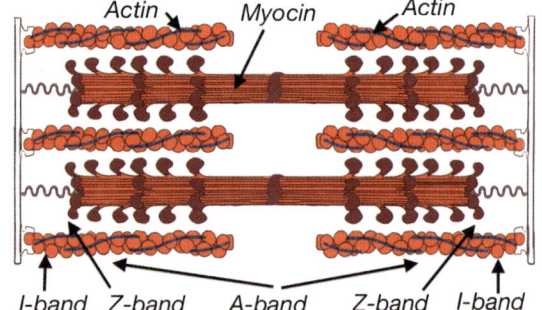

Contraction of a muscle tissue occurs when the myofilaments of its cells overlap. Small hook-shaped strands on the myosin protein latch onto the actin fibers to shorten the width of the cell. When muscles stretch, the strands unlatch and release the overlapping protein filaments.

When a muscle stretches, some fibers lengthen while others remain at rest, simply "going along for the ride". The final length achieved by stretching depends on the number of muscle fibers participating in the stretch. The more fibers engaged, the greater the length. A similar principle operates in muscle contraction. Muscle strength depends on the number of recruited fibers that contract.[2]

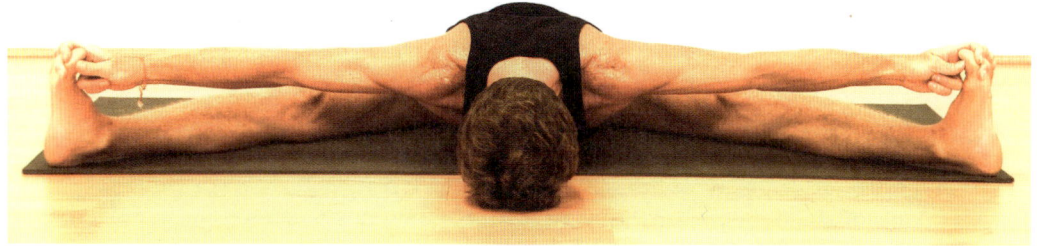

Stretching is forever

A muscle fiber is maximally stretched when all of its sarcomeres are fully elongated. The gel-like sarcoplasm of the cell expands into the additional space created by the stretch. This muscle cell expansion process is called *elastic* or *plastic elongation* and, in theory, can repeat indefinitely. If a stretch is held for a prolonged period of time on a regular basis, a permanent change occurs in the size of the muscle cells.[3]

Although muscle cells have a near unlimited capacity to expand, it is the myofascial sheathing around muscle tissue that is the actual determinant of the ability of a muscle to stretch or become permanently elongated. Since myofascia stretching is limited to 10% of its resting length, muscle tissue cannot exceed that point without traumatizing the myofascia.

The 10% rule

Among exercise professionals and trainers, it is common knowledge that physical activities such as running, stretching, and weightlifting can result in injury when the increase in demand is more than 10% of the base level of performance at any one time. This rule corresponds to the physiology of myofascia, for which the non-traumatic, maximum limit of tissue expansion is 10%.

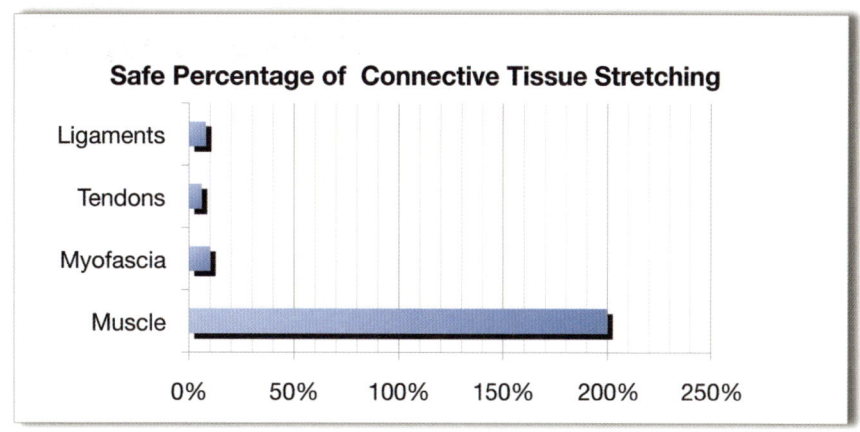

Speed, time and heat

When a muscle rapidly stretches and releases, no significant change occurs in the length of the tissues. The muscle returns to its original shape and length. When the stretch is slowed and held for an extended time, the myofascia expands in the direction of the stretch. The muscle tissue, now less confined, can fill into the space created. Bouncing or sporadically releasing a muscle while stretching triggers neurological reflexes that cause muscle fibers to contract, blocking any possibility of permanent elongation.

The amount of time necessary for elastic elongation to occur is not universal. The timeline is different for each individual, although, for the most part, benefits are derived after five minutes of stretching. Beyond five minutes, the benefits seem to level off. Long-held yoga postures, such as those practiced in *Yin Yoga*, can deliver permanent muscle elongation. For example, a five-minute, seated forward fold posture, performed regularly, can effectively increase the length of the hamstring muscles. Permanent tissue changes, however, come with a caveat. Prolonged stretching should only be performed while engaging constant and precise alignment. Since muscle elongation follows the line of force applied, correct alignment is necessary in order to prevent overstretching in unintended directions and the weakening of tendons, ligaments or already injured muscles.

Warming up muscles before stretching has great benefits. While warming up, significant amounts of heat are created by muscles' collagen-rich, myofascial sheathings as well as by the micro- folding of collagen in their tendons.

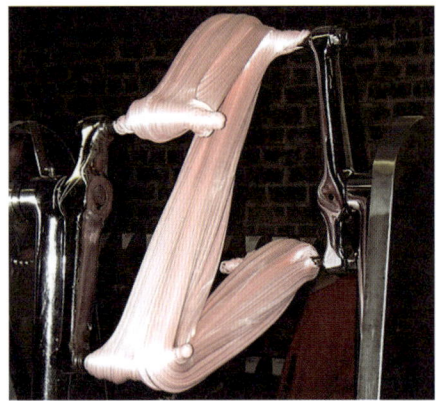

Like stretching taffy, muscles respond best to slow stretching performed over time and in a warmed up state.

Scar tissue

Scar tissue forms when reparative connective tissue fibers that grow into an injured area lay themselves out in a disorganized and random fashion. Scar tissue forms, not only on the skin but also within other connective tissue structures. Although scars are sometimes inevitable, stretching slowly, without bouncing and for extended periods of time, helps fibers align properly as they form. The more precise the alignment while stretching, the more organized are the new fibers, producing less scar tissue. Heat is beneficial for reducing the potential for the scar formation as well.

Skin deep

Skin sometimes becomes loose and non-elastic after significant weight loss or a muscle atrophy condition. The collagen in the skin, fascia and myofascia, once expanded by the body mass it enveloped, is permanently elongated and afterward, unable to retract to a smaller, tighter shape.

Strength, force and efficiency

Strength is generally understood to be the amount of force a muscle can exert regardless of its energetic cost. From a yogic viewpoint, muscle efficiency is more important than muscle strength. Efficiency measures the relative trade off between attaining maximum muscle performance and using the least amount of energy. Think Hummer vs. Prius.

Potential for muscle efficiency

Muscles reach maximum efficiency when stretched to 20% of their resting length. Similar to the lengthening a rubber band, stretching increases a muscle's kinetic energy. Beyond the "sweet spot" of 20%, efficiency decreases as a result of the proteins of the sarcomere being separated too far and unable to sufficiently overlap to provide maximum contraction.[5]

The long and short of it

Short muscles are generally more efficient than longer ones. For example, the masseter muscle of the jaw is one of the shortest and most efficient muscles in the body. In fact, at their beginning range of motion, many larger muscles are too inefficient to initiate movement by themselves. They rely on short, efficient muscles acting as "keys" to unlock the power of the large muscles.

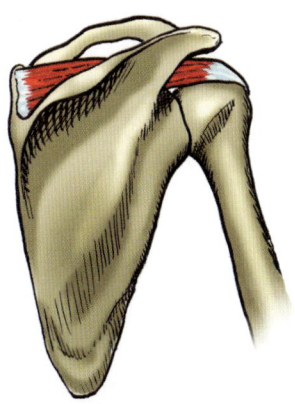

Supraspinatus

For example, the supraspinatus muscle has a key-type relationship with the deltoid muscle, initiating the action of shoulder abduction. This relationship is easily observed in someone with a rotator cuff injury who is unable to abduct their arm from the side of the body as a result of a tear in the supraspinatus. A similar relationship exists between the anconeus muscle and the triceps brachii in elbow extension, and with the popliteus and the hamstring muscles in flexion and rotation of the knee. In each case, the former, smaller muscle initiates the movement of the latter, larger one.

Muscles often shorten and reduce in size in older age and with some illnesses. The shortened fibers are the body's way to improve efficiency and compensate for loss of strength. As muscles shorten, their flexibility reduces. This phenomenon can be observed in the gait of our retired population, pejoratively referred to as the "senior" waddle.

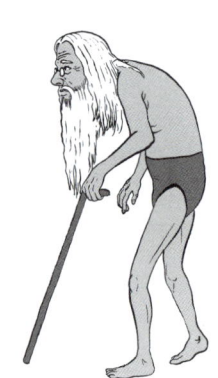

Overstretching

Stretching is not a simple matter of reaching the arms overhead. A degree of skill is required in order to avoid overstretching. As presented earlier in this chapter, overstretching can tear the myofascial sheathing around muscle tissue. Collagen-rich ligaments become permanently unstable after repetitive, prolonged stretching that exceeds their anatomical limits. Habitual overstretching, especially during the years of active body development, may result in hypermobile, unstable joints. This is a risk to be considered for children participating in dance and gymnastic activities. At any age or condition of health, the most skillful way to avoid overstretching is to implement the *integrative alignment* principles as presented in this book. The instruction to *draw bones together and extend muscles from their center* may be the best preventative for overstretching of tendons and ligaments (See Chapter 5 for more details.)

> Draw bones together and extend muscles apart when stretching to prevent overstretching

Mixing yoga with athletics...maybe!

If muscle efficiency is enhanced by muscle being short and compact, you might question whether yoga, or stretching in general, is appropriate for athletes. A question being explored in competitive sports training is whether stretching causes injury.

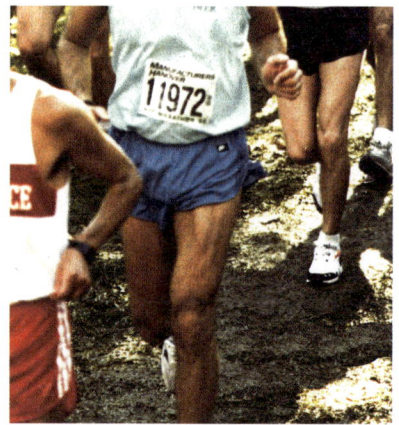

A number of coaches in Track and Field are discouraging their athletes from engaging in the static stretching; the type of long-held stretches done in yoga. They purport that static stretching reduces speed and power by lengthening muscles. Shorter muscles are more powerful due to a shorter "piston" distance transferring more energy across the joints.[6] These physiological considerations are valid, and extensive stretching before sports activity may not be beneficial.[7] And although this may seemingly warn against high-level competitive athletes practicing yoga, there are other factors to consider. An increase in flexibility, balance and agility obtained through yoga can overshadow the downside of a small loss of contractile power.

The increased body awareness that yoga provides the athlete may prevent traumatic sports injuries, which are probably the real challenges to a successful career and performance.

Scientific study of the effects of yoga is challenging. Current research provides no definitive answers. The typical tools of assessment, such as a prescribed number of minutes of practice or an isolated set of yoga postures, do not create a controlled experiment.[8] Countless variables challenge the scientific study of yoga. Were the postures performed with correct alignment? What level of intensity did the subjects bring to their practices? Were the test subjects aware of principles that prevent strain and injury? Was yoga approached as merely another exercise discipline? And, what are the physiological effects of the "spiritual" elements of mind-body interconnectiveness in the full yoga experience?

Offering an anecdote of my personal experience as a life-long athlete, and particularly in long distance running, I have found a balance between yoga practice and sport that seems to allow both activities to provide benefit. By practicing yoga for twice as long as I run, my muscles remain flexible, and running, though not competitive, remains injury-free. For a recreational athlete, a forty-five minute run, balanced by a ninety-minute yoga practice is a reasonable way to keep both activities safe and able to advance. Yoga is best practiced at times separate from other high-demand physical activities. Running and other sports activity frequently cause small tears in the muscle fibers; immediately practicing yoga or any extensive stretching is not recommended as the muscles recover. Since yoga practice itself can cause muscle micro-tears, it is not recommended immediately before intense sport activities.

The stretch reflex

Muscles and tendons can be subject to abrupt or rapid stretching. At other times, they may be forced to instantaneously contract, for instance, when suddenly loaded with weight. These quick changes put muscles and tendons at risk for injury. To protect muscles from potential injuries, embedded in muscle tissue and tendons are special, sensory nerve cells called *proprioceptors*. Through an intricate system that works like a trip wire, proprioceptors trigger a spinal reflex that rapidly relaxes a muscle before it can over-contract and become damaged. Located in the belly of muscles, the sensory neurons that prevent overstretching are called *muscle spindle cells*. They record changes in muscle length and the velocity of a stretch, sending signals to the spine. This is called the *stretch reflex* or the *myostatic reflex*. Reflexes are quick occurring because they respond directly from the spine without the need to wait for information from the brain.

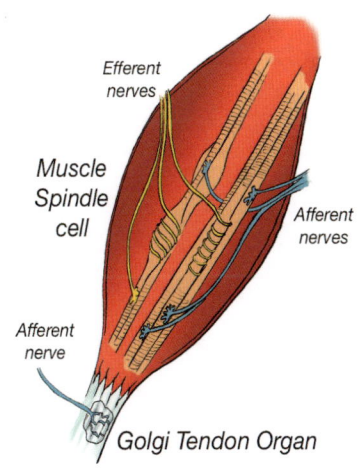

Muscle spindle cells prompt an overloaded muscle to contract and resist lengthening. The more sudden is the change in muscle length or load, the stronger the myostatic response. Besides this protective feature, muscle spindle cells also maintain basic muscular tone.

In the tendons, it is the *Golgi tendon organs* that signal muscles not to overstretch or contract beyond safe limits. Golgi tendon organs, or GTOs, are neurological devices interwoven in every ten to twenty strands of the collagenous end-fibers of muscle tendons. Triggered by a forceful, quick tendon contraction, the firing of the GTOs lessens the intensity of the contraction and the likelihood of injury. The GTOs send sensory nerve signals from the tendon directly to the spine, creating a reflex that rapidly inhibits muscle contraction.

Deep tendon and stretch reflexes

In a physical examination, a health care provider may take a small rubber-tipped hammer and gently strike a patient's knee or elbow. This test of *deep tendon reflexes* evaluates the path of the spinal nerves responsible for the contraction of the muscles that extend either the knee or elbow. The strike of the hammer on the muscle tendon stimulates the muscle's spindle cells to fire, which triggers a contractile response from the muscle. These innate reflexes have a useful place in human physiology, offering protection from injuries resulting from abrupt, changeable physical stresses that impact the body through daily activities.

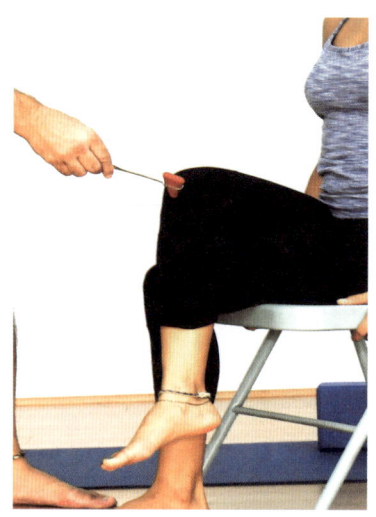

Habituation

If stretching continues over a prolonged period of time, the muscle spindle cells become accustomed to being stimulated and the alarm signals they send to the nervous system diminish. This suppression of neuromuscular reflexes is called *habituation*.

A yogi can use habituation as a tool to lengthen muscles without causing the reflexive firing of the stretch receptors. Yin and Restorative yoga utilize habituation effectively, taking advantage of the low-velocity stretching used in those approaches. While habituation can increase flexibility and have rehabilitative value, if used improperly there is potential risk of injury. Deep, habituated stretching makes muscles, tendons and ligaments vulnerable to injury if the body is poorly aligned. Tearing of the tissues can occur if sudden bouncing or changes of position take place while in the pose.

In strength training programs, there are disagreements regarding the effect of habituation on the Golgi tendon organs. Some experts believe that the Golgi tendon organs habituate muscles to the repetitive nature of weight lifting, making weight training less effective for strength building.

"It is theorized that overuse with forced repetitions on very heavy weight may teach muscles to prematurely fail. Strength training involves a neurological adaptation motor development, contraction efficiency as well as a morphological adaptation. Repeated use of forced repetitions on very heavy weight may prematurely activate the Golgi tendon organs." (exrx.net) [9]

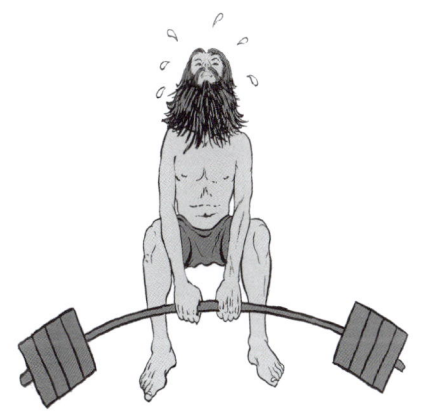

Other trainers and sport professionals disagree and contend that the Golgi tendon organs are "...nowhere near as powerful an inhibitor of muscle activation as many in the fitness industry believe." (Crago et al) [10]

This controversy may be important to those involved in serious bodybuilding pursuits in which every advantage received from training is explored. It poses little concern, however, for the yoga student striving to increase their general flexibility and overall strength.

Fast and slow twitch fibers

We are born with nearly equal numbers of fast-twitch and slow-twitch fibers in our muscle tissue. Fast-twitch fibers (type-two) are large and provide speed, power and strength. Fast-twitch fibers, however, fatigue easily. They contain fewer capillaries and their cells contain fewer mitochondria, the cell's powerhouse. Fast-twitch muscles are analogous to the "white meat" of flying fowl.

Slow-twitch fibers (type-one) are smaller than fast-twitch fibers but have higher endurance. They initiate muscle contractions and are able to continue well beyond the point where fast-twitch fibers fatigue.

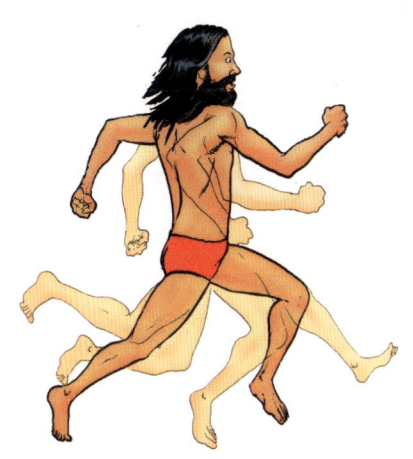

Slow-twitch fibers correspond to the "dark meat" of fowl muscle tissue. Their cells are dense with mitochondria and they have a high blood flow, thus making them darker in color. Slow-twitch fibers receive more oxygen, produce less waste, and are more efficient. For these reasons, type-one fibers are most suitable for humans in older age.

Muscles and aging

At the level of individual muscle fibers, strength and endurance does not significantly decrease with age. Once activated, the cell proteins in the sarcomeres overlap to the same degree in advanced age as they have throughout one's life. Muscles, however, demonstrate clear changes with age. Older muscles require a longer recovery time between episodes of exertion and tend to re-fire more slowly. This process is known as *contraction fatigue.*

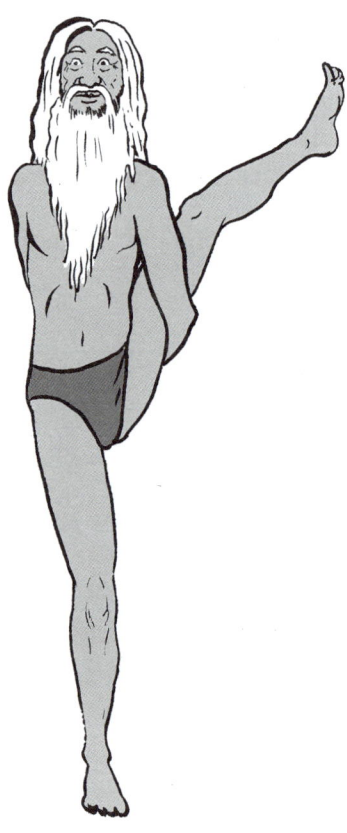

The overall mass of muscle decreases with aging, a condition referred to as *sarcopenia*. Muscle mass loss is usually greater in the lower extremities than the upper body. Between the ages of twenty and eighty, the average person experiences a 25% decrease in the overall number of muscle fibers. The primary fibers lost are motor units, the fibers that directly communicate with the nervous system. Muscle loss from aging almost exclusively occurs in the fast-twitch fibers, whereas their slow-twitch counterparts undergo little change. Muscle loss, therefore, increases the percentage of slow-twitch to fast-twitch fibers. It has been theorized that slow-twitch motor neurons may actually replace or rescue and repair the lost motor units in aged muscles.[11]

> *Technically Speaking*
> A motor unit consists of the motor neuron (nerve) and muscle fibers upon which it acts. A motor neuron may control between 100 to 10,000 individual fibers.

The value of yoga for aging muscles

As we age, yoga offers countless benefits for the entire body. For muscles specifically, yoga improves pliability and increases strength. Building a large mass of muscle in the early years of life helps preserve fast-twitch fibers. Building muscle also stimulates muscle's ability to self-repair, thereby increasing muscle fiber longevity.[12]

Building muscle mass is called *muscle hypertrophy*. Yoga, along with most physical activities, stimulates hypertrophy. Arm balances and single-leg balancing postures are recommended to be included in a daily practice to significantly increase the mass and strength of muscle.

Since asana practice provides these benefits, the younger a yoga student is when they begin to build strength, the greater the number of fibers they have at their disposal in later years. Building more muscle mass at an earlier time of life provides a higher baseline of muscle density before the effects of aging and its muscle mass loss inevitably set in.

Yoga, as a practice for aging, helps to maintain posture and balance. Balancing poses develop core strength, challenge agility and keep the nervous system stimulated. The flexibility derived from yoga postures keeps muscles adaptable and responsive to the activities of daily life.

Yoga is valuable to the elderly for its ability to increase blood circulation and improve arterial health. A gentle, yet flowing vinyasa series increases cardiovascular capacity and brings greater blood flow to the muscles. Being a muscle, the heart benefits greatly from yoga's nasal breathing techniques. Nose breathing is shown to be healthier for the heart muscle than the more explosive type of breathing typically experienced during intensive sport activities. More details on this topic are presented in Chapter 25.

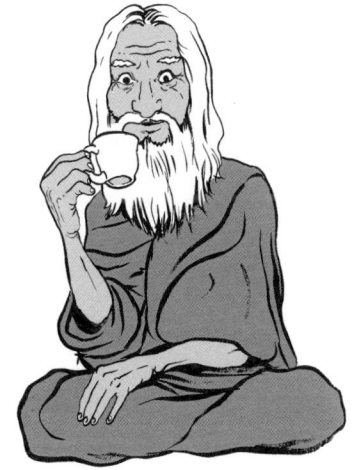

In practical terms, if a certain mass of muscle is required to lift the morning teacup, having extra fibers to spare ensures more soothing cups of tea enjoyed much longer in life!

10 Anatomy and Physiology Cartilage and Bone

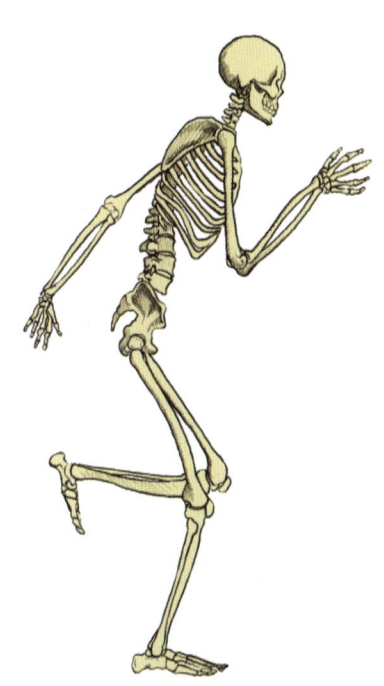

This final chapter on anatomy and physiology reviews one of the most easily identified parts of the human body, the skeleton. Bones and cartilage are classified as connective tissue. They form the framework on which muscles attach and internal organs are suspended. The skeleton also protects internal organs from external injury. The infant skeleton consists of over 270 soft bones that are made up of mostly cartilage. Cartilage converts to bone through a process of calcification and fusion that continues into our early twenties, leaving a tally of 206 bones in the adult skeleton. Bones are a basic component of all mechanical activities of the body. Yoga practice places great emphasis on the skeleton and makes no bones about that!

Cartilage

Cartilage is found throughout the body in various forms. Flexible cartilage is the major constituent of the ears, nose and bronchial tubes. A more firm and fibrous form of cartilage composes the outer rings of the intervertebral discs. Hyaline cartilage, a firm, dense and pearly blue tissue, covers the joint (articular) surfaces of bone. Cartilage is produced by *chondroblasts*, specialized cells that release chemicals called protoglycans that infiltrate collagen fibers and transform them into cartilage tissue.

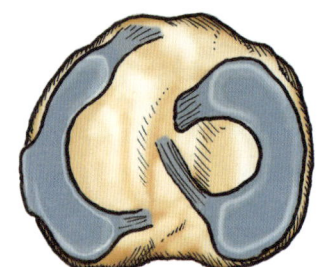

Medial Meniscus of knee

Lateral Meniscus

There is essentially no blood supply to adult cartilage. The sequestering of cartilage from blood keeps it free of minerals. If blood were present in cartilage, it would deposit minerals and mineral salts of calcium, silicon and boron. Cartilage exposed to these minerals converts into bone.

Although not desirable for the adult skeleton, cartilage-to-bone conversion is essential for bone growth and maturation in children. The proliferation of blood vessels into the child's cartilage-rich skeletal system slowly orchestrates its transition into bone.[1]

As an infant develops muscle tone, cartilage-to-bone conversion is stimulated by the electro-mechanical energy produced by muscle contractions. This process occurs when, as a baby first begins to stand, its lower back muscles more fully contract, stimulating the spiny processes of the lumbar vertebrae to mold and form into bone.

Because of the absence of blood supply, cartilage imbibes nutrients directly from the synovial fluid that lubricates joint surfaces. Short, squeeze-and-release compressions created by joint movement provide a pumping action that cleanses cartilage, allowing vital nutrients to enter and waste products to leave. This lavage method of supplying cartilage with nutrients is, unfortunately, slow and inefficient. It does, however, prevent cartilage from coming into direct contact with blood. With its rudimentary and inefficient circulation, the healing process of cartilage is substandard. Damaged cartilage rarely heals without consequences, such as the formation of scar tissue.

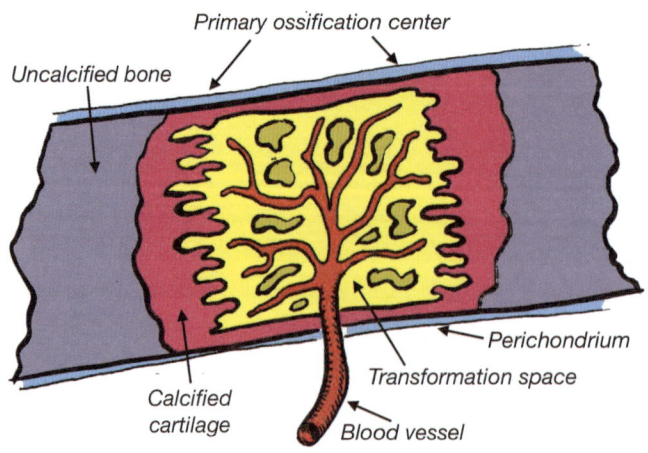

Hyaline Cartilage

Hyaline cartilage encapsulates the ends of bones, helping to smooth movement by reducing friction between joint surfaces. The blue-colored hyaline cartilage corresponds to the gristle found on the ends of bones eaten by our carnivorous cohorts.[2]

Hyaline cartilage has an important role as a barrier between the rich blood supply located in the *periosteum*, the outer layer of bone, and the synovial membranes on the inner linings of the joint. After an injury during which blood vessels dilate and cause excessive swelling, blood can enter the joint. This can cause calcification of the joint cartilage, arthritic spurring and the deformation of joint surfaces. Swelling is the body's method of immobilizing an injured joint. All too often, the impatient yoga student will force their injured, swollen joints to move before they have properly healed, causing the hyaline cartilage to shear and tear.

Bone

Mature bone is a living tissue. It is as strong as cast iron yet flexible and lightweight. Bone has good tensile strength (resists stretching), but buckles when excessively compressed. Bone is constructed of collagen fibers infiltrated by an ideal balance of organic proteins and inorganic minerals forming a strong, flexible matrix. There are two types of bone, compact and spongy (cancellous). Compact bone forms the shafts of long bones and the outer surfaces of all of the bones of the skeletal system. Spongy bone is located in the heads of long bones and in irregular bones, such as vertebrae and the skull. A series of canals course through bone's many layers, carrying blood vessels and nerves. The blood supplies minerals and other essential nutrients to the bone. The nerves enable sensation and provide electrical stimulation to the bone, which helps maintain density.

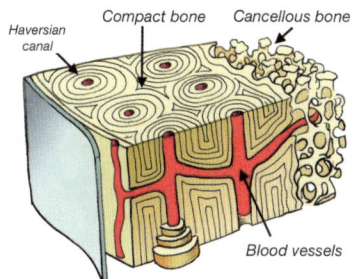

Technically Speaking

Bone matrix is made up of bone fibrils formed from a suspension of *hydroxyapatite*, a complex form of phosphate and calcium- $Ca_5(PO_4)_3OH$. The matrix is then infused with micro-crystals mineralized with calcium, boron, silicon and other trace minerals. Bone is ceramic by nature and can withstand moderate compression and shearing stresses, while providing excellent tensile stretch. The bone fibrils that form the bone matrix align in relation to the forces placed upon them by gravity, weight, and muscular tension.

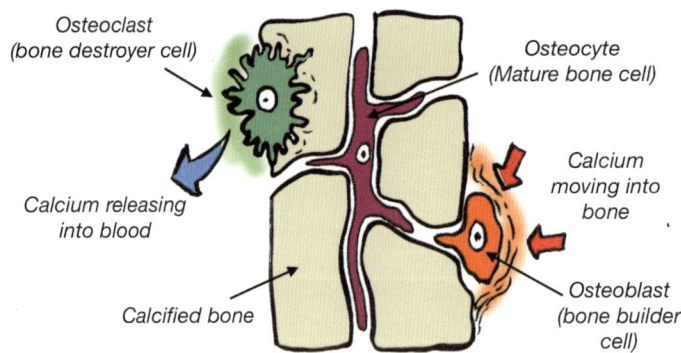

Bone Density

Calcium and other inorganic mineral ions are constantly in circulation throughout the body. The calcium located in the femur bone one week might be found in the stomach two weeks later manufacturing digestive acids. As described previously in relation to cartilage, minerals such as calcium can easily penetrate soft tissue collagen and form bone, often in undesired places. Bone spurs that accompany arthritic joints are an example of this process.

The primary promoter of bone density is mechanical forces on the bone itself. In normal physiology, bone is constantly breaking down, rebuilding and remodeling to accommodate the changing tensions and stresses to which bone is subjected. Nerves continually measure mechanical stresses that pass through bone. The autonomic nervous system coordinates the action between the *osteoblasts*, cells that build bone, and the bone destroying cells, the *osteoclasts*. The cells in stable bone tissue are called *osteocytes*.

Bone becomes markedly thickened where there is great muscular contraction. In athletes and professionals with physical occupations that create muscle imbalances, bone density often becomes uneven. If injury or disease causes disproportionate weakness in muscles around a bone, osteoclast activity will dissolve bone on the weakened side, while the osteoblasts will build bone on the side that remains strong.

Yoga practice can improve bone density. Muscle contraction, gravity and heel strike forces all deliver mechanical signals to bone to maintain density. The Anusara yoga instruction to *"hug the muscles to the bone"* creates significant mechanical tension on bone. In cases of advanced bone loss, an entire yoga practice may consist of simple isometric contractions that hug the muscles to the bone while holding basic sitting and standing postures. Correct alignment and the principle of **Samasthiti** (balanced tension) are essential tools for practitioners needing to increase bone density. In cases of scoliosis, where the spine abnormally curves and the musculature becomes imbalanced, precise alignment and Samasthiti are an essential focus during yoga practice.

Resistance training (weight lifting) is one of the best methods for delivering mechanical tension to the bone and increasing its density. Mineral mass measures highest in the femurs of weightlifters although considerably less in swimmers. During prolonged periods without mechanical stimulation, such as during bed rest, there can be a 1% bone loss per week.[3]

Osteoporosis and Osteopenia

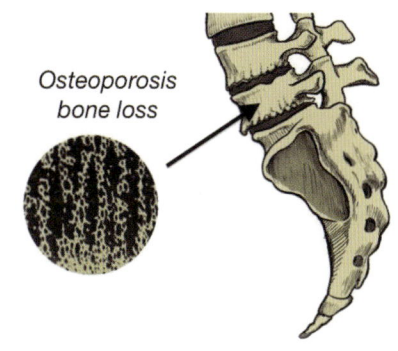

Osteoporosis bone loss

Osteopenia is a serious and practically epidemic bone condition in first world cultures. It is characterized by the deterioration or destruction of the protein-matrix of bone. As a result, minerals are without a place to embed. Calcium supplements offer little benefit to bone tissue when its matrix is lost. When mineral concentration is measurably reduced, the condition is called *osteoporosis*. All too often these two bone-loss conditions result in structural collapse of bone in the form of compression fractures.

Hormonal changes, particularly reduction in estrogen and adrenal hormone levels, result in bone loss. Hormones regulate the levels of minerals in the bloodstream and their absorption into all tissues of the body.

Bone's absorptive qualities

As described, the collagen proteins of bone can easily absorb trace minerals. This metabolic process ensures that bone receives micronutrients needed to maintain its density.

Substances besides those that build healthy bone structure may also become absorbed unwittingly into bone tissue. As we know from dental treatments, fluoride minerals can be readily absorbed by teeth. After treatments, levels of fluoride in bone tissue have been shown to increase, as well. Although fluoride makes teeth and bones stronger, it causes bone tissue to be more brittle.[4] Heavy metals and toxic chemicals, from nicotine to DDT, have been found in bone tissue, absorbed and stored in the collagen proteins of the bone matrix.

When bone loss occurs, as is commonly seen with aging, a release of these sequestered metals and toxins can send them back into the blood stream, potentially triggering serious illnesses.

Avoiding heavy metals, such as lead and mercury, is an obvious preventative to this scenario. A diet high in organic fruits, vegetables and whole grains helps remove toxic substances that are already present. Starting a healthy, high-fiber dietary regimen early in life can protect the body from toxic substance storage in bone.

Bone re-modeling and the value of good posture

Mechanical forces and electrical stimulation not only affect bone density, but also modify and remold bone's actual shape. Laboratory experiments have demonstrated the ease with which the shape of bone can be manipulated. In a patently non-yogic experiment, rabbits had the bones of their legs placed in vice-like, movable casts that were slowly twisted during a six to eight week period. Bones were forced to remodel from straight to curved. The procedure was then reversed and the bones returned to being straight.[5] Adaptation of this principle is used in orthopedics for treating fractured bones. Mechanical and electrical devices have helped heal bone fractures utilizing the same physiological properties demonstrated in the rabbit lab tests.

Yoga and yoga therapy can also influence bone re-modeling. The physical forces on bone during asana, such as gravity and muscle contraction, can re-shape bone. If the forces are correctly distributed and integrated through alignment, bone can re-model into a stronger, more desirable form. Although no scientific studies have confirmed yoga's ability to re-model bone, many experienced yoga teachers and students can attest to yoga's effectiveness in this area. Anecdotes are frequently heard of yoga practitioners applying alignment principles to help straighten bowed legs, and achieving positive results with a dedicated, long-term practice.

During the aging process, yoga provides an excellent opportunity to maintain bone density and the overall organic health of our human frame. Here too, long-term practitioners have first-hand experience that upholds the value of yoga and its ability to assist bone health and repair.

11 Align By Design

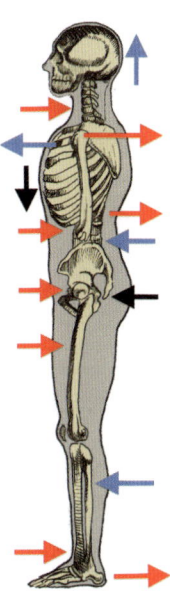

There is wide variation in the appearance of the human form. Vast differences are apparent in our sizes and shapes, hues and colors. Body types range from that of the sleek and flexible savanna dwellers on the African continent to the large-boned population originating from European peasant stock. Differences between individuals can also be found in our internal anatomy. The presence or absence of certain muscles, nerves and blood vessels fluctuates in the human population. The location of ligaments and tendons, at times, seems haphazard and makeshift. And yet, the genetic make-up between all humans is virtually identical. Less than one tenth of one percent of human DNA varies between the most diverse members of our species.

When it comes to understanding the mechanical properties all human bodies hold in common, the variations in anatomy between individuals prove to be relatively inconsequential.

Yoga practice is appropriate for everyone and suitable for all body types. Despite the vast differences in capabilities among individuals, there is only one "owner's manual" for the body. All yoga students follow the same *universal blueprint* that outlines the basic design of the body and how best to establish alignment.[1] Even more importantly, it is not necessary to learn a new set of alignment instructions for each and every asana. The principles of alignment apply to the body, not to the form of the asana. Asana is simply the expression of alignment. Of course, adjustments and modifications are made to the asana to account for subtle anatomical differences between students or to accommodate injuries. These adjustments, however, pertain to how the poses are performed and do not modify or nullify the underlying alignment principles. Students are best protected from potential injury when alignment is stringently followed.

Technically Speaking

One anatomical variation of the body occurs in the vertebral joints. For a small number of people, these joints, which are called *facets*, face in opposing directions. This anomaly is referred to as *asymmetrical facets*. When the affected vertebra moves, an undesired twist of the segment may occur. It requires radiological imaging to detect the presence of asymmetrical facets. Should a yogi have this design anomaly in their spine, knowing its location and configuration is important. The student can adjust his practice to prevent excessive twist and torque on these distressed segments. Implementing the principles of integrative alignment skillfully, especially Samasthiti, can effectively minimize aberrant movements and avert the damage that this anatomical anomaly can cause to the spine.

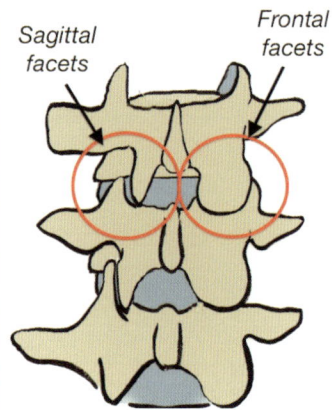

Need GPS?

Do you know the directions of movements that bring posture into its correct alignment? Every part of the body, large and small, is designed to move in a specific direction to come into alignment. Alignment may require an actual physical movement or may call for an isometric muscular contraction with an energetic intention. Movements that bring the body more precisely into alignment have positive, therapeutic qualities. Movements that shift the body further from ideal alignment become dangerous and set up the conditions for injury.

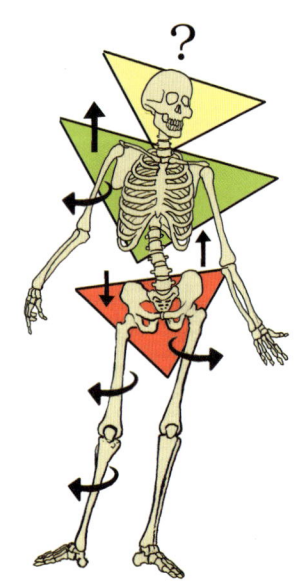

> The principles of alignment are applied to the body, not to the asana.
> Asana is the expression of body alignment.

The Alignment Grid [3]

The most fundamental posture in yoga is **Tadasana**, the Mountain Pose. As its name implies, Mountain Pose embodies a state of groundedness. *Samasthiti,* the quality of balanced tension, is expressed fully in Tadasana.

All essential elements of alignment used for all other asana exist within Tadasana. Although Tadasana is perhaps the first posture a novice student will learn, it requires practice and skill to master all of its subtle actions. The precision a student applies to Tadasana often reflects the intention that that student will bring to their entire practice.

The actions that move every asana into alignment follow the directions depicted in the Alignment Grid.

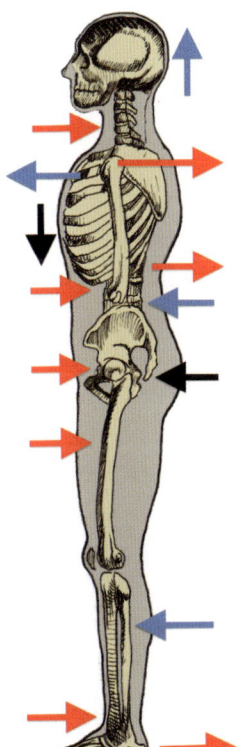

- Heels draw back
- Ankle creases draw back
- Shins move forward
- From the side, hip socket (greater trochanter) is vertical over ankle
- Thighs draw back
- Hip creases and navel draw back
- Low back at L4 - L5 level moves forward to form egg-sized curve
- Coccyx *scoops* forward
- Lower rib cage draws back
- Each side of the rib cage lengthens
- Chest extends forward
- Inner and outer armpits, with equal effort, draw the shoulders back
- Tip of breastbone (xiphoid) drops down and scoops toward navel
- Throat draws back
- Roof of mouth is horizontal with the center of the ear canal
- The base of skull lifts vertically

Every movement we make is coordinated and interconnected with all others. An action that increases alignment does not offset a prior action or disrupt any previously aligned region; instead it further contributes to an integrated posture.

Simple triple "S" alignment (skull, scapulae, sacrum)

The posterior portions of the skull, shoulder blades (scapulae) and sacrum all align vertically.[2] This triple S configuration aligns the body's central axis and configures the spinal curves to provide their greatest strength and weight bearing. A useful way for students to practice this alignment is to sit or stand with their backs against a wall as they attempt to press the skull, scapulae and sacrum equally to the wall. This exercise is a simple, yet excellent therapy for improving postural alignment.

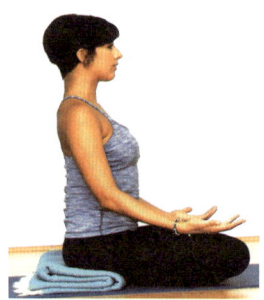
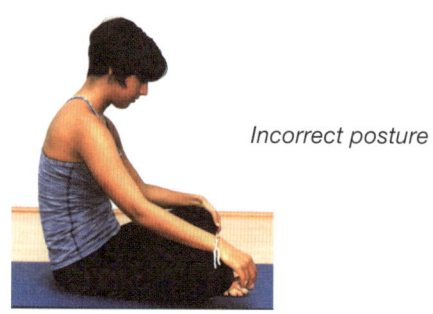

Incorrect posture

In **Ardha Matsyendrasana** (Seated Twist), the alignment principles are the same as in Tadasana. Often, students incorrectly let their shoulders and head drop forward and the upper back round in order to bring the front elbow forward of the knee or to clasp the hands. Those actions should not be forced if it causes alignment to be abandoned. If the shoulders drop forward and the central axis cannot be maintained, the pose will cause injury.

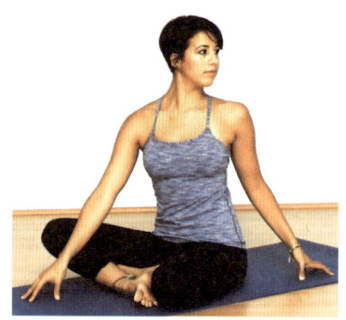

Lock and Load: Step-by-step stabilization for alignment

Stability begins by setting the foundation of the pose. Then, step-by-step, subsequent alignment actions lock into place. With this method, each alignment action serves as the foundation for the next. For example, moving the shins forward and locking them in place creates leverage for the thighs to draw back against. Another example is drawing the lower rib cage back creates a stable foundation and leverage for the chest as it extends forward. Applying this progressive, "lock and load" approach helps develop the skill of implementing the Alignment Grid and a better understanding of integrative alignment.

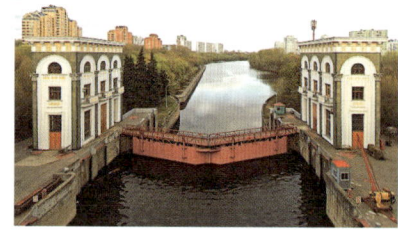

The floating ribs

The lowest two sets of ribs are called *floating* ribs because they have no structural attachments on the anterior body, connection only to the skeleton with joints on the vertebral column posteriorly. The floating ribs cover and protect the kidneys from trauma.

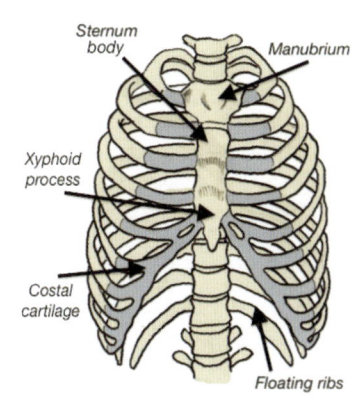

To bring the floating ribs into integrative alignment, three directions of movement are engaged. The lower rib cage *draws back*, *widens on the back*, and *lifts*. This action is difficult for many yoga students, especially for the more flexible students. B.K.S. Iyengar instructs his students to broaden the kidneys across the back body. John Friend addresses this action with his principle of *Kidney Loop*.[4]

Greater details on lower rib cage alignment are presented in Chapter 15.

Design and function

The sacrum is centered between the two hipbones, and the sternum (breastbone) locates centrally in the anterior rib cage. From the side view, both the sacrum and the sternum have a similar curve and appearance. Each also has a small tail at its tip - the coccyx on the sacrum and the xiphoid process at the bottom of the sternum.

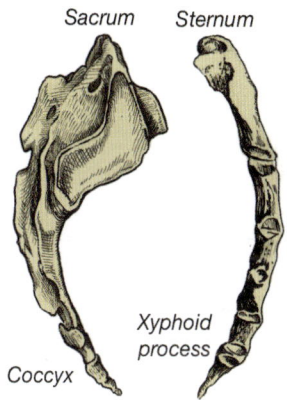

Scoop, Scoop, Draw in the Navel, Keeps the low back stable!

A major challenge in asana practice is integrative alignment between the pelvis and the lower torso. This simple method effectively establishes alignment, which is essential for safe function of the lumbar spine. Scoop the tip of the tailbone forward and scoop the tip of the breastbone inward toward the navel. Then draw the navel softly inward. Keep the thighs drawn back. The front of the body does not contract, collapse or shorten.

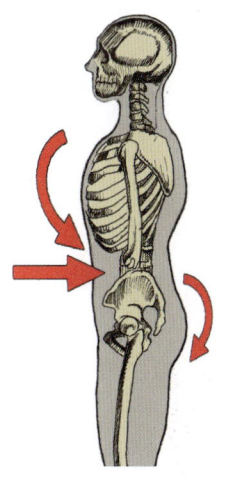

The scooping actions are soft, yet deliberate. The muscles of the pelvis do not firmly contract. As will be explored in subsequent chapters, the scooping actions correspond to what some yoga traditions refer to as engaging the bandhas, or the yogic energy locks.

> Anusara yoga teacher Jaye Martin describes the quality of the action of *drawing in the navel* as imagining a ripe strawberry placed in the belly button being drawn inward about a half inch, gently so as not to crush it.

Zip it!

A useful visualization for integrating the lower torso and pelvis is offered by senior Iyengar yoga teacher Joan White. White suggests that the student imagine zipping up a pair of pants. This has the same effect as a *forward tailbone scoop*. Borrowing White's metaphor, the student can also zip down from the xiphoid process to the navel as visualization for scooping the tip of the breastbone.

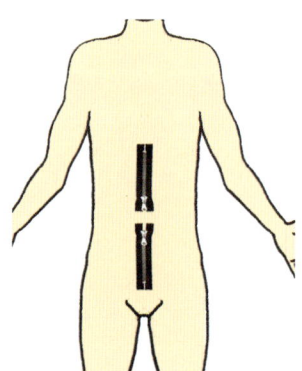

Beauty in its simplicity

As this book emphasizes, there is no need for yoga students to learn a complex list of alignment instructions for each individual asana. Every yoga pose follows the same set of directions. Once students are comfortable with applying the Alignment Grid and other supporting principles, mental effort transforms into ease and fluidity.

New styles and hybrids of yoga are emerging rapidly. Some of these new yoga incarnations are brilliant, while others lack the intention of alignment altogether. Students will remain safe with these new approaches by remembering that all alignment is in reference to the body, not to the poses. Yoga is the practice of retaining alignment in every variation of form and posture.

Just in case...

... you want a quick, simplified version of alignment that can be easily remembered or taught, below are two fundamental principles that establish alignment in every asana. Although simple, they still require effort and intention to apply. With practice, the two instructions below allow a beginner student to display the sophistication and refinement of an advanced practitioner.

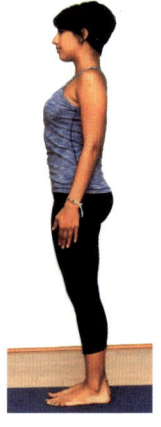

The chest is in front and the shoulders are in back. Shoulder blades hug close to the spine on back.

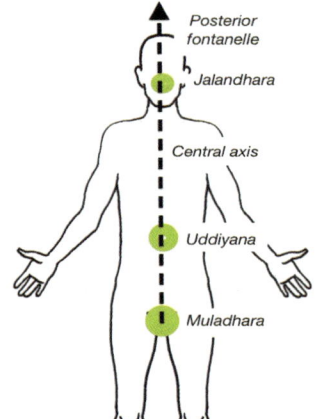

Align the bandhas through the body's central axis

12 Anatomy of the Pelvis and Sacroiliac Joints

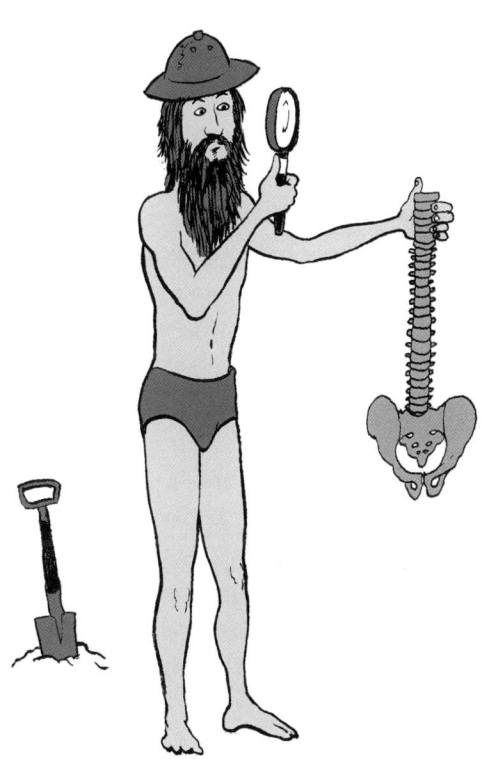

Archeologists love to unearth pelvic bones. The smallest remnants provide a treasure trove of information about the specific life and behavior of their owner and human ancestry in general. A prehistoric pelvis can reveal untold details that relate to the human evolutionary journey. Did this ancestor live mostly in trees or on the land? Was it bi-pedal? What was its gait like? What degree of uprightness did this species reach? Besides these questions, the pelvis reveals the sex of the individual and, if female, how she gave birth (parturition). The pelvis is not only a fascinating part of the human frame but plays a central role in body mechanics.

The pelvis is a bowl-like structure constructed of three bones: two outer hipbones (os coxae) and the sacrum at the center. It forms a ring that protects the organs of the lower abdomen. The hip joints emerge from the lower, outer portion of the pelvis. The sacrum is positioned as an inverted triangle with its broad base at the top of the pelvis, providing the foundation for the vertebral spine.

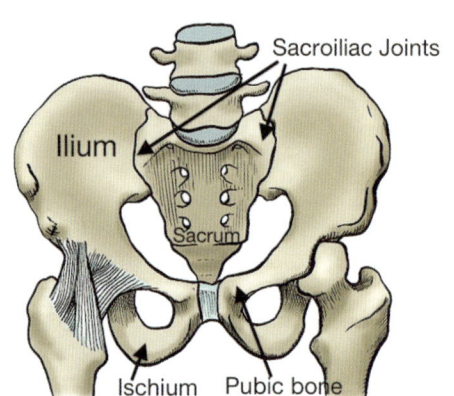

The acetabulum

The construction of each hipbone is broken down further into three anatomically separate bones - the ischium, ilium, and pubis. All three bones join together at the center of the hip joint, forming a deep, cup-shaped hip socket called the acetabulum. The joining of the three bones specifically at the hip socket's center enables gravity and the pounding forces of heel strike to be evenly distributed throughout the pelvis.

The acetabulum does not completely form into one solid bone for most individuals until the age of 20 to 25.[1] Bone formation in women often completes earlier, depending upon their age at the start of menstruation.[2] Beginning a yoga practice at an age before the hip sockets completely form may be beneficial for increasing flexibility by molding the acetabulum into a broader shape. Adults starting a yoga practice after their bones are completely formed, however, should not be discouraged. As we have seen, bones retain a subtle ability to re-model throughout a lifetime. As bones and joints age, it is more likely that the changes will be degenerative, resulting from daily wear and tear. Bones and joints, however, maintain their potential to remodel into healthier, more flexible shapes. A well-aligned yoga practice can direct the many forces on bone to build density, mass and shape.

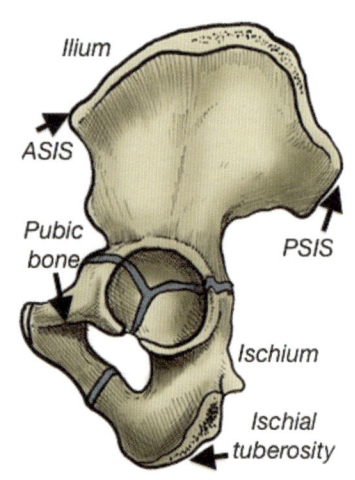

Encapsulating the acetabulum is a tight collar formed from a strip of articular cartilage that secures the head of the femur bone to the joint. The femur head is centered in the joint to achieve stability and support for weight bearing while minimizing the amount of *joint play* or wobble. This snug arrangement in the hip socket has a "vacuum effect" that suctions the head of the femur into the hip socket. In comparison, the shoulder joint has one to two inches of joint play along its central axis of rotation, allowing significantly greater ranges of motion but compromising its stability.

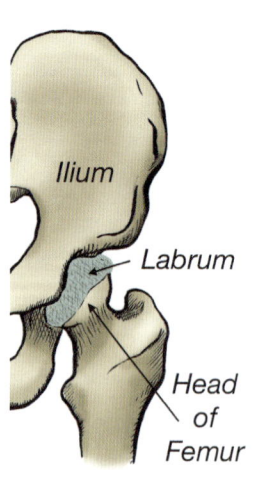

The "sitting" bones

The German word *Sitz* translates into seat. It is often used to reference the curved, lower surface of the pelvis used for sitting. Anatomically, the *sitz bones* refer to the *ischial tuberosities*.

The pelvis rocks!

The curved-bottom ischial tuberosities function similarly to rocking chair runners. Rocking forward on the ischial tuberosities tips the pelvic floor and sacral base forward. This causes the body's central axis to angle forward and the lumbar curve to deepen. Conversely, rocking back on the ischial tuberosities brings the pelvic floor and sacral base more horizontal. Rocking back moves the central axis posterior and causes the lumbar curve to flatten. In response to rocking back on the ischial tuberosities, the upper back and shoulders will often round. Good alignment in asana requires finding the "sweet spot" on the ischial tuberosities that aligns the body's central axis vertically through the perineum and the thoracic diaphragm.

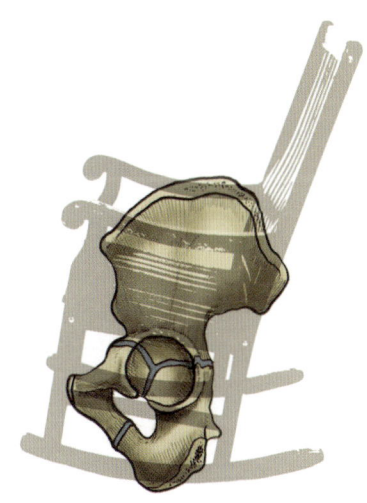

Tight hamstring muscles can significantly limit forward pelvic rocking and prevent the lumbar curve from properly forming. Students with tight hamstrings can sit on a support or blanket to tilt the pelvis into a more anterior position and enable it to rock more freely. The closer toward the pubic bones the student sits, the deeper the lumbar curve.[3]

Sacroiliac joints: the posterior joints of the pelvis

The two iliac bones adjoin respective sides of the sacrum to form the sacroiliac joints. The sacroiliac joints (SI joints) are large and irregular in shape, designed to be powerful weight bearing joints for the spine and torso. Early anatomists believed that the sacroiliac joints were immovable. It is now well established that they do move, although only in a limited fashion. Although subtle, essentially all mechanical movements of the pelvis occur only at the sacroiliac joints.

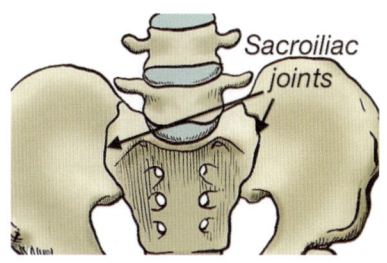

The primary function of the sacroiliac joints is not to provide gross movements but to absorb and distribute the various shocks and forces that the human frame must constantly endure. The SI joints use a subtle, ratchet-like and recoiling action to open and close as they move. Mechanical dysfunction of the sacroiliac joints occurs somewhat easily and is a common cause of lower back pain.

A yoga practice that utilizes pelvic integrative alignment principles can prevent many injuries. These principles, which are presented in the following chapter, serve also as essential tools for the healthy rehabilitation of injured sacroiliac joints. The sacroiliac joints move in two basic directions, *nutation* and *counter-nutation*. Nutation is an anterior, tip-and-glide movement, its name derived from the Greek, *to nod*. The posterior direction of this movement is called counter-nutation. Experts debate the full range of nutation/counter-nutation but most settle on a distance of approximately 6mm.

Pubis symphysis: the anterior joint of the pelvis

The two pubic bones form the anterior ring of the pelvis. At their juncture is a hard, fibrocartilage disc located at the anterior midline called the *symphysis pubis*. Also referred to as the pubic symphysis, this joint has minimal movement in a normal, non-pregnant state. Mechanical movement from the pubic symphysis should be avoided. If injured, the pubis symphysis may become chronically hypermobile, producing deep pain and chronic pelvic instability.

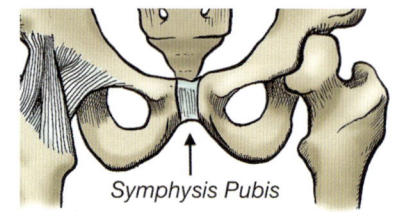
Symphysis Pubis

Pelvic torsion is produced in closed hip postures when one hipbone rotates forward and the other back. Precaution should be taken in extreme, counter-rotating hip poses, such as **Hanumanasana** (Forward Split), which will create shearing forces on the pubic symphysis disc. Keep the hips square and firmly scoop the tailbone forward to protect the pelvis from torsion and shearing forces. Engage muscular tension evenly through both hips.

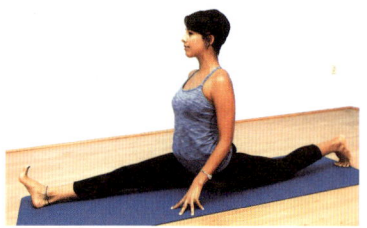

It's shocking!

Every step transfers the upward force of heel strike through the legs and pelvis, continuing through the rest of the body. Heel strike forces are typically measured using a bite plate to record changes in pressure on the jaw. A vertical, up-and-down jump produces forces that can reach levels 10 times the weight of the body. Gravity, the other major force on the human frame, compresses the body with a steady, downward vector impacting the pelvis and sacroiliac joints.

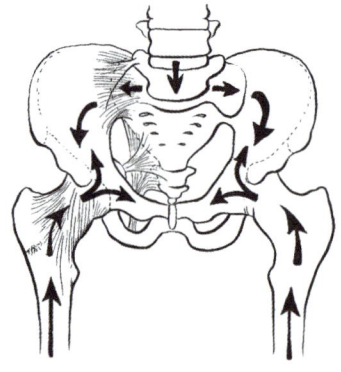

The forces of heel strike and gravity converge in the pelvis. The energy they create reverberates and spreads around the pelvic rim. The forces circulate in a manner similar to a finger running around a glass goblet and emitting a vibratory hum.

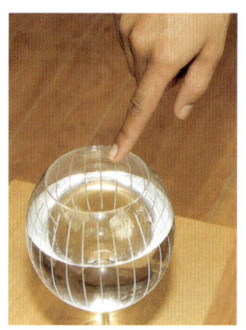

The sacroiliac joints act as the pressure release valve for the build up of forces in the pelvis. As energy builds up around the pelvic bowl, the sacroiliac joints subtly recoil and discharge the pressure. Should either sacroiliac joint become immobilized, forces fail to dissipate and transfer to the next most freely movable region, the lower discs of the spine. It is also common for one sacroiliac joint to become less mobile than the other, producing additional twist and torque on the lower discs each time they receive a shock or force.

These torsional stresses on the lumbar discs are a frequent cause of disc herniation and if they become chronic, spinal deterioration.[4]

Sacroiliac function

One reason anatomists first assumed the sacroiliac joints were immovable is that they are purely ligamentous joints with no muscles that directly move the sacrum in relation to the ilium. Today it is well accepted that the sacroiliac joints do move. Research has also uncovered that the biceps femoris muscle can move the sacrum via a remnant of tendon tissue that connects to the sacrotuberous ligament. The legs, acting as long, efficient levers, can turn small actions into significant movements of the SI joints.[5] More details are provided in Chapter 20.

Trap door

During the birth processes of labor and delivery, hormonal changes increase the elasticity of the ligaments. The sacroiliac ligaments respond by increasing nutation from the typical 6mm to 22mm or more. The sacroiliac joints are able to separate widely, allowing the sacrum to drop open like a trap door for the baby's entrance to this world.

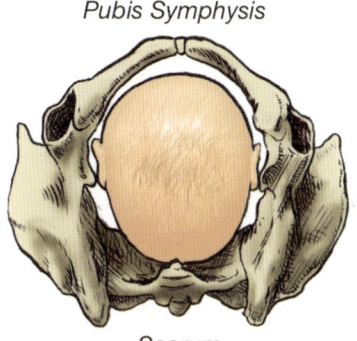

Pubis Symphysis

Sacrum

Open and shut case

The inner surfaces of both the sacrum and ilium are rough and irregular. The small bumps on their interfaces match up and align, similarly to intermeshing teeth on a gear or sprocket.

Iyengar-tradition yoga instructor Roger Cole equates the sacroiliac joint surfaces to a ceramic dish that is broken in two.

"The broken edge of each piece has a rough surface, but because they match one another exactly, you can fit the two pieces back together precisely. The bumps on one surface fit into the depressions on the other."[6]

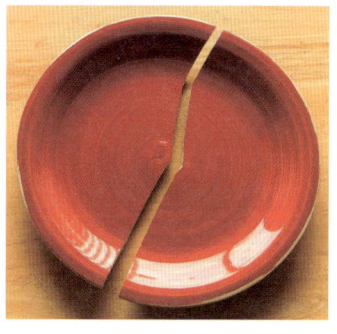

The sacroiliac joints move in a ratcheting-type fashion. The joints first open, separating their irregular surfaces. This allows movement to occur. After the sacroiliac joints have moved to the desired degree, the joints close, locking in and re-establishing stability.

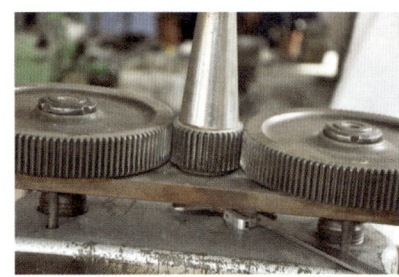

Insult and injury

The sacroiliac joints can become injured during yoga practice. Asana's constant transitioning between movement and stability places significant mechanical demand on the sacroiliac joints. Injuries can occur during either the open or closed phase of sacroiliac movement.

To illustrate this concept, the following examples are presented:

- If the pelvis is forced to move before the sacroiliac joints have opened, the locked joints cannot provide the necessary movement and the surrounding soft tissues are strained.

- If the sacroiliac joints do not adequately spread open before the closing phase begins, the sacrum becomes bruised as it jams against the closed joint.

- Injury can occur when the sacroiliac joints need to be stable for weight-bearing but are stuck in their open position. If the joints are unable to fully close, they remain unstable. Excessive strain is placed on the sacroiliac ligaments as they attempt to compensate for the instability of the joint.

In making his analogy, Roger Cole also offers a hypothesis for injury:

> "If you misalign the two pieces (of the ceramic dish) in any direction, the bumps on one will clash with the bumps on the other. The surfaces of the sacrum and ilium have similar bumps and depressions that fit together but clash with one another if you shift the bones out of place in any direction… the pressure of bump on bump (may be) the source of sacroiliac pain. If it continues over a long period of time, it may eventually cause the cartilage and then the bone to deteriorate, causing more pain."[7]

The question arises, how does the yoga practitioner control the opening and closing of the sacroiliac joints? The next chapter describes the procedure in detail. Opening and closing the sacroiliac joints is part of a broader methodology that works with the pelvis as one mechanical system, aptly called *pelvic integration*.

Sacral pump

Although the sacroiliac joint is primarily designed for weight-bearing, shock absorption and minor movement, it does have another, more subtle function that is critical for the nervous system and, therefore, for the overall health of the body.

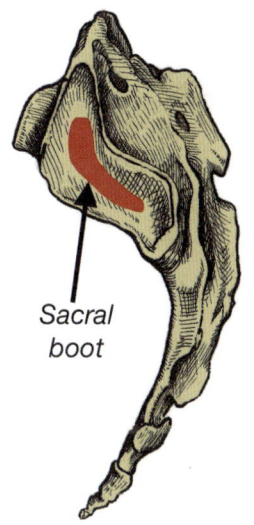

Sacral boot

On the rough, inside surface of the sacroiliac joint is a small, smooth portion that is shaped in the form of a boot. The boot is situated at the level of the second sacral segment. This is also the level where the outer covering of the spinal cord, the dura mater, attaches to the spinal canal. Above this attachment point begins a small, tapered channel that pools the cerebrospinal fluid, the vital liquid that nourishes the brain and nervous system.[8]

Because the dural sleeve of the spinal cord attaches to the boot of the sacrum, movements of the sacroiliac joint tug the dura and pump cerebrospinal fluid up the spine to the brain. This pumping action is called the *primary sacral respiratory mechanism*.[9] Therapeutic modalities, such as Sacro Occipital Technique, Cranial Release Technique and Craniosacral Therapy pay particular attention to this pumping mechanism. An array of bodily ailments, which include headaches and back pain, has been associated with inadequate sacral pumping.

Something else to chew on

Many holistic approaches to body therapy recognize the subtle but powerful neuro-mechanical relationship between the tempromandibular joints (TMJ) and the sacroiliac joints. Therapeutic approaches can be used to evaluate and restore imbalances that may develop between these two regions. The interconnection between the jaw and the sacroiliac joints may seem unlikely but can often be observed with weight bearing activities. The sacroiliac joints engage when lifting a heavy object, often accompanied by clenching of the jaw.

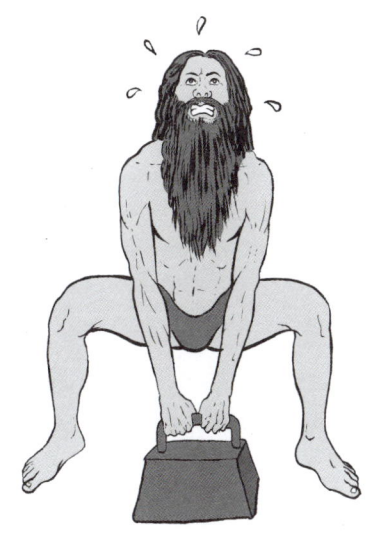

Equator of the body – the sacrum–coccyx juncture

When passing over the equator in a boat or plane, no clear lines or signposts mark the location. But, from one side to the other, an invisible shift in polarized energy takes place, pulling subtly in opposite directions. This demarcation affects the earth as a whole. The human body has a similar, energetic equator. It is located at the sacral-coccyx joint, where the bottom tip of the sacrum joins the upper portion of the coccyx.

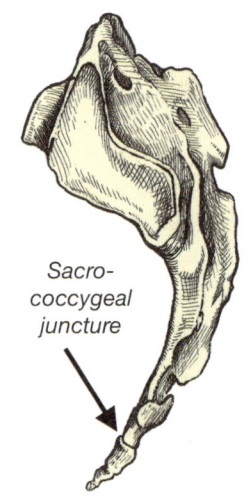

Sacro-coccygeal juncture

Above the sacro-coccygeal juncture, all muscular tension in the body draws energetically and isometrically in a superior direction toward the head. From the coccyx down, all energy and muscular tension draws toward the feet.[10]

This energetic equator also crosses horizontally through the center of the hip joint. This corresponds with the yoga alignment instruction for the legs to contract lengthwise, from the hip sockets, energetically and isometrically, down toward the heels.

In **Uttanasana** (Forward Fold), the sacrum is the highest point of the posture. A teacup, or perhaps for those less daring, a foam yoga block, can be placed and balanced on top of the sacrum safely when practicing the pose.

Energetically, the buttock muscles lift and draw toward the head while the tailbone scoops downward. From the center of the hip sockets, the pose draws down toward the feet, an action that protects the hamstring muscles from injury. The sacrum ideally occupies the highest point of the pose. This is the desired position for other forward bending postures as well, including **Parivrtta Trikonasana** (Revolved Triangle Pose), **Prasarita Padottanasana** (Wide-angle Forward Bend), **Parsvottanasana** (Pyramid), and **Adho Mukha Svanasana** (Downward Facing Dog).

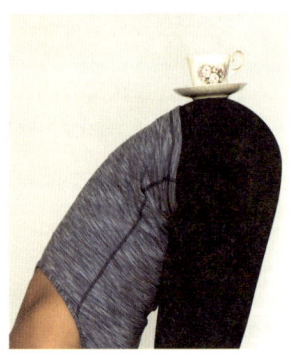

It is important to remember that it is not how far the posture physically moves that makes it safe and effective. Not all students have the physical capabilities or have developed the skills needed to take poses as deeply as desired. As long as students have the understanding and demonstrate the intent to move in accordance with the equatorial transition point of the body, the alignment of the posture is energetically integrated and the pose is safe and beneficial.

13 Pelvis and Sacroiliac Joints Alignment Principles

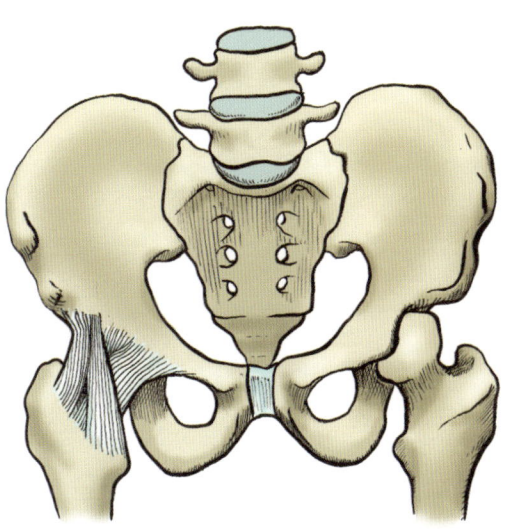

*As goes the pelvis, so goes the spine.
And with that, goes everything else!*

The pelvis is the structural foundation of the spine. The floor of the pelvis is called the *perineum*, a trampoline-like structure constructed from dense myofascia and muscle. A wide, pliable pelvic floor is the best foundation for the body, both physically and energetically. The perineum provides an adjustable base for the body's energetic core, the central axis, which rises vertically through the body's "diaphragms" until it exits the posterior fontanel of the skull. The perineum is believed to be a remnant of muscles used to wag a tail earlier in our evolutionary path. Engaging the perineal muscles during yoga practice may stir up some primordial "memories" for students!

Move from the Mula

The Root chakra, known as the *Muladhara*, is located at the center of the perineum, between the anal sphincter and urethra. Contracting the perineum engages the *Mula bandha*, the Root chakra energy lock. The contraction is not a forceful tightening of the anus or the genitals but a gentle lift of the central perineum.

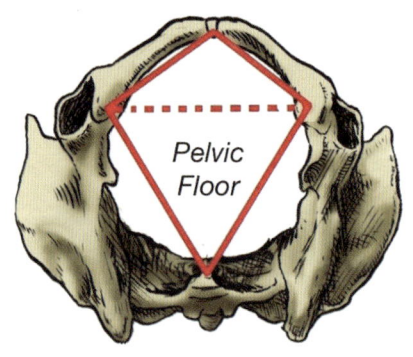

Move into asana by first generating the gentle lifting action of the Mula bandha. The next action is to align the thoracic diaphragm vertically over the perineum, allowing the body's core alignment to establish along the central axis. This action is performed as a subtle rocking and shifting that does not alter nor distort the general position of the pelvis.

Tight hips and legs can limit movement in the pelvis, restricting the engagement of Mula bandha and the ability to effortlessly shift the spine's axis. Yoga postures that increase the range of motion of the hips and those that stretch the hamstring muscles will promote freedom of movement throughout the body by making Mula bandha engagement more accessible.

When initiating **Utthita Trikonasana** (Triangle pose), the pelvis side bends directly from the Mula. This method keeps the central axis aligned and the spine lengthened. Moving from the Mula into Trikonasana helps lift the front ilium and prevents compression of the hip socket. Samasthiti, or *equal tension,* is more easily maintained when movement initiates with Mula bandha.

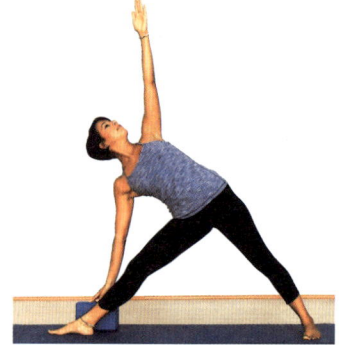

How do I tell thee? Let me count the ways

Yoga teachers tend to amass a collection of metaphors and analogies to describe alignment and explain structural relationships to students. For the sacroiliac joints, there is no shortage. Doug Keller teaches how to move the pelvis by describing the two front hip points (the ASIS's) moving inward and out. Various schools of yoga use a concept of pelvic rocking and tilting. Richard Freeman instructs his students to lift the S-2 vertebra toward the navel as a way to align and stabilize the sacrum. Joan White uses the analogy of "zippering up" the front of a pair of pants as a way to stabilize the sacrum. Most often, the metaphors presented in this book are modifications of alignment principles developed in Anusara yoga. The Anusara concepts should not be considered style-specific; instead they offer a user-friendly lexicon that is complementary to all yoga traditions and styles. Specifically, this chapter uses the Anusara concepts of *inner spiral* and *scooping the tailbone* to direct how to move and align the sacroiliac joints. The term *inward hip release* is used in place of the Anusara term *inner spiral* to describe a broader application of this mechanical process.

As discussed in Chapter 12, the sacroiliac joints perform essentially all of the movement within the pelvis. The sacroiliac joints move with a subtle, nodding action called nutation. The sacroiliac joints first open to allow movement and then close to create stability. Yoga practice must adhere to the proscribed functions of the sacroiliac joints in order to avoid injury.

Pelvic integrative alignment

The principles of *pelvic integrative alignment* manage the function of the sacroiliac joints, the lumbar spine, the hips, pelvis, and legs. Their presentation in this chapter is specific to the sacroiliac joints. Pelvic integrative alignment consists of a two-step procedure used in every asana to safely operate the sacroiliac joints. The first step is *inward hip release*. It opens the sacroiliac joints, creating the space that is necessary for mobility. The second step, equally important, is *forward tailbone scoop*. *Forward tailbone scoop* stabilizes the sacroiliac joints. Both steps work together and are essential components of sacroiliac joint function. Greater exploration of pelvic alignment principles is found in Chapter 14.

Step one – Inward hip release

Moving from the upper inner thighs (groin), the legs *roll in*, *draw back* and *spread apart*. The legs are used as long levers to initiate the action. *Inward hip release*, the first step in engaging the sacroiliac joints, opens the joints and widens the pelvic floor.[1]

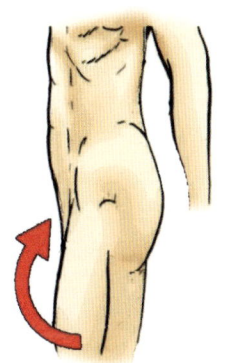

Step two – Forward tailbone scoop

Forward tailbone scoop is performed exactly as its name describes: the tailbone scoops forward under the pelvis in the direction of the pubic bones.[2] This second step of pelvic integrative alignment closes and stabilizes the sacroiliac joints and externally rotates the hip. In some instances, *forward tailbone scoop* is a firm action; in others, it occurs simply as the subtle engagement of Mula bandha.

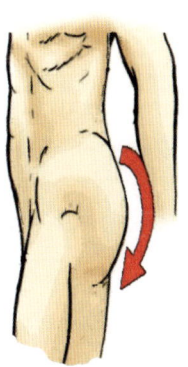

> Prevent injuries by using the principles of *inward hip release* and *forward tailbone scoop* correctly and consistently in every asana.

Baddha Konasana and the bruised sacroiliac joint

In the full pose of **Baddha Konasana** (Bound Angle), the hips externally rotate and abduct. These movements of the hips activate *forward tailbone scoop*, causing the sacroiliac joints to close. To perform Bound Angle safely, first engage *inward hip release*. Draw the buttocks flesh diagonally toward the posterior. Flex the hip, rotate it inward, and bring the thigh toward the midline of the body (adduction). Keep as much internal rotation as possible in the joints as the knees gently drop to the sides, opening the hips toward the floor. These seemingly counter-intuitive actions open the sacroiliac joints and, importantly, create the space where the tailbone can scoop. Aggressively attempting Bound Angle without first engaging *inward hip release* can bruise the sacroiliac joints. This type of injury is a common cause of pain in the buttock region.

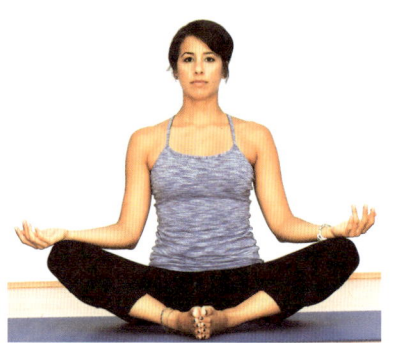

Causes of sacroiliac injuries

The sacroiliac joints "open and close" while transitioning between "movement and stability" and are often put into positions where they are vulnerable to injury. The sacroiliac joints can become *stuck* (joint fixation) at any point between fully opened and fully closed, the way a door might get stuck along the swing of its path. More often, sacroiliac fixation occurs toward the closed-joint position, causing the joint's movement to reduce or stop. Asana practice and yoga therapy techniques are more effective restoring lost mobility, as in this situation, than when joints are lax and require stabilization.

Less often, the sacroiliac joints are in the unstable, open position. When open, the joints are unable to support the torso. The surrounding musculature, predominantly the iliopsoas muscle, responds in an effort to provide additional support. As a result, the muscles become tight, shortened and often fatigued as they attempt to support and stabilize the joints. Inflammation of overstretched tissues around the sacroiliac joints, which often accompanies their instability, can cause symptoms of back and pelvic pain. The relative strength and tension of the muscles of the pelvic region can be evaluated and used as indicators of underlying joint instability.

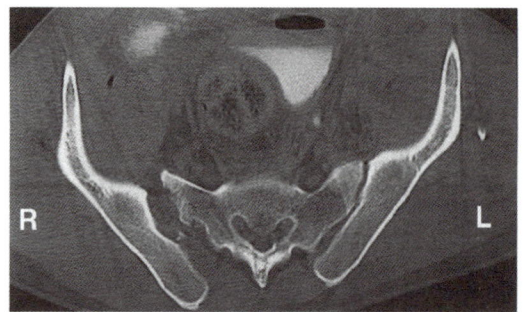

Radiographic image looking from above at a traumatic separation of the right Sacroiliac joint

Evaluating the function of the sacroiliac joints

General testing of sacroiliac function can be performed and provide useful information to guide asana practice safely.

Marching in place

When one leg lifts, the sacroiliac joint on that side opens and the ilium rotates posterior. The sacroiliac joint on the standing-leg side does not move but remains stable.

To test:

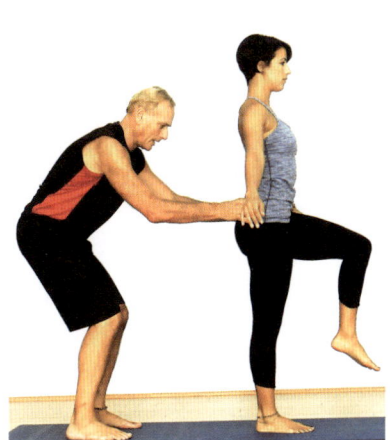

- The assistant stands behind the student, choosing one sacroiliac joint to test.
- The assistant places one thumb on the posterior superior iliac spine (PSIS) of the side being tested and the other thumb horizontally across on the sacrum.
- The student slowly marches in place.
- When the leg lifts on the ilium side, the assistant's thumb drops slightly, indicating a normal posterior rotation of the ilium.
- When the opposite leg lifts, neither thumb moves, indicating the sacroiliac joint is stable. The thumb on the sacrum remains unmoved in normal circumstances.
- Sacroiliac instability: If the joint is unstable, the thumb on the sacrum will drop, indicating that the joint cannot support the additional demand caused by the lifting of the leg.
- Sacroiliac immobility: If the sacroiliac joint is locked, the thumb on the ilium, instead of dropping, will rise as the leg lifts, demonstrating that the ilium cannot rotate posterior.
- If the standing leg collapses while testing the lifted leg side, the sacroiliac joint on the standing leg side is most likely unstable and the musculature weak.
- The test is repeated on each side.[3]

With practice, this test will not be as complicated as it might first appear. It is a general test but it is reliable. False interpretations are possible should there be muscle weakness or imbalance in the hip region that is unrelated to the sacroiliac joints, although this is a less common occurrence.

Observing the sway

A less predictable but interesting method of sacroiliac evaluation is to observe the direction in which the pelvis sways when the yogi stands in the stillness of **Tadasana** (Mountain Pose) with eyes closed.

If the sacroiliac joints are locked, the pose may exhibit a subtle rocking forward and backward. This may be the body's way to generate sacral pumping of cerebrospinal fluid that is compromised when the sacrum is unable to move freely.[4]

If the sway is a side-to-side movement, this is indicative of open and unstable sacroiliac joints. The sideways swaying is an attempt by the pelvis to re-establish better contact with the weight-bearing portion of the joints.[5]

With both eyes closed, the pelvic sway that signifies healthy sacroiliac joints combines both forward-and-back and side-to-side movements. If no sway is observed, this may indicate other possible conditions, such as a lumbar disc herniation.

These unconscious swaying motions are controlled through a function of the nervous system called *proprioception* that works with our sense of spatial orientation.

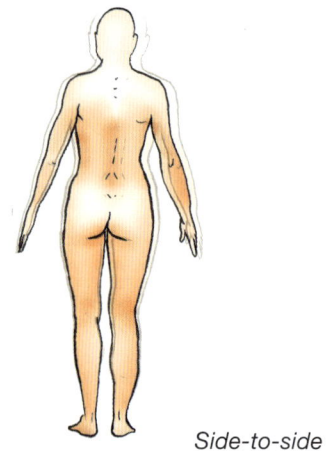
Side-to-side sway

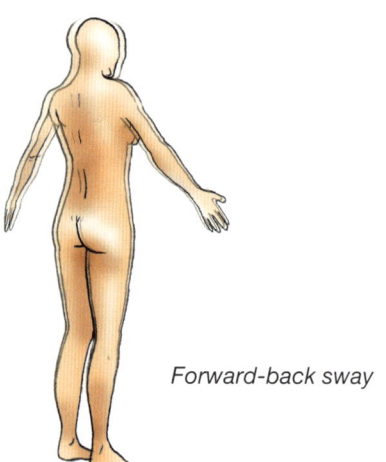
Forward-back sway

In this chapter and subsequent ones, information is presented regarding the causes of injuries and how various structural conditions affect the health of the body. Some basic evaluation protocols and yoga therapies are provided that have shown significant benefit in improving many of these conditions.

It must be re-emphasized that the therapeutic discussions in this book are educational and may offer guidance in administering self-assistance. They are not intended to negate, replace or discourage any evaluation or treatment from any qualified health care provider. Nor are they intended to be an absolute cure for anything.

That said, most health professionals are unaware of the therapeutic properties of yoga or how to utilize them. These techniques, if carefully applied, are safe and may provide a breakthrough in the cases of some challenging conditions. When practicing asana or utilizing yoga therapy methods, the key guide to determining the appropriateness of any action is the lack or diminishment of pain. If an asana or therapy is truly offering therapeutic value, pain will diminish during its administration as ease and comfort increases.

Sacroiliac Therapeutics

Imbalances between *inward hip release* and *forward tailbone scoop* can be addressed using yoga asana therapeutically. Once the type of sacroiliac imbalance is determined, stuck either open or closed, the yoga student can modify their practice to include asana that focus on the action that needs greater assistance or restoration. The following examples demonstrate how postures can specifically address sacroiliac joint issues. Because *inward hip release* and *forward tailbone scoop* are required in every asana, a yoga practice that adheres to precise alignment will be therapeutic by itself.

Therapeutic Supportive Bridge: Setu Bandha

Place a yoga block under the pelvis while in Bridge Pose.

If the sacroiliac joints are locked in a closed position, place the narrow part of the block vertically under the sacrum *only*. In this position, the hip bones can slowly release while the sacrum is held stable, eventually restoring movement to the sacroiliac joints.

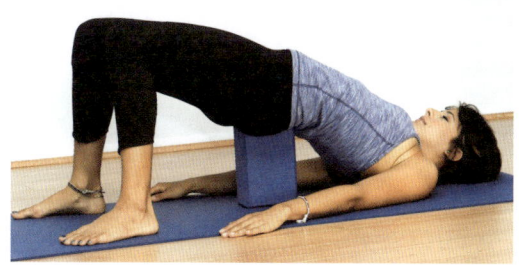

If the sacroiliac joints are unstable, place the wide part of the block horizontally, entirely across both sacroiliac joints. In this position, the block stabilizes the joints. The time spent holding this pose proprioceptively stimulates the ligaments and musculature to strengthen and provide greater stabilization.

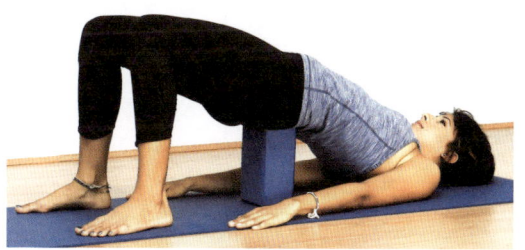

If it is too painful or difficult to lift onto the highest positions on the block, the lower counterparts can be used with equal effectiveness.

The Supported Bridge is a corrective therapy but also another means of evaluating the sacroiliac joints. The relative comfort of the two block positions can determine whether the sacroiliac joints are locked or unstable. Choose either the narrow or wide end of the block and hold the Supported Bridge for approximately 30 seconds. Repeat in the other position. The correct position for the yoga block produces comfort, while the incorrect block placement will be less comfortable or cause pain. Pain indicates that the block is aggravating a dysfunctional condition, either increasing the mobility of unstable joints or compressing joints that are already locked.

Additional tip for bridge pose: The knees do not splay outward but remain in line with the center of the hip joint. Knees splayed outward shorten the hip flexor muscles and compress the sacroiliac joints.

Asana that open fixated sacroiliac joints

The basic form of some yoga postures will emphasize *inward hip release* and can be used therapeutically to open the sacroiliac joints when they are locked.

Gomukhasana   Cow Face Pose

In **Gomukhasana**, the leg position is set into place with one knee nestled over the other. This produces significant leverage in the legs to spread open the sacroiliac joints. The effect is more pronounced in the SI joint of the top leg. *Inward hip release* initiates as the posture is established. *Forward tailbone scoop* is engaged to complete the pose. Incorporating Gomukhasana into a regular practice will keep the sacroiliac joints open and the hips functioning healthily.

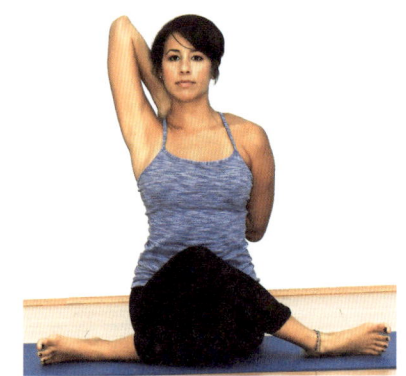

Garudasana   Eagle Pose

The position of the legs in **Garudasana** is excellent for releasing locked sacroiliac joints. The wrap-around leg configuration of the pose provides powerful leverage that opens the joints and increases their mobility. Here again, the effect of the pose is experienced greater in the sacroiliac joint of the top leg. The therapeutic focus in Eagle pose derives from *inward hip release*, however, as in all asana, *forward tailbone scoop* is also engaged to complete both steps of pelvic integrative alignment.

Procedure:

"Eagle legs" is most effective when performed as a restorative pose, lying on the back and avoiding the additional challenges of balance. The feet stay active and press out through all four corners, especially through the inner heels.

A spinal twist can also be added to the pose. To keep the central axis aligned in the twist and reduce back strain, shift the hips 8-10 inches toward the side of the top leg before dropping the legs across to the opposite side. An egg-sized curve in the lumbar spine is maintained. The upper rib cage rotates toward the floor in the opposite direction of the legs.

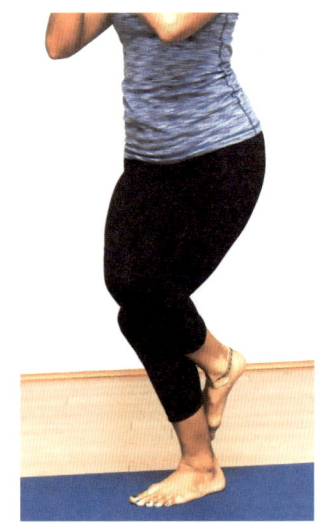

> Regardless of how severe sacroiliac joint fixation may be, every yoga posture and therapy incorporates some degree of *forward tailbone scoop* to avoid overstretching the joints.

Twists when the sacroiliac joints are unstable

Placing a block between the knees in a supine lumbar twist minimizes the torque created by the legs and, with that, the strain on the sacroiliac joints. With the block between the knees, the hips cannot internally rotate and the sacroiliac joints remain in a neutral position. The practitioner can still receive the benefits of twists, even when the sacroiliac joints are weak.

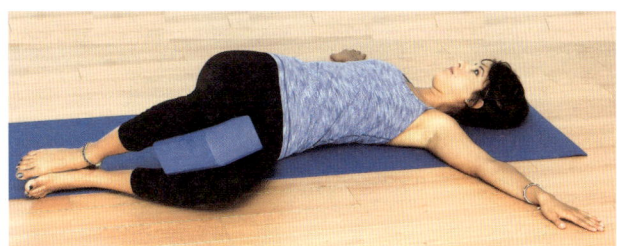

Asana and yoga therapy for stabilizing open sacroiliac joints

When the sacroiliac joints are stuck in an open position, they are unstable and unable to provide weight-bearing support. Postures that draw the sacroiliac joints together will be therapeutic. *Forward tailbone scoop* is the specific therapeutic tool used to stabilize the sacroiliac joints. And because all asana require both steps of pelvic integrative alignment, *inward hip release* will still be slightly engaged to initiate the asana or therapy.

Sacroiliac strap stabilization

Support the unstable sacroiliac joints by tightening a yoga strap across the center of the joints and encircling the pelvis. The strap horizontally crosses the greater trochanters at the level of approximately two finger distances above the pubic bones, measured on the front of the body. In actuality, the strap provides only minor mechanical stabilization to the joints but the healing effects of proprioceptive stimulation to the damaged ligament tissues are significant.

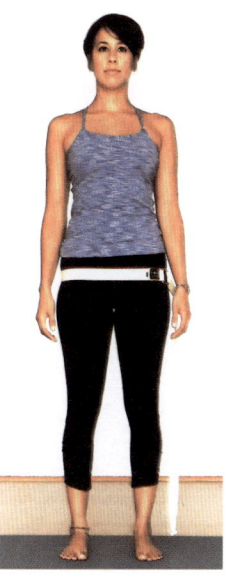

Supta Baddha Konasana   Reclined Bound Angle

This restorative pose stabilizes the sacroiliac joints, allowing them to gently compress. Hold the posture for five minutes or more, with or without back support. *Inward hip release* is performed when initiating the pose and *forward tailbone scoop* is held while in the full pose.

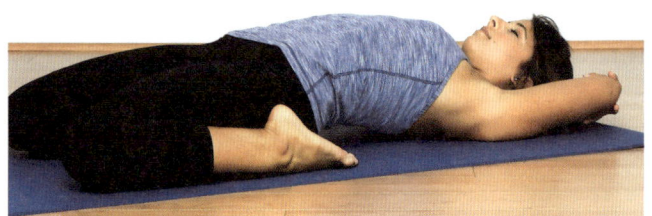

Supta Virasana with sacral block

The traditional forms of **Virasana** (Hero Pose) and **Supta Virasana** (Reclined Hero Pose), when performed without a block under the sacrum, are poses that increase *inward hip release*. When a block is positioned under the sacroiliac joints and body weight firmly rests on it, the joints are stabilized. The block also provides a supported *forward tailbone scoop.* Any sized block can be used for this restorative posture as long as it provides a solid foundation. The block also helps reduce overarching and compression of the lumbar spine.

Even for non-injured yoga students, the full form of Supta Virasana is challenging. Tight quadriceps muscles often contribute to its difficulty, and the lower back tends to overarch. To protect the lower back, *forward tailbone scoop* must be firmly engaged. Support by a block in Virasana and Supta Virasana is highly recommended for all students when the sacrum cannot fully reach the floor.

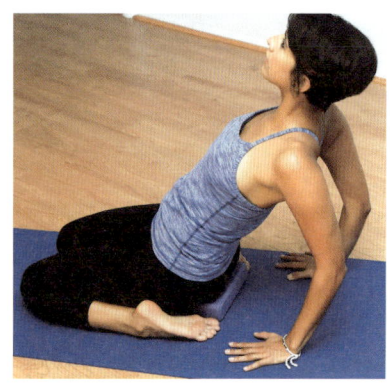

If the sacrum does not rest on either the floor or a block in Virasana poses, the postures become sacroiliac joint openers instead of stabilizers, and this may be adverse to the desired affect.

14 Integrative Alignment of the Pelvis

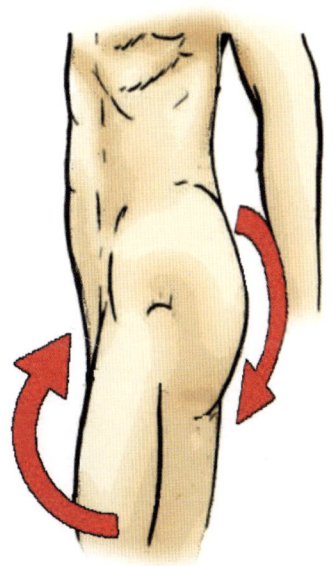

Chapter 13 introduced the principles of *pelvic integrative alignment* in their application specifically to sacroiliac joint function. This chapter expands on the details of this methodology and its effect on the pelvis as a whole. Pelvic integrative alignment elaborates on the teachings of B.K.S. Iyengar and the subsequent innovations and modifications developed in Anusara yoga. It offers a sophisticated, precise, yet user-friendly approach to alignment.

Inward Hip Release

Inward hip release is the first step of pelvic integrative alignment. It creates mobility by loosening the ligaments of the hips and opening the sacroiliac joints. *Inward hip release* consists of three separate but interdependent actions that originate from the upper thighs (groin). They are most effective when performed in the following order:

- Upper, inner thighs (groin) *roll in*[1]
- Front of the thighs *draw back*[2]
- Upper, inner thighs (groin) *spread apart*

When *inward hip release* is performed, it is normal for the buttocks to stick out - lifting and spreading apart in an oblique, posterior direction. The knees remain forward-facing and do not roll inward. With practice, moving the upper femur without disturbing the position of the knee and lower leg will become easily achievable.

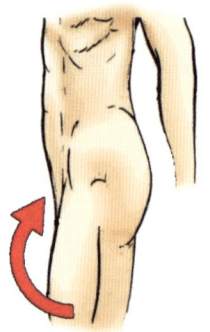
Inward Hip Release

Major anatomical effects of *inward hip release*

- The primary ligaments of the hips micro-pleat and loosen, increasing mobility in the hip joints.

- The sacroiliac joints spread open, increasing their mobility.

- The pelvic floor widens, stretching the musculature of the perineum and creating added space needed for *forward tailbone scoop*.

- The psoas major muscle stretches, increasing the curve of the lumbar spine.[3]

- *Thighs back* causes the pelvis to flex and creates what is referred to as *anterior tilt*. Pelvic flexion tips the top of the sacrum forward, angling the foundation on which the spine rests and causing the curve of the lumbar spine to deepen.

- Inner thighs *spread apart*. This action aligns the fibers of the hamstring muscles lengthwise, which increases their flexibility and strength and improves their recovery from injury. This action is also beneficial to the rehabilitation of knee injuries.

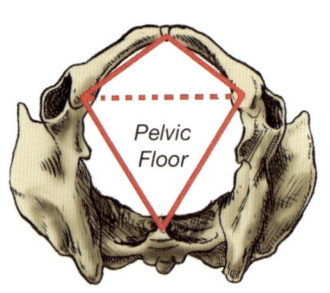
Pelvic Floor

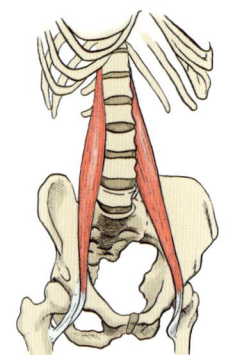
Psoas Muscle

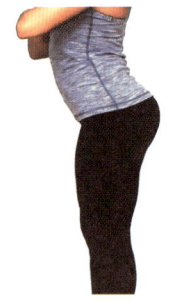
Anterior Tilt

> Roll-in, back, and apart is the "mantra" for *inward hip release*.

Forward tailbone scoop

Forward tailbone scoop is the second step of pelvic integration. After *inward hip release* opens and mobilizes the sacroiliac joints and loosens the hips, *forward tailbone scoop* closes the sacroiliacs and firms the hip ligaments, bringing stability to the pelvis for managing the demands of weight-bearing. Forward tailbone scoop also stabilizes the lumbar curve, preventing hyperextension and compression of the lumbar spinal discs.[4]

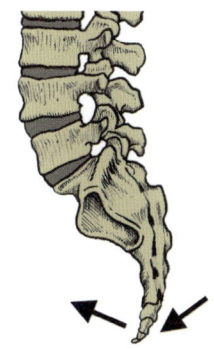

The "tailbone" refers specifically to the *coccyx,* the lowest three segments of the spine. At birth, the coccyx consists of three separate vertebrae, but these form into one solid bone as the spine matures during adolescence. The action of *forward tailbone scoop* draws the coccyx forward toward the pubis. Forward tailbone scoop creates pelvic extension, also called *posterior tilt*.

Forward tailbone scoop is usually a firm, deliberate action. Its movement is in balance with *inward hip release* and does not overpower it. A useful instruction for students as they engage *forward tailbone scoop* is to resist the thighs' inclination to shift forward.

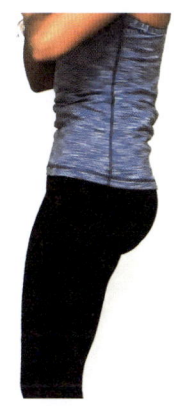

Posterior tilt

Forward tailbone scoop accomplishes many important actions:
- Closes the sacroiliac joints and stabilizes the pelvis.
- Externally rotates and stabilizes the hips
- Limits the degree of lumbar curve, preventing over-arching and compression of the lumbar discs.
- When performed subtly, the perineum gently lifts to engage the Mula bandha.
- Moves the pelvis into posterior tilt, or pelvic extension.

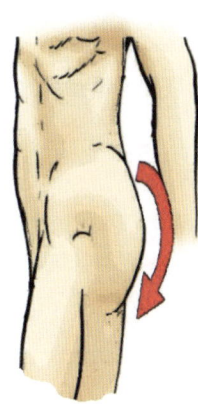

> Yoga teacher Betsey Downing, PhD., asserts that the difference between the terms "scoop" and "tuck" is significant. Tucking implies a tightening and contraction where scooping suggests a more lengthened and spacious action.

Finding the sweet spot

How does the yoga student find that just right "sweet spot" between *inward hip release* and *forward tailbone scoop*?

In straight-legged postures, the sweet spot that balances *inward hip release* and *forward tailbone scoop* is the point at which the greater trochanters of the hips align directly over the ankles. The knees are not forced, but will naturally find their alignment close to the same vertical line. The sweet spot of pelvic integration creates an egg-sized curve in the lower lumbar spine. The lower ribs do not jut forward, but are drawn toward the back of the body.

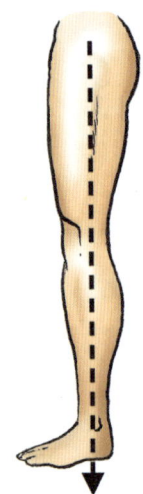

The greater trochanter aligns over the ankle when the pelvis is balanced.

Each student finds the sweet spot of balance between *inward hip release* and *forward tailbone scoop* differently. Some yoga students have a naturally lifted and protruding buttocks while others are flatter. As an example, students with a "big booty" usually exhibit an abundance of *inward hip release* in their normal posture. For them, the need to first engage *inward hip release* is minimal. For balanced alignment in the pelvis, these students would focus mainly on the singular action of *spreading thighs apart* and place greater effort on *forward tailbone scoop*.

Conversely, flat-butted yogis would need to deeply engage *inward hip release*, especially the action of *thighs back*. These students would engage *forward tailbone scoop* only slightly because that step of pelvic integration is well pronounced in their normal posture.

Students with tight hips that have limited ability to internally rotate would focus on *inward hip release* throughout every asana, giving special attention to the first cue to *roll-in* the upper, inner thighs.

The Human Pez® dispenser

The first attempts to use pelvic integrative alignment principles can be challenging. The actual physical movements may be quite elusive. An effective learning tool used by many teachers is to place a yoga block between the legs at the upper groin. This may conjure the image of a human Pez™ dispenser.

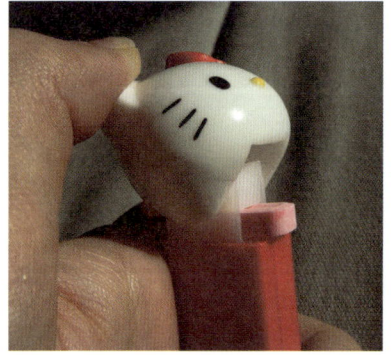

FOURTEEN: INTEGRATIVE ALIGNMENT OF THE PELVIS

Procedure:

To experience the first alignment step of *inward hip release*, the student, while standing, places a block between the inner thighs so that the block presses directly against the lesser trochanter of each femur. Using the musculature of the legs and pelvis, the student rolls the block in and back, an action that resembles the defensive response to a feigned kick to the groin. This action produces the *roll-in and drawing back* of the thighs while the position of the block creates the spreading apart aspect of *inward hip release*.

To experience *forward tailbone scoop*, the student firmly places their fingers on the front of the block. As they engage *forward tailbone scoop,* the fingers prevent the block from being forced forward and bringing the thighs with it.

Balance between the two actions is complete when the *forward tailbone scoop* is engaged as fully as possible without the greater trochanters moving forward of the ankles.

When *inward hip release* and *forward tailbone scoop* become second nature, these actions flow in a subtle and seamless manner. Pelvic integration brings an underlying intelligence to the foundation of every asana. When yoga is practiced with confidence and clarity, it is also much more fun!

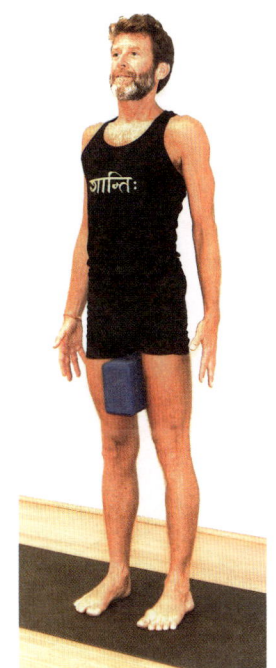

Pelvic positions

Neutral pelvis - ASIS and PSIS are horizontal (approximate)

Anterior pelvis - ASIS drops below the PSIS

Posterior pelvis - PSIS drops below the ASIS

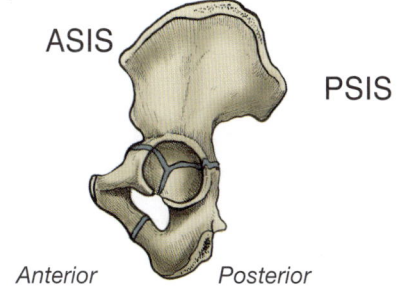

Backward Butt Walking

Another procedure that teaches yoga students how to engage *inward hip release* and can also be used as therapy for limited hip rotation is the backward butt walk. Sit in **Dandasana** with both hips squared toward the front of the yoga mat. Lift one hip off the mat and, from the upper inner groin, internally rotate the thigh as it is placed back down a few inches further behind its original position. Place the pelvis down on the mat as far forward on the ischial tuberosity as can be done comfortably. Shift your weight over to the opposite pelvis and repeat the procedure. Slowly continue the backward walking until the back of the mat is reached.

This procedure engages all three actions of *inward hip release*. The thigh draws back and internally rotates as the hipbone moves back a few inches. As weight is shifted from one hip to the other, the thigh spreads apart.

This is also a fun teaching tool!

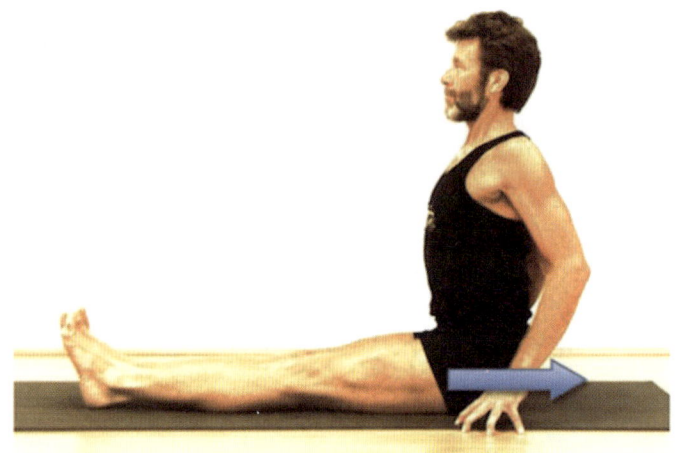

15 The Middle Way

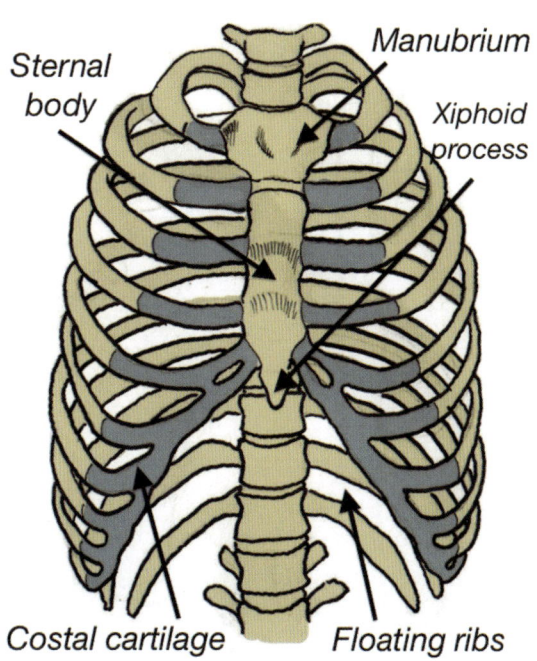

Although this chapter is short and its focus specific, the position of the lower rib cage is of great importance to the structural integrity of the entire body. At first glance, the lower rib cage seems to be an unlikely place to focus attention in the overall approach to alignment. Yet, without stabilizing the lower rib cage, the pelvis and shoulder girdle cannot achieve integrative alignment with each other. *Lower rib cage integration* is an important action to take in every asana

Lower rib cage integration – a simple concept but a challenging action

Lower rib cage integration is a simple alignment principle: draw the lower ribs posterior, widening them across the back body.

Anatomically, the lower ribs have no attachments to other bones or cartilage on the front body. Their only structural attachment is posteriorly to the spine column. The level of the floating ribs, particularly the twelfth thoracic vertebra, acts as a fulcrum that supports the upper torso and serves as the spine's major swivel point. Many yogis, including those considered most limber, find it challenging to move the lower portion of the rib cage interdependently. The tendency is for the shoulders to roll forward and the chest to drop as compensatory movements to drawing the ribs back. Similarly, the lower rib cage often juts forward in a see-saw type of response when the yogi draws his shoulders back. If the lower ribs jut forward, structural support of the torso is compromised. The lumbar spinal curve increases as the ribs jut forward, setting up potential compression of the lower spinal discs.[3] Learning to isolate the movement of the lower rib cage from other regions takes practice and patience.

Method to engage lower rib cage integration

- Lift and lengthen the right and left sides of the body, from the iliac crests to the armpits, creating space between the ribs.
- The bottom tip of the breastbone scoops down toward the navel.
- The lower ribs draw back, lift and spread wide across the back.
- The navel draws into the abdomen without forcibly contracting the abdominal musculature.

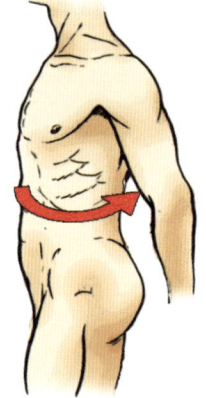

Visualizing lower rib cage integration

"Zipper" the bottom tip of the breastbone (xiphoid process) down towards the navel while gently drawing the navel into the abdomen. This zipping action, as previously presented in Chapter 11, is used in conjunction with the upward zipping action similar to zipping up a pair of pants.[1]

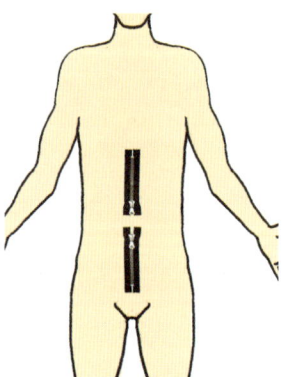

> When aligning the lower rib cage, the front of the body does not shorten or collapse.

Scoop the breastbone, Scoop the tailbone, Draw in the navel

This principle is presented repetitively throughout this book as it is fundamental to integrating the upper and lower torso. It is an essential practice for keeping the lower rib cage from jutting forward, especially in backbend postures.

If a quicker, simpler action is necessary, simply draw inward the lower abdominal muscles from the level of two inches below the navel.

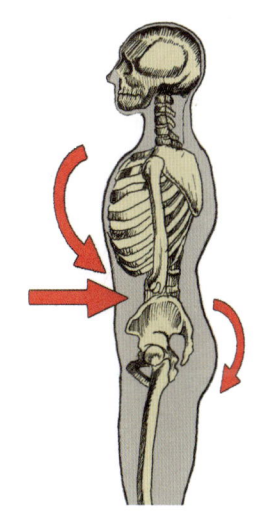

In **Urdvha Dhanurasana** (Upward Bow), press from the bottom tips of the shoulder blades, located at the level of the T-7 vertebra, upward to extend the thoracic spine and fully open the chest. Draw lower portion of the rib cage back by scooping the breastbone toward the navel and drawing the navel inward. Firmly scoop the tailbone forward to prevent lower back compression. Without these actions, the curve of the lumbar spine would angle sharply instead of lengthening into a smooth arc.

Urdvha Dhanurasana is often referred to as the Wheel Pose. More accurately, it is a "Half Wheel", with the imagined lower portion of the wheel continuing below the plane of the floor. Ideally, the rim of the wheel curves evenly along the spine while the "spokes" of the wheel remain equal in length.

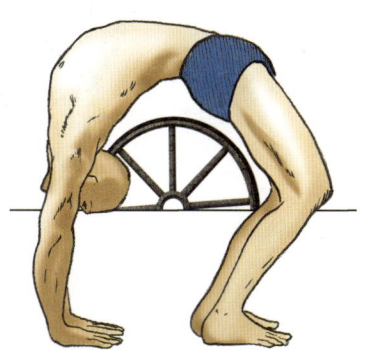

Technically Speaking

The method of lower rib cage integration is derived from Anusara yoga's *Kidney Loop* that instructs yogis to draw back and lift the lower ribs in a looping fashion onto the lower back. Iyengar yoga teachings emphasize the spreading of the kidneys across the lower back.

In **Ustrasasna** (Camel Pose), the lower rib cage must firmly draw back and not jut forward. The lower ribs widen on the back and the navel firmly draws in. *Forward tailbone scoop* is an important action to engage to avoid compressing the lumbar spine. A vertical line, centered through the greater trochanter of the hips aligns directly over the knees. The hips and thighs do not press forward.

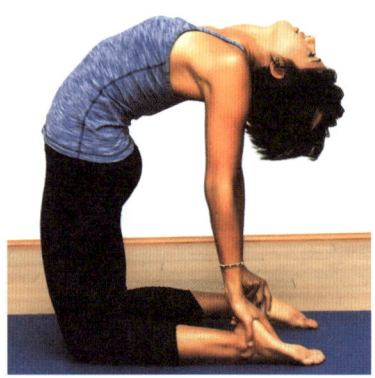

In **Bhujangasana** (Cobra Pose), the lower rib cage draws posterior while the tailbone scoops toward the floor. The navel is drawn in. Additional alignment instructions for Cobra Pose:

- Keep the elbows in line with the side body rib cage.
- Draw the throat back without lifting the chin. Instead, subtly lift the back of the skull.

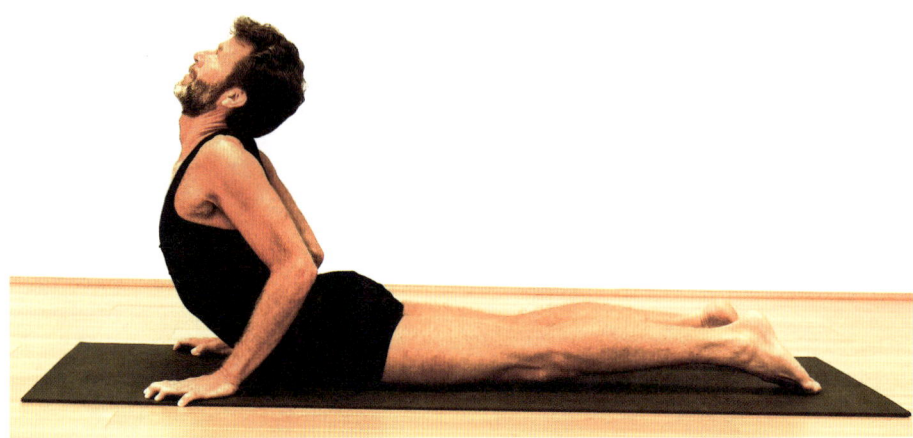

Paired actions

When the throat is drawn back, the body reflexively draws the lower ribs and thighs back.

16 The Alignment of Sitting

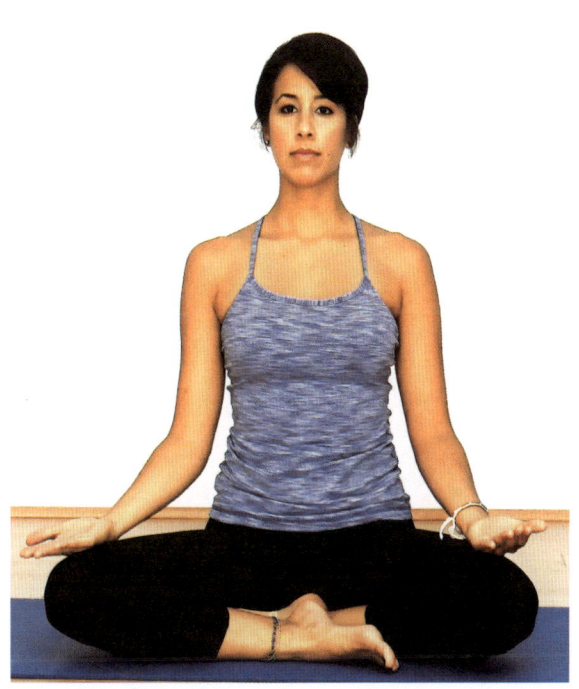

"Where we start is where we're going!"[1]

Yoga classes often begin with students instructed to take a basic seated posture, either cross-legged in **Sukhasana** or aligning heel-to-heel-to-pubis in **Siddhasana**. While some students can barely sit still, restlessly waiting for yoga class "to start", others are fully engaged, aware that their yoga practice began long before their mat was unrolled. This seemingly insignificant seated posture represents the ultimate intention of yoga asana.

The rigors of asana practice put the body through a series of complex and ever challenging postures. Asana practice conditions the yoga student to perform the simple act of sitting with undemanding effort. Eventually, the ability to maintain alignment for long periods of time is attained. The ability to sit with effortless precision is an essential prerequisite for performing the more advanced forms of yoga: meditation and Pranayama. The seated posture is where students start and where they are ultimately going.

Following are the alignment cues for seated posture in full detail. The instructions pertain not only to sitting but all poses, postures and positions the body will assume.

- Sit at a height where the knees do not rise above the hips.
- Sit forward on the pelvic floor so the perineum is in firm contact with the sitting surface.
- The lower lumbar spine forms a small, egg sized curve.
- The perineum, thoracic diaphragm, and soft palate align vertically, forming the central axis of the body that rises through the posterior fontanelle of the skull.
- The back of the sacrum, the shoulder blades and the back of the skull align vertically.
- The perineum, the 3rd lumbar vertebra, the diaphragm, the base of the heart, and the roof of mouth align horizontally with the floor.
- The roof of the mouth remains level and in line horizontally with the center of the ears.
- The bottom tip of the breastbone scoops inward without causing the chest to collapse.
- The side-body ribs lift and the armpits deepen without the shoulders shrugging.
- The collarbones square and widen to the outer edges of the shoulders.
- The shoulders simultaneously draw back both from the armpits and the outer surfaces.
- The shoulder blades slide on the back toward the spine.
- The inferior tips of the shoulder blades gently press forward onto the back ribs.
- The head and neck balance effortlessly on a broadened foundation formed by the shoulders.
- The triceps muscles roll inward to bring the elbows in line with the side body rib cage.
- Along every body surface, the principle of Samasthiti is engaged, maintaining a subtle awareness of balanced muscular and energetic tension.

17 The Hip Joint

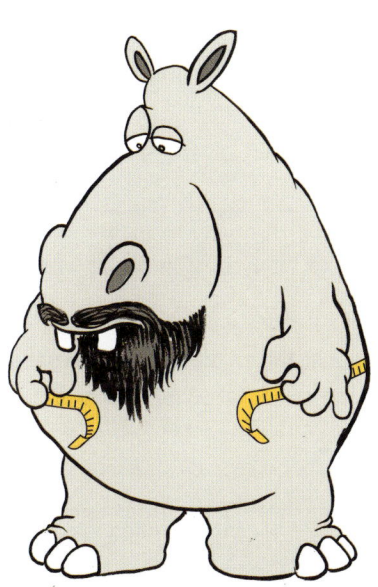

Are you *hip* to this?

When a yoga teacher instructs a class to stand with feet hip-width apart, some students slap the sides of their pelvis and shudder a silent, "Oh no!" while reluctantly widening their stance. The good news is that our "nightmare hips" are not what the teacher has in mind. The intended position is at least two to four inches in from the lateral surfaces of the body. *Hip-width apart* refers to the distance between the hip sockets (acetabulum), not the broad outer crests of the iliac bones. The acetabulum is the point of convergence of the three bones that form each hipbone. With the legs directly below this point, a stable standing foundation is established for the pelvis.

How far apart are the feet when spaced hip-width apart?

The short answer is 4 to 6 inches.

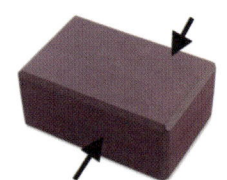

The longer answer considers two anatomical references for determining the distance between the feet.

- The distance between the hip joints corresponds to the width of the head, between the ears. For most students this distance approximates the width of a standard yoga block: six inches across.

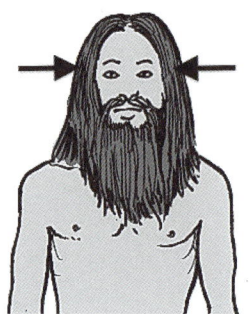

- The distance between the ischial tuberosities. When the heels kick back toward the buttock, the point of contact is the ischial tuberosities. The ischial tuberosities align with the center of the acetabulum. For most students, this distance is between four to six inches across.

A stance constructed according to anatomical parameters is stable and can best manage the many forces and tensions transferring through the lower extremities. Some yoga traditions instruct students to stand with their feet closer than hip-width, perhaps even touching. This position, which is based on style more than anatomy, may become problematic for the knees. Stances wider than 4-6 inches reduce strain on the hamstring muscles in forward bend poses.

> **Traditional alignment is not always anatomically based**
>
> Confusion arises between the stylized appearance of asana and forms that are based on anatomy and body mechanics. Unfortunately, some "traditional" asana instructions are ineffective and unsafe. Some traditions of yoga were formulated before the current principles of anatomy and biomechanics became readily available. Other traditions attempt to create a certain esthetic appearance in the postures, trying to express something more ideological than physiological. Students are often sentimental about their first yoga teachings and become complacent or uncomfortable learning something new. Ultimately, it may come down to something quite arbitrary and personal. The original guru may simply have had long arms or narrow hips. Possibly, he was able to hold his big toe in Triangle Pose and expected all of his students to do the same!

A snug fit

The head of the femur fits securely into the acetabulum, surrounded by a thick cartilage collar called the *labrum*. This snug fit has a strong vacuum effect on the femur head, making hip dislocation difficult without first tearing the cartilage to release the suction. Additional support for the joint comes from the hip ligaments.[1]

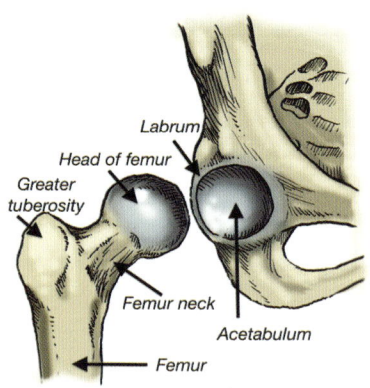

The swing of things

The hips are designed to pivot between the two femur bones in a fashion similar to the swinging of an upside-down bucket between its handles. This configuration is beneficial for the knees, which swing toward the midline of the body as they flex, an action necessary for walking and body balance.

The ideal angle for the neck of the femur bone to resist hip dislocation is approximately 120-125°. Females with wider pelvises may have femoral necks with reduced angles that reach to nearly a right angle.

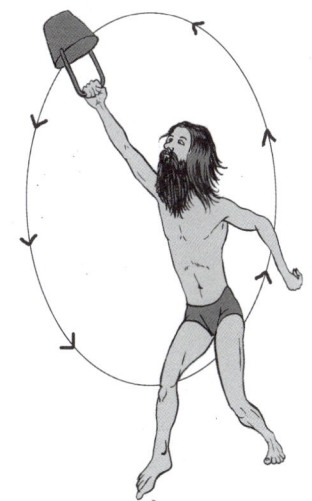

Hips move in three axes of motion

Hip ranges of motion occur along axes in three planes - *sagittal*, *frontal* and *vertical*. In the sagittal plane (front to back), the hips flex and extend. In the frontal or coronal plane (side-to-side), the hips move toward the midline (*adduction*) and away from the midline (*abduction*). Down its vertical axis, the hips rotate internally and externally.

Mind the gap

The region of the front hip and upper thigh is called the *femoral triangle*. It is an area dense with massive muscles and tendons. To effectively move this area, a deep, spacious *hip crease* must be created. The hip crease is the gap formed between the front of the upper thigh and the anterior spine of the pelvis, or ASIS. To accomplish this, draw the femur back and lift the ASIS away from the femur. This action occurs in all asana but is important in poses involving deep hip flexion such as **Uttanasana** (Forward Bend). When creating space, place emphasis on widening the lateral aspect between the femur and the ASIS to further refine this action and provide more freedom of movement.

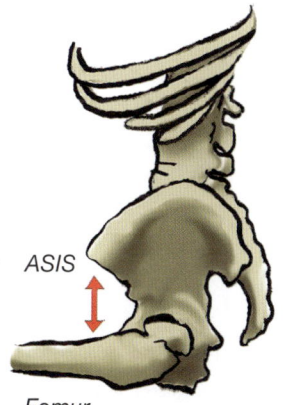

Femur

Using a prop to widen the gap

A partially rolled blanket or yoga mat can be placed deeply into the anterior space between the femur and the ASIS when performing a standing or sitting forward bend. This prop creates a physical opening of the gap and helps release myofascial tension in the upper thighs. It also produces the tactile stimulation to the body that assists the sensory nervous system in "remembering" to open the gap.

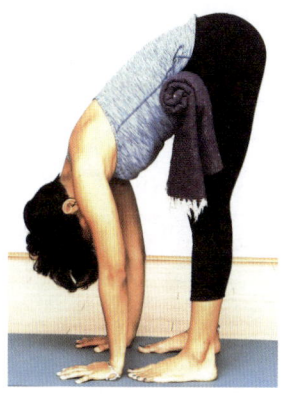

Avoid the pinch

Laterally bending the hip (abduction) when the leg faces forward causes the greater trochanter of the femur to press into the upper rim of the acetabulum and lower iliac ridge, irritating the bone and surrounding soft tissue. To avoid this trauma, first externally rotate the femur before abducting the hip. This will divert the greater trochanter posterior to the ilium and avoid the pinch.

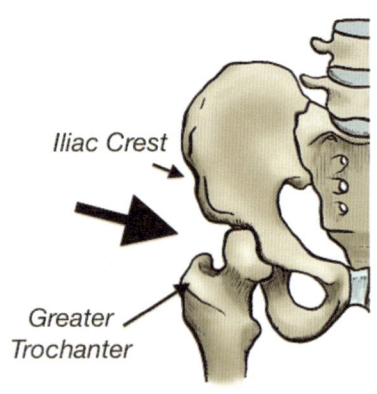

In most *open hip* poses, such as **Trikonasana** (Triangle Pose), the front hip externally rotates in order for the greater trochanter to clear the ilium as the leg abducts. Before externally rotating the hip, draw the thigh back and deepen the hip crease. This increases mobility and reduces the potential for injury. When externally rotating the hip, the leg turns equally to maintain the alignment of the center of the hip with the knee and ankle.

Ligaments Loosen	Ligaments Tighten
•Flexion	•Extension
•Internal rotation	•External rotation
•Adduction	•Abduction

Hips in action

For the hips, the micro-pleating system of ligaments plays an important role in asana alignment and, ultimately, in preventing injuries (details on ligament function are found in Chapter 7). The hip of the rear leg in standing, *closed-hip* postures internally rotates in order to loosen the ligaments and allow the hips to square forward.[2] Warrior One and Revolved Triangle are two examples of such poses where freedom of movement in the rear hip determines success of the pose. *Inward hip release* is engaged in the rear leg of most asana.

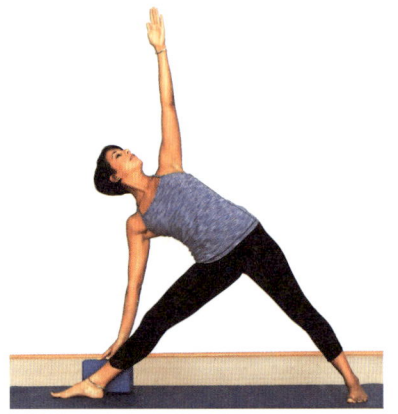

The front leg in most standing poses externally rotates and abducts, causing the ligaments to become taut and enabled to provide stability. *Forward tailbone scoop* is engaged in the front hip of most asana.

Baddha Konasana   Bound Angle

In Bound Angle, the hips widen and release toward the floor. The directions of movement are external rotation and abduction, two actions that cause the hip ligaments to tighten and become restricted. To counteract the limitations imposed by the ligaments, engage *inward hip release* at the start of the pose by lifting the gluteal muscles back and apart.

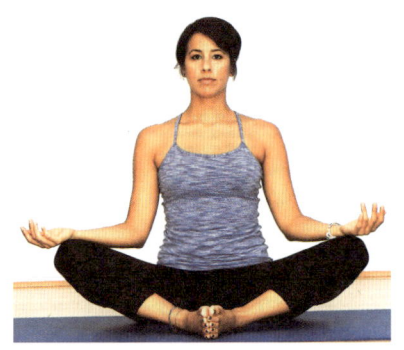

At the same time, internally rotate the upper inner thigh. As the legs release outward, *inward hip release* continues to be "energetically" engaged.

Prasarita Padottanasana   Wide-Angle Forward Bend

With the hips in full abduction in this pose, the focus is placed on *inward hip release* to loosen the ligaments and avoid the pinch at the greater trochanter. External rotation is not engaged and the feet face forward. *Forward tailbone scoop* is added when forward flexion reaches 90° to prevent damage to hamstring muscle attachment on the ischium.

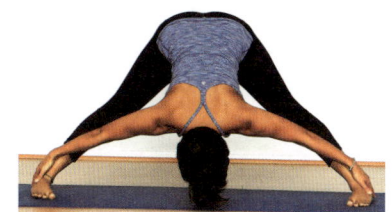

The Pinwheel

Pinwheel Pose is challenging for yoga students who have limited hip internal rotation. The effectiveness of this pose is realized when the hips, knees, and ankle joints all form 90° angles.

Attempt to sit squarely with weight balanced on the ischial tuberosities while maintaining a vertical spine. It may be difficult to bring both ischial tuberosities to the floor, but it is important not to force them down. Support can be placed under the pelvis or knees to minimize strain on the joints. To increase joint mobility and release tension in the ligaments and tendons, gently "piston" the internally rotated leg into its hip socket, adding side-to-side, figure-eight movements.

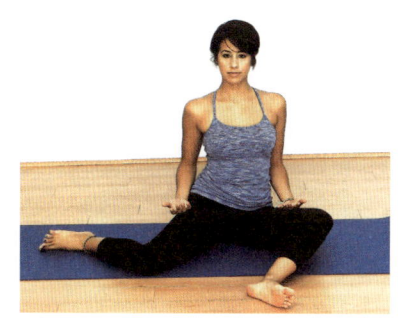

The effects of Pinwheel Pose on the hip of the leg that drops toward the midline (internally rotated hip) are more pronounced than on the other hip. When performed with precise, conscious awareness, Pinwheel is a useful therapy for arthritic conditions of the hip.

Agnistambhasana   Firelogs pose

Firelogs Pose is a challenging hip-opening pose. The shin of one leg is placed over the other, as if stacking fire wood. For the pose to be effective, the ankle of the top foot rests on top of the kneecap of the lower leg. The sole of the foot aligns as wide as the knee or beyond. The Achilles' tendon behind the ankle remains smooth and "wrinkle-free".

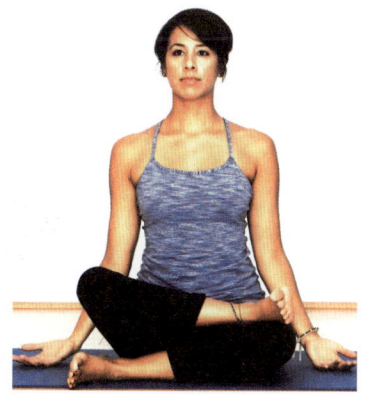

A significant degree of hip external rotation occurs in Firelogs pose. To allow the hips to open deeply and safely, *inward hip release* is engaged throughout the asana. To protect the knees and ankles from torsion strain, the feet press out through the inner heels. This action also releases the hips and further opens the pose.

In an externally biased world, internal rotation is highly valued

In many of our daily activities, the legs tend to splay apart, externally rotating and abducting the hips and thighs. Sinking into a car seat or collapsing on a soft sofa causes the legs to spread apart and the hip flexor muscles to shorten, particularly the iliopsoas group. The hips externally rotate when yogis habitually stand with their knees locked in hyperextension with their thighs rolled out and forward. This stance is often exaggerated when students are fatigued or standing lazily. It requires less muscular effort to take this posture because the calf muscles alone can essentially hold the entire skeleton upright if the hips and legs lock into an externally rotated position.

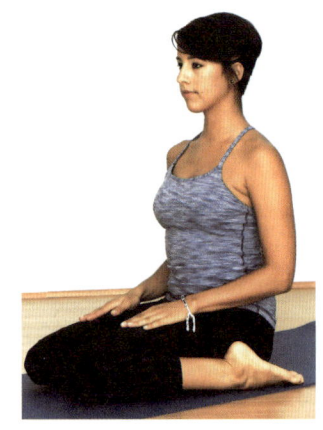

Virasana

External rotation overdevelops the musculature of students of ballet, martial arts, and athletics that require turned out stances. An additional challenge to attaining greater degrees of internal rotation is the naturally occurring torque in the myofascia of the upper thighs.

With all of the external rotation in our lives, internal rotation gets little opportunity for development. Few yoga asana emphasize internal rotation of the hips. The Pinwheel pose is an excellent one. **Virasana** (Hero Pose) and **Supta Virasana** (Reclined Hero Pose) are two additional postures that increase internal rotation when the knees remain hip-width apart. Supta Virasana has the additional challenge of minimizing strain on the lower back and knees when deepening in the pose.

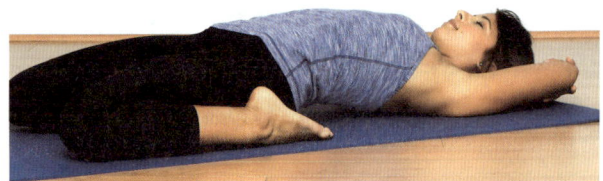

Supta Virasana

18 Hip Extension

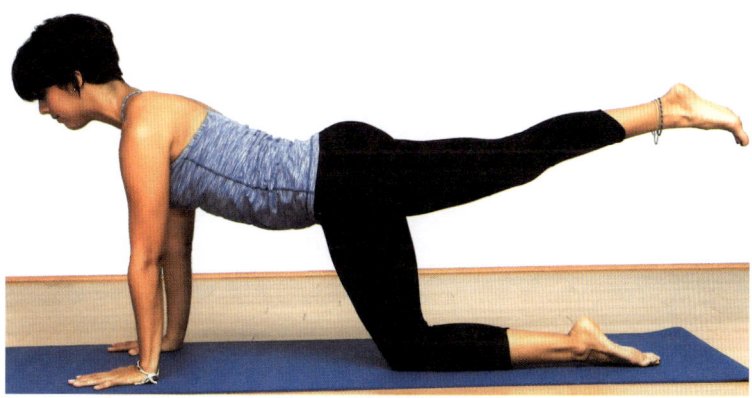

As presented in the previous chapter, healthy functioning hips are essential for a safe asana practice and overall physical wellbeing. Anyone challenged by pain or arthritis in the hip joints needs no reminder of the fundamental role hips play in performing daily activities.

Mechanically, more than seventeen muscles move each hip joint in a total of six different directions.[1] One of these directions is extension: movement of the leg posterior to the hip bone. It may seem simple enough but clearly there must be something significant about hip extension to warrant its own chapter in this book!

Limited range of motion

Hip extension is deceptively limited. Often attempts at hip extension merely extend the lumbar spine. If students are carefully observed during yoga practice, true hip extension will be seen to be practically non-existent. In fact, anatomists once argued that the hips, like the knees and elbows, do not extend.

Experiencing the limits of hip extension

Lie on your stomach (supine) with both legs straight. Reach under the front of the hip and determine the amount of space between the hip joint and the floor. The space reveals that, even at rest, the hip maintains a slight degree of flexion. Keep the hipbone in contact with the floor and lift the thigh without arching the lower back. Most students will discover that it is very difficult to raise the leg into extension without either the hip lifting or the back arching.

The physiological range of hip extension is:
- 10° with knee bent
- 20° with knee straight
- 30° in a passive (assisted) stretch

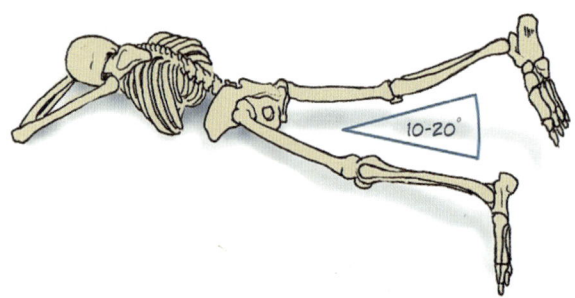

The degree of hip extension is determined by the following factors:
- The shape of the acetabulum. A shallow articular surface with a less developed brim allows greater range of motion. See Chapter 11 for an anatomical review of the acetabulum.
- The strength of the hip extensors, especially the gluteus maximus and hamstring muscles.
- The resistance created by the antagonistic hip flexor muscles. The flexibility of the quadriceps and iliopsoas play a major role in the degree of available extension. When the hip flexor muscles are short and tight, hip extension is impeded.
- The percentage of elastic-type collagen fibers in the genetically-determined composition of the hip ligaments.

> *Antagonist* muscles are muscles that oppose each other's action.
> They are often paired and located opposite one another along a joint.
> *Synergists* are muscles that work together.

Limited hip extension causes lumbar spine injury

Hip extension is routinely forced beyond its normal capability. The limitations of hip extension, when combined with students' exuberance to advance their practice, can lead to injuries. Most frequently, resulting injuries are to the lumbar spine.

Because lumbar extension is readily accessible and hip extension so limited, students often hyperextend the lumbar spine before any attempt is made to first engage hip extension. Hyperextending the lumbar spine compresses the discs and nerves of the lower back. It can bruise the vertebrae and, worse, result in disc herniation. Chronic back pain often results from repetitive lumbar hyperextension. Tight musculature in the legs is often the precursor to lower back injury due to its effect on hip extension. For the flexible yogi who routinely overstretches, pain may not appear for many years; however, spinal degeneration may start long before any symptoms begin.

Hyperextension trauma can also occur at the front of the hip socket. Repetitive overstretching in hip extension weakens the ilio-femoral ligament that stabilizes the head of the femur and keeps it from slipping forward of the socket. Once this ligament is overstretched, the hip becomes permanently unstable. Degenerative hip disease is a common result of hip instability.

Natarajasana (Dancing Shiva Pose) is an asana that challenges the limits of hip extension and puts the lumbar spine at risk. After reaching their maximum range of hip extension, yoga students of all levels often force the lumbar spine to hyperextend and create trauma to the lower back. Engaging the integrative alignment principle of *Scoop the tailbone, Scoop the breastbone, Draw in the navel* reduces the likelihood of trauma in the pose.

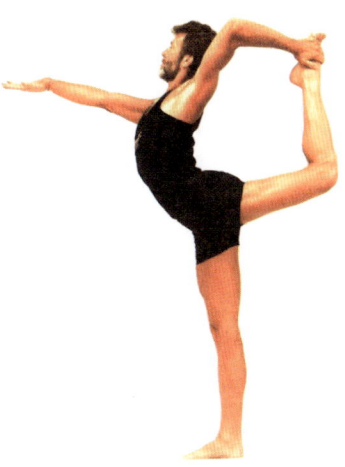

Natarajasana

Comparison of hip flexion and extension

Hip flexion ranges:
- 90° with straight leg
- 120° with bent knee
- 120° passive straight leg stretch
- 140° passive with knee bent

Hip extension ranges:
- 10° with knee bent
- 20° with knee straight
- 30° in a passive stretch

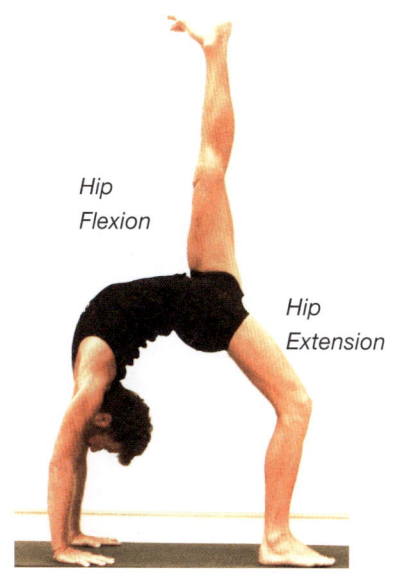

Hip Flexion

Hip Extension

Muscles of hip extension

The gluteus maximus and hamstring muscles are the major muscles involved in hip extension. When demand is low, such as during the back swing of the leg in the normal gait (walking), the hamstring muscles provide most of the power for hip extension. When demand increases, such as when running, climbing, or lifting the leg into extension, the gluteus maximus engages.

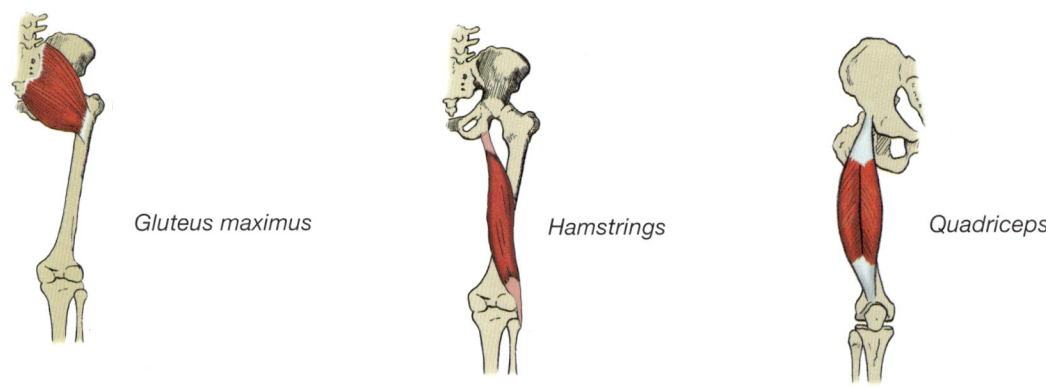

Gluteus maximus   *Hamstrings*   *Quadriceps*

Quadriceps stretch

The quadriceps muscles are hip flexors and antagonists to the hamstring muscles. Tight, inflexible quadriceps muscles are common because of limited hip extension. Conversely, tight quadriceps muscles limit the degree of hip extension that is possible. Stretching the quadriceps provides the dual benefit of increasing hip extension and improving hamstring flexibility.

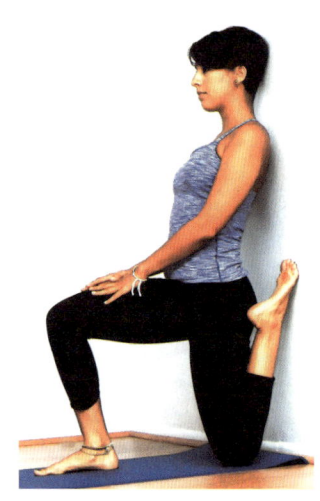

To stretch the quadriceps:
1. Place the rear knee as close to the wall as possible with the leg bent into **Virasana** (Hero Pose).
2. Straighten the torso to the alignment of **Tadasana**.
3. Keep the lumbar spine from hyperextending and the sacroiliac joints stable with *Scoop the tailbone, Scoop the breastbone, Draw in the navel*.
4. As ability to stretch in the pose progresses, bring the sacrum, shoulder blades, and skull to touch the wall.

For an added stretch, bring the pelvis forward and bend the front knee more deeply to engage **Anjaneyasana** (Crescent Lunge). The rear hip will experience more extension in this position.

Iliopsoas muscle stretch

Because the range of hip extension is limited, the iliopsoas, which is the major hip flexor and antagonist to the hip extensors, has less opportunity to stretch. Iliopsoas contraction is almost constantly occurring in most postures but a deep stretch of this muscle is more difficult. Stretching the iliopsoas is an important factor to help increase the range of hip extension.

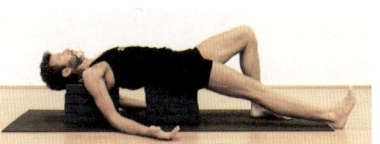

In a supine position, drop one leg over the edge of a table or a set of raised yoga blocks. The dropped leg extends the hip and its iliopsoas stretches. The torso must firmly maintain **Tadasana** alignment. To prevent lumbar hyperextension and sacroiliac strain, engage *Scoop the tailbone, Scoop the breastbone, Draw in the navel*. The leg that is dropped, considered the rear leg of the posture, actively engages *inward hip release* with the thigh rolled-in and drawn back.[2] This stretch can also be performed with a block under the sacrum and both legs stretched toward the floor.

Extenuating circumstances

Two major challenges yoga students face in hip extension asana are keeping the thighs drawn back and resisting lumbar spine hyperextension. These two actions not only prevent injury but ultimately enable asana to go deeper. *Scoop the tailbone, Scoop the breastbone, Draw in the navel* is the mantra for all hip extension poses.

When observing the angle formed between the thigh and the hip during extension, it becomes evident that only a small degree of hip extension actually occurs, despite the deep appearance many poses can achieve. The challenges of hip extension are obvious in the poses below and in postures such as **Virabhadrasana I** (Warrior One) and **Anjaneyasana** (Crescent Lunge).

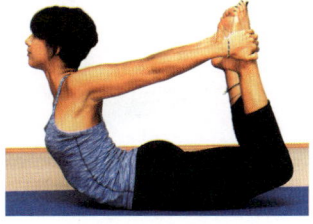
Dhanurasana

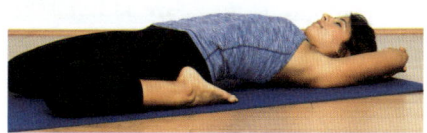
Supta Virasana

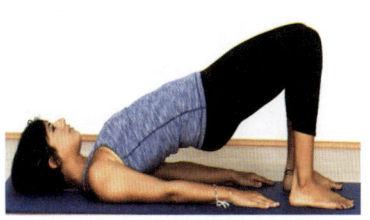
Setu Bandha Sarvangasana

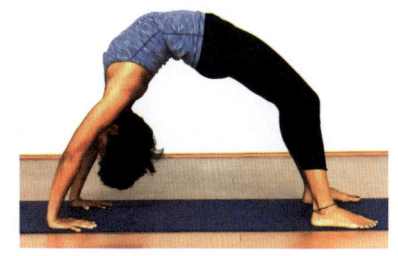
Urdva Danurasana

Why thigh muscles are massive and tend toward inflexibility

Another name for a joint is an *articulation*. When a muscle crosses over two joints, it is called a *bi-articular* muscle. The role of most bi-articular muscles is to transfer the power of muscle contraction across two or more joints. When a muscle's primary duty is to deliver power, it is most efficient when it is short, massive and remains under tension.

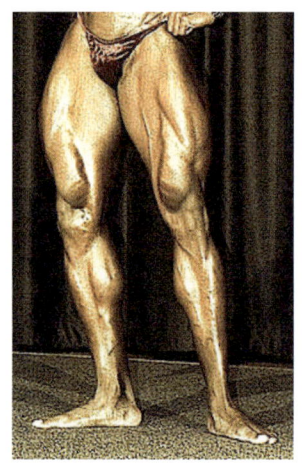

The muscles of the thighs are bi-articular muscles that transfer powerful, contractile forces of locomotion from the hips to the knees. Because of the demand for power transfer on the quadriceps and hamstring muscles, flexibility is often compromised. Runners and those engaged in sports that require surges of explosive movement, such as football and basketball are often challenged in their flexibility. Power lifting can also cause thigh muscles to become massive and less flexible, though some interesting recent studies have produced contradictory results.[3]

Hip extension and the anterior pelvis

When the pelvis tilts forward (anterior), the angle between the thigh and the pelvis reduces, moving the position of the hip from neutral into flexion. Anterior pelvic tilt "borrows" a few degrees of flexion that can be used in asana as *relative extension* before the limitations of true extension are reached. Tilting the pelvis anterior, however, cannot be wildly exploited. Although it provides "extra" hip motion, it also increases the base angle of the sacrum and with that, an increase in the lumbar curve.

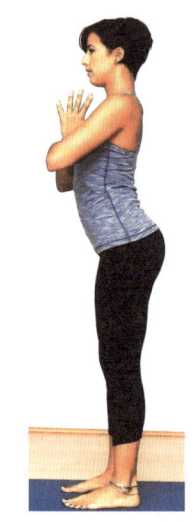

These "extra" degrees of flexion can be used in **One-legged Downward Facing Dog** to facilitate lifting the leg before reaching the natural limitations of hip extension. This small adjustment does not increase the true hip extension but will make it easier to lift the leg and keep the pelvis square.

Either Mula bandha or *forward tailbone scoop* is important to engage to balance the action of anterior pelvic tilt and protect the lumbar spine from hyperextension injury.

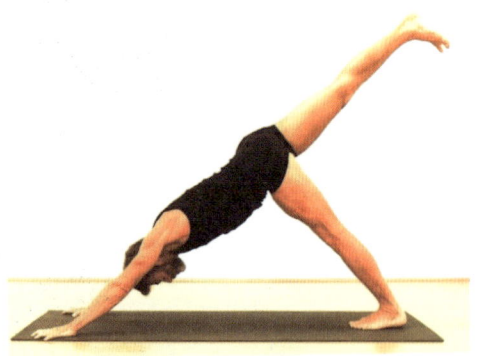

19 Alignment of the Legs

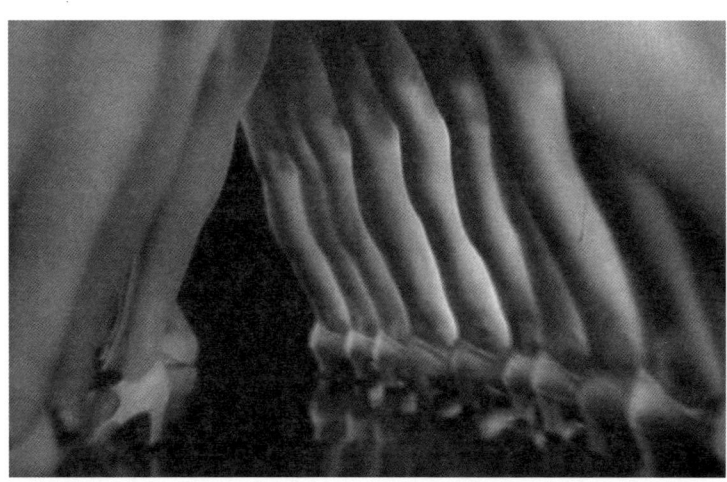

The legs are the masters of the pelvis

Perhaps you have heard a yoga teacher make this claim. They may have further described the legs as the foundation for the hips and pelvis, and with that consideration, affect alignment throughout the body.

Although the legs provide a stable foundation, they are not stiff and static. The legs constantly integrate and balance muscular tension while adapting to the pounding shock of the heel strike forces. Balancing these mechanical stresses in each leg through a vertical axis of the hip, knee, and ankle, provides safety and maximum mobility.

Alignment of the legs significantly enhances yoga practice. A few benefits are:
- Stabilization of the knees and limiting potential damage from hyperextension.
- Strengthening the arches of the feet and preventing the ankle joints and arches from collapsing.
- Aligns the muscle fibers of the leg muscles, especially the hamstrings, increasing their efficiency and flexibility.
- Correct leg alignment is essential for healing hamstring injuries.

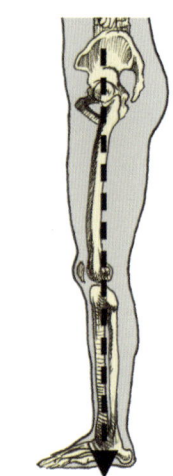

General alignment of the legs

From the side view of the leg:
- Hips align over the ankles.
- Greater trochanter of the femur aligns vertically over the lateral malleolus (ankle bone).
- The femur aligns vertically with the tibia. This takes into account substantial differences in muscular thickness between the front thigh muscles and front shin muscles that may make the thigh appear forward of the shin.

From the front view of the body:
- Center of the hip socket aligns with the center of ankle.
- The knee aligns with the hip and ankle but may deviate medially or laterally. The alignment of the knee is not forced but remains unlocked with a subtle micro-bend.

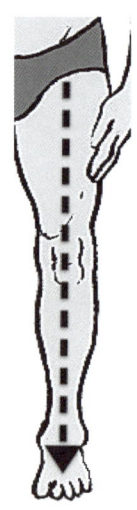

The Q-angle

Viewing the leg from the front, the femur does not descend along a perfect vertical line. Instead, it forms an angle 3° lateral of true vertical, which may vary, based on hip width differences. Wider hips require a wider angle.

A measurement used to assess the potential for knee injury from excessive angling of the leg is known as the quadriceps, or *Q-angle*. It indicates whether the forces of muscle contraction will be balanced above and below the knee. If the tendon of the quadriceps muscle is not positioned correctly, the forces pulling across the knee can cause damage. Good mechanical alignment is present when the Q-angle does not exceed 15° in men or 20° in women. The lower the angle, the safer the knee and the higher the efficiency of the quadriceps.

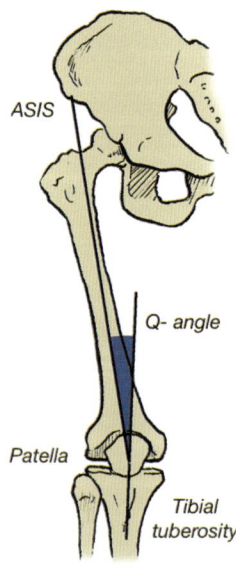

Compensation for a large Q-angle

- The primary way to compensate for a large Q-angle is to widen the stance. Add 1-3 inches of distance between the feet to significantly reduce the angle.
- Slightly bend and widen the knees, then re-straighten while maintaining the new width.
- Engage the gluteus medius and tensa fascia lata (TFL) muscles to isometrically abduct and externally rotate the upper femurs. This action reduces the deviation of knees toward the midline (knock-knees).
- Spread apart the inner groin.

Technical details for the Q-angle

The Q-angle compares the contractile tension of the rectus femoris muscle with tension created by the patellar tendon on the tibia. The Q-angle is measured in the frontal plane by establishing two ascending lines - one from the tibial tubercle to the middle of the patella and the other from the middle of the patella to the ASIS.

If the angle increases beyond the normal range, the patella will track improperly in the groove formed between the femoral condyles where it is seated. This can result in pain and eventual damage to the knee joint. *Patellofemoral arthralgia* and degenerative joint disease are complications arising from a chronically increased Q-angle.

The Q-angle often increases as a result of collapsed arches and excessive foot pronation. This causes the tibia to medially rotate and the tibia to twist, what is called *tibial torsion*. The result is excessive strain on the knee and the quadriceps tendon. If pronation of the foot is severe, orthotic correction may be appropriate.

The specifics of leg alignment

As with all alignment instructions, alignment of the legs may require actual movements or be engaged as only an isometric or energetic action. The instructions apply to all asana, not only standing postures. Exceptions, if any, would be noted otherwise.

The legs align in three planes of the body - sagittal, frontal, and axial.

- Sagittal: anterior/posterior plane (front-to-back)
- Frontal: medial/lateral plane (side-to-side, also called the *coronal* plane)
- Axial: central plane (vertical, or top-to-bottom)

The legs engage counter-balancing actions between the thigh and shin. This approach makes the legs stronger, more stable, but also more flexible. The actions are named simply by the description of what they do:
- Shins forward-thighs back
- Shins in-thighs apart
- Lengthwise contraction (from hip to heel)

Shins forward-thighs back

In the sagittal plane, align the femur bone vertically over the tibia by pressing the shin forward and the thigh back. To better facilitate this action, micro-bend the knee. It is easiest to first press the shin forward, holding it stable while the thigh draws back without altering the position of the shin or knee.

Shins forward-thighs back can often be elusive for both beginner and experienced students. Some practitioners have developed the habit of reversing the directions the shin and thigh move, unaware of this unsafe practice until it is brought to their attention. Once a habit, it takes effort to overcome and correct. This reversed leg alignment with the shins back instead of forward makes it easier to exploit the power of the calf muscles, an advantage when the legs are fatigued. As mentioned in Chapter 17, the calf muscles alone provide exceptional support for the legs. Reversing *Shins forward-thighs back*, however, will hyperextend the knees, causing the knees' posterior cruciate ligaments to overstretch and the knee cartilage (menisci) to compress.

Shins forward-thighs back is a fundamental action when applying yoga as therapy for the knees. More details are presented in Chapter 21.

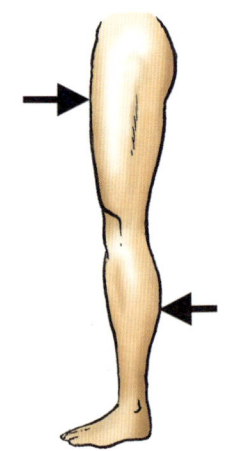

Shins forward-Thighs back

Shins in-thighs apart

Shins in-thighs apart[1] aligns the legs in the frontal plane. It provides excellent stability in the knees, increases hamstring flexibility and improves flattened foot arches.

The *shins in* portion of the action contracts the peroneus muscles, located on the outer shin.

Thighs apart contracts the muscles located on the outer hip and thigh, particularly the tensa fascia lata and the gluteus medius. *Thighs apart* is used in *inward hip release*.[2]

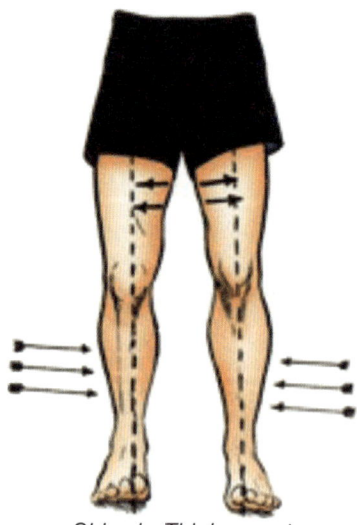

Shins in-Thighs apart

Lengthwise contraction

Lengthwise contraction is an isometric contraction through the long axis of the leg. The leg musculature contracts from the center of the hip socket, through the ankle to a point just in front of the heel bone (calcaneus). *Lengthwise contraction* occurs in both directions, "rooting" down from the hip to the foot and drawing up through the leg, from the foot to the hip. The reversed direction, contracting upwards, becomes more obvious in non-weight-bearing postures such as **Paschimottanasana** (Seated Forward Bend).

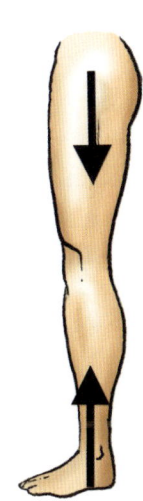

Engaging *Forward tailbone scoop* contributes to the action of *lengthwise contraction*. As described in chapter 12, the center of each hip socket is on the same horizontal plane as the sacral-coccyx juncture, the body's equator. As the tailbone scoops forward, all musculature contracts lengthwise toward the feet.

Are you pulling my leg?

If these instructions seem somewhat abstract or confusing, that may be natural! Merely reading along and trying to visualize each step of alignment is a challenging task. With physical practice and experiencing each instruction in one's own body, however, they become fully understandable. Mastering the principles of leg alignment will change the very nature of your entire asana practice, not only standing poses.

The asana and yoga therapies presented on the next few pages put the principles of leg alignment into practice. Practicing each alignment cue, one at a time, and integrating them into a few basic postures is the best way to master these principles.

Roman sandal strapping

Shin forward-Thigh back

Wrapping a strap behind the calf when performing straight leg stretches helps keep the shin forward while contracting lengthwise through the leg. Using this strap modification is especially beneficial for students who hyperextend the knees.

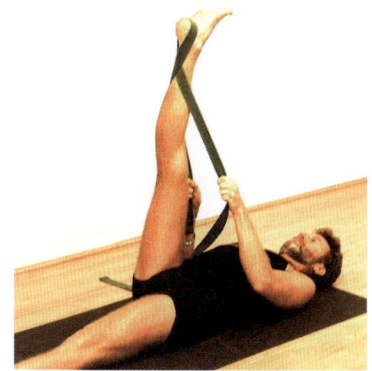

Vrksasana   Tree Pose

Shins in-thighs apart

- Press the heel of the bent leg firmly into the upper, inner femur of the standing leg. If possible, press directly into the *lesser trochanter*, the hip flexors' insertion point. The outward pressure of the foot provides *thighs apart* in the standing leg. The counter-balancing action of *shins in* instinctively engages. As balance in the pose is held, the peroneus muscle group located on the lateral shin contracts, which can be observed by its mild fluttering.
- Students unable to press their heel into the thigh should avoid the knee and press into the inner shin. In this case, press the shin into the bottom of the lifted foot, effectively engaging *shins in*.

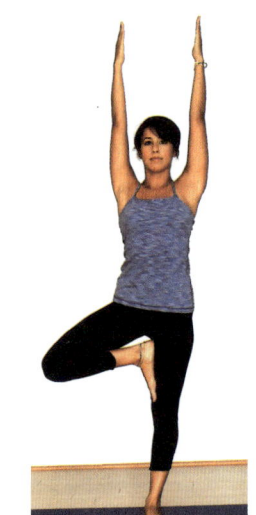

Trikonasana with block

Shins in-thighs apart

- A block is placed firmly against the outside of the front shin to reinforce the action of *shins in*. The student widens the thigh laterally for *thighs apart*.
- In **Trikonasana** (Triangle Pose), some yoga traditions place the front hand to the inside of the leg; other styles place it to the outside. The value in placing the hand to the outside with forearm or a block pressing into the shin is to reinforce *shins in*.

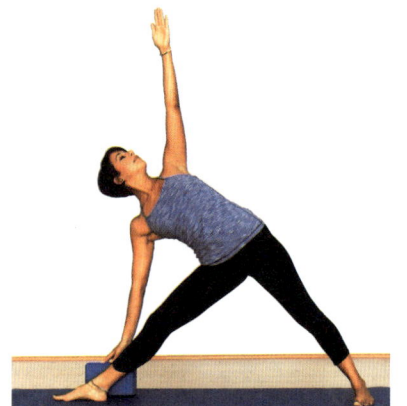

Tadasana   Mountain Pose with props

Shins in-thighs apart

- Squeeze a block between the shins, creating the action of *shins in*.
- Spread the thighs apart against the resistance provided by a yoga strap that is stretched across the mid thighs.
- The block and strap positions can be reversed to shift the focus to engaging the *thighs apart* action.

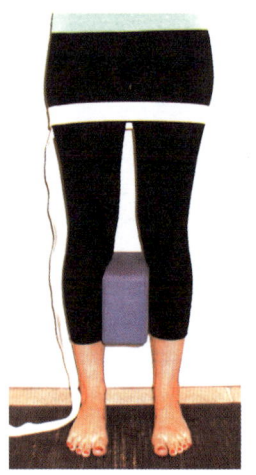

Trikonasana with rear leg assist

Shins in-thighs apart

- The student sets the position of the rear leg of the pose, aligning the greater trochanter over the ankle.
- The assistant stands in tandem behind the student, using his rear foot to stabilize the student's rear foot.
- From behind, the assistant places his hand securely on the inner musculature of the student's rear upper thigh. At the same time, the assistant uses his other hand to press directly into the mid shin. The two-hand press toward the midline of the leg creates a firm counter-resistance. The student will experience the *shins in-thighs apart* action from the assist and can explore moving deeper into the pose.

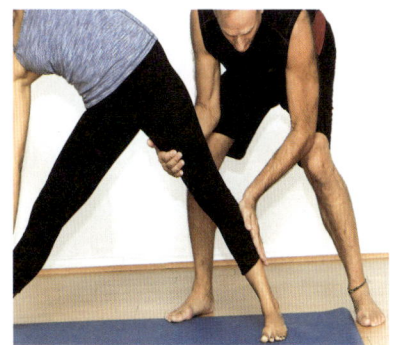

Utkatasana – Active Chair Pose

Shins forward-thighs back

- Move into the Chair Pose and lift the heels while the pressing the *shins forward.* Knees do not move beyond the front of the toes.
- Return the heels to the floor while keeping the *shins forward.*
- Draw the *thighs back,* bringing the head of the femur bones deep into their sockets.
- Lift the front of the pelvis away from the femur, creating more space in the hip crease.

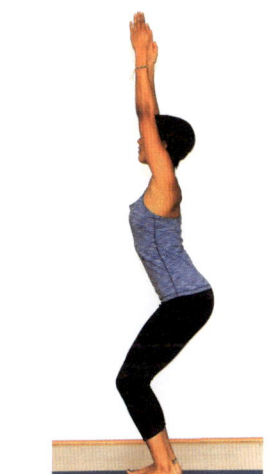

Tadasana stabilization assist

Shins forward-thighs back

- Slightly bend both knees while maintaining a firm foundation in the feet.
- Assist only one leg at a time, supporting behind the calf in a *shins forward* position.
- The student slowly straightens both legs, engaging *thighs back* against the firm resistance provided by the assistant.

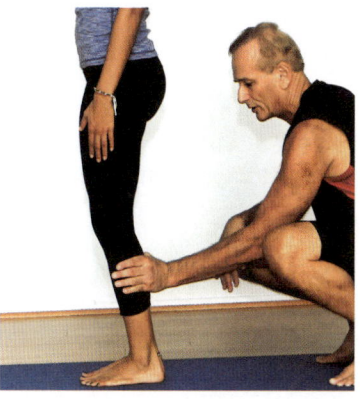

Trikonasana   Triangle Pose with block

Shins forward-thighs back

- Angle a block to support behind the fleshy portion of the calf, stabilizing the shin from moving posterior.
- From this position, firmly draw the *thigh back*.
- This procedure is beneficial for rehabilitation of knee hyperextension injuries. Injured hamstring muscles can be safely stretched in this supported position. The supported calf position enables the quadriceps to be more easily engaged to build strength in the injured leg.
- As a rehabilitative therapy for injury to the anterior cruciate ligaments of the knee, the calf can be pressed back into the block while the thigh is kept stable.

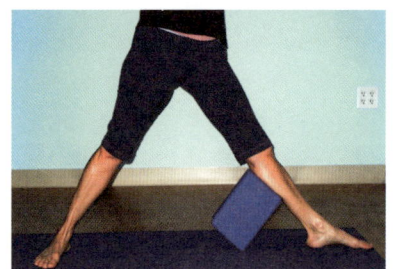

Reciprocal inhibition

The quadriceps and hamstring muscles are *antagonists* because they work in opposition to one another. When one contracts, the other is inhibited from contracting and relaxes. This is called *reciprocal inhibition*. Similar oppositional relationships between major muscles exist throughout the body. Reciprocal inhibition is necessary for all major joint movements to occur. It is controlled by the nervous system through feedback loops that control muscle contraction.

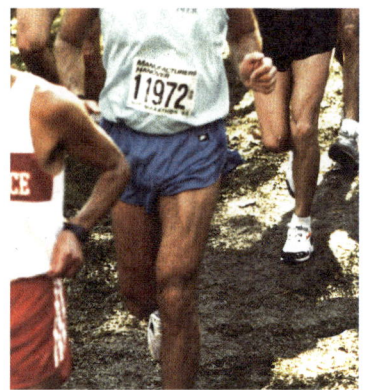

Muscles that stretch or contract in synchrony with each other are called *synergists*. Optimal stretching is achieved when the synergists stretch and the antagonists contract. As an example, when stretching the hamstring muscles, their antagonists, the quadriceps muscles, contract, while the synergists, the gastrocnemius and soleus (calf muscles), stretch.

Lift your kneecaps!

In a forward bend pose such as **Uttanasana**, the quadriceps muscles contract, causing the kneecaps to lift. The quadriceps are antagonists to the hamstring muscles and create reciprocal inhibition when they contract, helping the hamstring muscles release deeper into the stretch. Reciprocal inhibition is a valuable therapeutic tool to reduce muscle spasm.

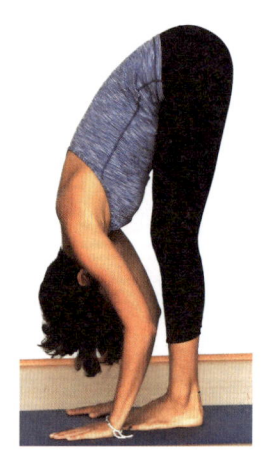

Adho Mukha Svanasana (Downward Facing Dog) stretches the hamstring muscles. As the heels press toward the floor, the calf muscles stretch as synergists to the hamstring muscles. The quadriceps, the antagonist muscles to the hamstrings, contract as they lift the kneecaps.

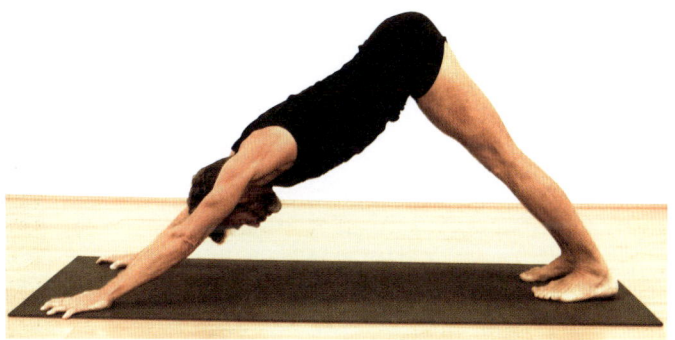

Co-activation

In case this topic is not completely confusing by now, there is another action that opposing muscles can do, called *co-activation*. Co-activation occurs when a muscle switches its performance from being an antagonist to that of a synergist and contributes strength to the muscle. Co-activation also plays a role in preventing large, powerful muscles from overpowering the fine motor movements produced by smaller muscles.[3]

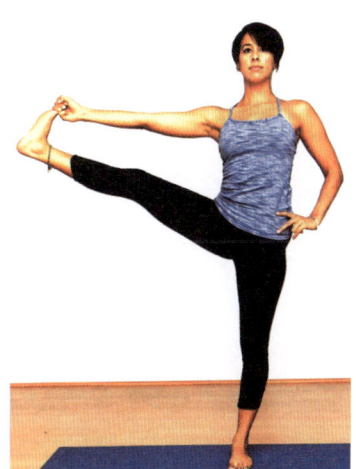

All three hamstring muscles co-activate with the quadriceps muscles beginning at 9° before full extension of the knee. The hamstring muscles can contribute up to 20% to the strength of quadriceps extension (measured at the knee joint).[4] Co-activation by the hamstring muscles helps to stabilize the knee and prevent hyperextension. Co-activation distributes pressure across the knee joint more evenly and reduces strain on the anterior cruciate ligaments. Co-activation protects the tibia from dislocating if a quick, severe contraction of the quadriceps muscles occurs during the end stage of knee extension.[5]

Need a lift?

When first learning to stand, walk, or run, there is rarely someone available to coach us in the finer details of locomotion. Early in life, we establish postural habits that become the patterns we follow throughout our lives. The development of our bones and muscles follow what these patterns of movement dictate.

A common, but unfavorable habit is to thrust the hip forward when taking each step. This distortion in gait causes the hip flexors to shorten, the thighs to roll out, and the pelvis and lumbar spinal curve to flatten. This habit is common for a few reasons. When the quadriceps muscles become weak or fatigued, instead of lifting the knee to take a step, the person can use momentum to swing the hip forward. Another cause of hip thrusting is a weak, short, or tight iliopsoas muscle. The iliopsoas is the major muscle of hip flexion. Another cause of failure to fully lift the knee is tight or inflexible hamstring muscles that restrict the quadriceps muscles as they contract to raise the knee.

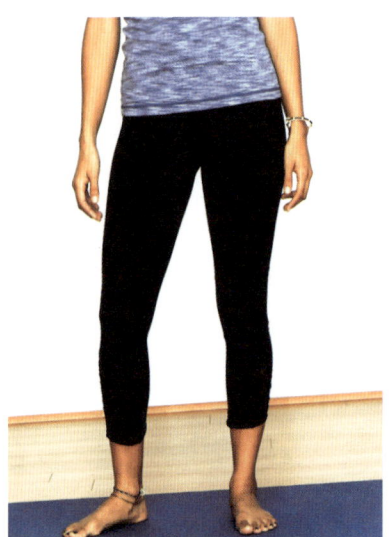

To correctly initiate each step, first draw the femur into the socket. This action deepens the hip crease and engages the quadriceps muscles to lift the knee. With the femur heads drawn back and the hip creases deepened, the hips are better able to remain square and aligned. The lumbar spine will also remain stable and maintain the desired egg-sized curve. *Shins in-thighs apart* can be engaged with every step to protect the knee from twisting and being damaged by the shock of heel strike forces.

20 The Hamstring Muscles

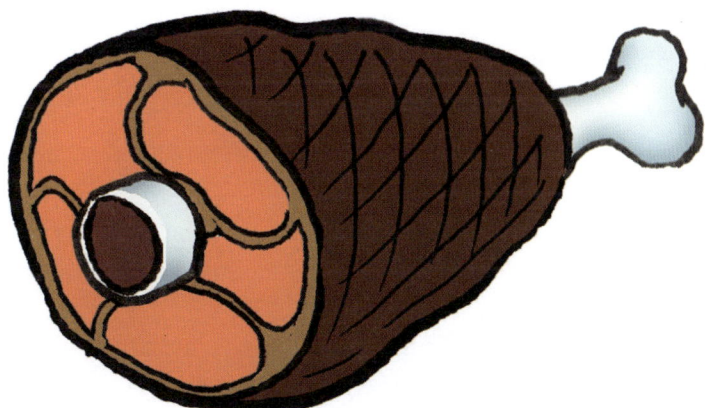

In Wikipedia's definition of hamstring, *ham* refers to a cut of meat taken from the thigh of the back leg of an animal, a pig in particular.[1] The *string* refers to the tendon from which the hindquarter is hung on a hook while the ham cures. Non meat-eaters, such as myself, may find this interesting. Hamstring or "being hamstrung" also describes the rendering of someone or something powerless, ineffective, crippled or thwarted.[2] As a yogi with tight hamstring muscles, I find this interesting too. Being a long-distance runner, I relate to the latter meaning and, after a long, challenging race, I have felt like the former!

For less flexible yoga practitioners, tight hamstring muscles tend to be the prime culprits in thwarting aspiring practices. Most evident in straight-legged, forward bends, hamstring limitation not only hinders hip flexion but directly restricts the mobility of the pelvis. And as goes the pelvis, so goes the rest....

More ham, less string – muscle to tendon ratio

Muscles can stretch to nearly 200% of their resting length, while tendons only safely achieve a 4-8% stretch from their starting point. A predictor for hamstring flexibility is the ratio between the lengths of muscle and tendon. If the hamstring muscles have long, cable-like tendons, which are good for power transfer, but small muscle bellies, they simply have less muscle tissue available for stretching. Students with long hamstring tendons can access more muscle belly by bending the knees and flexing the torso over the thighs. The thighs press back to straighten legs with less tendon strain.

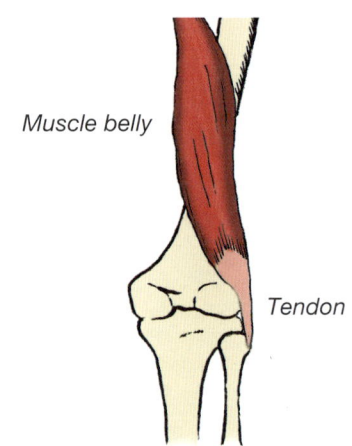

The function of the hamstring

The hamstring muscles are bi-articular muscles, crossing both the hip and knee joints. Their function is to extend the hip and flex the knee. The degree of flexion in the knee determines the strength, efficiency, and flexibility of the hamstring muscles. The hamstrings perform better when the knee is flexed. As the leg straightens and the hamstrings lengthen, strength and efficiency decreases (after 20% increase in length) and flexibility becomes more challenged.

Basic anatomy of the hamstring muscles

The hamstring muscles are a three-muscle group that is commonly referred to as one large muscle. They comprise the *semimembranosus*, *semitendinosus*, and the *biceps femoris*. The biceps femoris has two parts, the *long head* and the *short head*. The hamstring muscles are located on the posterior thigh, originating at the ischial tuberosities of the pelvis and inserting below the knee, medially on the tibia and laterally on the fibula.

Semimembranosus

The semimembranosus originates at the ischial tuberosity and inserts medially on the posterior tibia. It flexes the knee and medially rotates the tibia. The semimembranosus extends, adducts and medially rotates the femur. The semimembranosus provides important stabilization of the posterior and medial aspects of the knee. When the leg is stationary, the semimembranosus stabilizes the pelvis posteriorly and extends the hip joint.

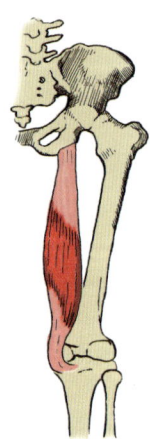

Semitendinosus

Along with its companion above, the semitendinosus originates at the ischial tuberosity. It inserts medially on the tibial condyle, having a common insertion with the gracilis and sartorius muscles. The semitendinosus, like the semimembranosus, flexes the knee and rotates the tibia medially. From the hip, it too extends, adducts and medially rotates the femur. The semitendinosus protects the knee from torque and shearing forces when the knee rotates. It stabilizes the knee and prevents *valgus deviation*, the knock-knee misalignment of the knee.

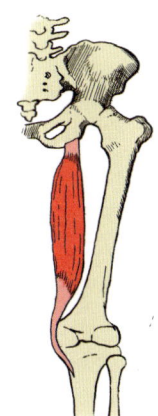

Biceps femoris, long head

The long head of the biceps femoris muscle also originates at the ischial tuberosity. It crosses the rear thigh to insert laterally on the fibula. Muscle fibers from the biceps femoris embed into the lateral collateral ligament and the deep fascia along the outer knee. The biceps femoris flexes and externally rotates the knee. It extends and adducts the hip, but unlike the medial hamstring muscles, it laterally rotates the femur. With its fibers embedded into the ligaments and fascia of the knee, the biceps femoris can be squeezed to laterally stabilize the knee.

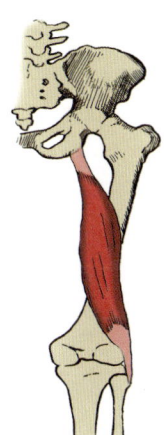

Biceps femoris– short head

The short head of the biceps femoris originates mid-shaft on the femur and, with the long head, inserts with a common tendon on the lateral tibia. It is not considered a true hamstring since it crosses only the knee and not the hip and, therefore, is not bi-articular. It also has a different nerve supply than the rest of the hamstring muscles.

When the knee is fully extended, the short head acts as the "key" that unlocks the knee and allows it to flex. The long head of the biceps femoris is insufficient in the position of full knee extension and depends upon the short head to initiate flexion.

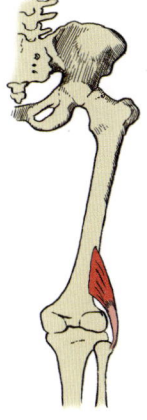

Why do tight hamstring muscles cause back pain?

Limited hamstring muscle flexibility is a common pre-condition for lower back pain. All three hamstring muscles attach to the ischial tuberosity of the pelvis. When the hamstring muscles are tight and shortened, the back of the pelvis is held down and its ability to flex is restricted. If the pelvis cannot flex, the top of the sacrum (sacral base) cannot tip and angle forward (anterior) to help form the lumbar curve. Tight hamstring muscles also make it more difficult to engage *inward hip release* (upper thighs roll in, draw back and spread apart), resulting in inadequately opened and less mobile sacroiliac joints. The mechanical limitations caused by tight hamstring muscles are most evident in forward-bending poses. Injury to the hamstring tendons and surrounding soft tissue can easily occur when forward-bending asana are forced beyond safe limits.

Tips and refinements for the hamstring muscles

- In forward-bending postures, use a wider stance to reduce hamstring strain. Regardless of how wide the stance, precautions should be taken to keep the knees from rolling or dropping inward.

- Engage *Shins In-Thighs Apart* to align the hamstring muscle fibers. *Shins In-Thighs Apart* increases hamstring flexibility, efficiency and safety. It also provides therapeutic value for healing hamstring and upper leg myofascial injuries.

- Engage *lengthwise contraction* from the hips to the heels to reduce hamstring strain. This action can be engaged with *forward tailbone scoop* and posterior pelvis tilt. These three actions function together to reduce the pull on the hamstring attachments at the ischial tuberosity, protecting the hamstring muscles from tearing at this very vulnerable spot.

- To prevent hamstring overstretching and knee hyperextension, "hug" the hamstring muscles firmly to the femur and squeeze the muscles into the sides of the knee. Also, contract the quadriceps, the hamstring's antagonist, to activate reciprocal inhibition (see Chapter 19 for details).

- Stretch the hip flexors and practice hip opening poses prior to hamstring stretching.

> **Technically Speaking**
>
> As introduced in Chapter 12, the sacroiliac joints are stabilized to resist forward flexion (nutation) by an obscure anatomical feature of the biceps femoris muscle.[3] In our human evolutionary past, the biceps femoris tendon once connected directly to the sacrum. The sacrotuberous ligament was once the upper portion of the biceps femoris tendon before evolving into a new, separate tissue. The two structures remain interconnected. Because of this, the legs can act as long levers and affect the motion of the sacroiliac joint. Although many muscles indirectly move the sacroiliac joint, this remote connection is the only instance of direct muscle movement.

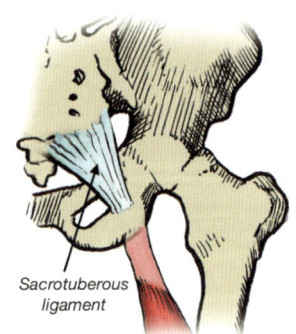

Sacrotuberous ligament

Extend the hips, not the knee

In **Urdvha Dhanurasana** (Upward Bow) and its precursor pose, **Setu Bandha Sarvangasana** (Bridge Pose), lift the pelvis by contracting the hamstring muscles to initiate hip extension. The pelvis does not lift by contracting the quadriceps to extend the knees. **Eka Pada Urdvha Dhanurasana** (One-legged Upward Bow) is a challenging pose for many reasons. As the legs straighten, both strength and flexibility decrease.

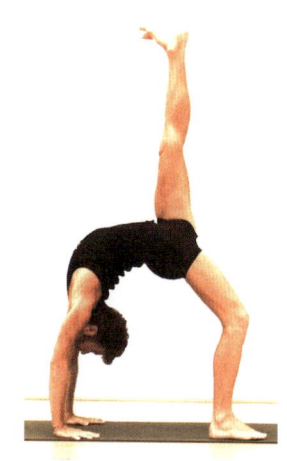

Uttanasana – a two stage procedure

Forward bending postures, such as **Uttanasana** (Standing Forward Fold), are essentially poses of hip flexion. In theory, the torso remains in **Tadasana** as it flexes forward over the legs, hinging from the hip joints. Hamstring inflexibility is the primary limiting factor in Uttanasana, restricting the hips from hinging fully and causing the torso to become rounded. When the hips are flexed and the legs fully extended, the hamstring muscles are most susceptible to injury.

Forward bends can be divided into two distinct stages. In stage one, the hips and pelvis flex but the torso remains in Tadasana. The natural curves of the spine are maintained and the central axis is fully aligned. The shoulders do not round forward. In stage one, *inward hip release* directs the movement of the asana. *Inward hip release* tones the psoas muscle, enabling it to assist in forming the lumbar curve. The femurs have a natural tendency to externally rotate. This is due to the inherent pull of the biceps femoris and the natural external torque of the myofascia of the upper thigh. Because the femurs tend toward external rotation, *inward hip release* is an important action to engage. The *thighs apart* portion of *inward hip release* also widens the hamstring muscles at their attachments, increasing flexibility and safety when stretching.

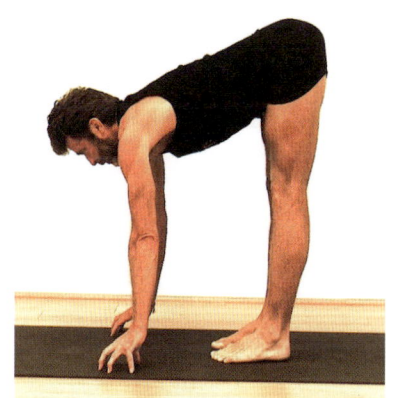

Stage two engages at approximately 90° of forward flexion, characterized by the activation of *forward tailbone scoop*. Scooping the tailbone reduces tension on the hamstring attachments by lowering the ischial tuberosities, essentially shortening the distance the muscle is being stretched. *Forward tailbone scoop* also stabilizes the sacroiliac joints and prevents their injury. A common error that students commit is engaging only the first stage of forward flexion. Failing to activate *forward tailbone scoop* can result in inflammation or tearing of the hamstring tendon or muscles.

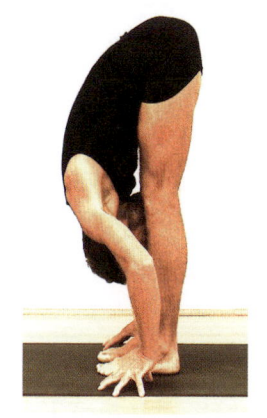

Sitting hamstring stretch

The yoga poses **Paschimottanasana** (Sitting Forward Fold) and **Janu Sirsasana** (Knee Head Pose) are popular, seated hip-flexion postures. Hamstring inflexibility is the limiting factor for most yoga students in these poses.

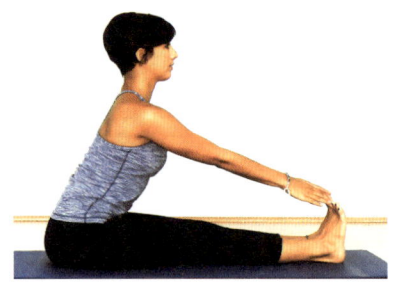

As in standing hip-flexion poses, the same two stages of forward flexion are followed. Additionally, when forward-folding asana are performed on the floor, the heel presses down and muscular tension is drawn up, from the heel to the hip socket. The entire leg medially rotates to bring the bulk of the hamstring and calf muscles into firm contact with the floor. The knee, however, does not rotate and the kneecap remains in alignment, facing upward. The muscles and flesh of the buttocks are manually spread back and apart to allow better contact of the pelvis with the floor. The broader the contact with the floor, the more effective will be the stretch. *Inward hip release* and full contact with the floor produces a visible toning of the quadriceps, especially around the knee.

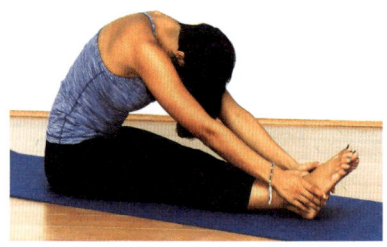

Sitting on blankets is beneficial when the hamstring muscles are tight. Sitting on props, however, compromises full contact of the leg with the floor. If the back of the leg lifts significantly off the floor, a blanket can be placed under the thigh to create better contact. This set-up is similar to the hamstring rehabilitation set-up that is presented at the end of this chapter.

Rounding the upper back and dropping the shoulders forward is counterproductive, increasing strain on the lumbar spine and its musculature.

"The poison is the cure"[4]

This mantra of homeopathy also serves as the underlying principle for yoga therapy. The hamstring muscles are often injured while stretching. Stretching, however, is essential for their successful rehabilitation. The cause of injury, stretching, becomes the cure when performed with precision and uncompromising attention to alignment.

> Integrative alignment is fundamental to all therapeutic and restorative postures. Long-held postures are especially effective in the healing of damaged connective tissue. Postural alignment allows tissues to rebuild according to their anatomical design, not to a distorted form.

Rehabilitative stretching of the hamstrings

Should the hamstring muscles become torn or injured at their attachment on the ischial tuberosity, a yoga strap can be used as therapy and to prevent further injury. A strap or belt is tightened around the upper thigh, as high into the groin as comfortable. The strap crosses the hamstring attachment, overriding the injured tendon and anchoring the hamstrings to the femur from an uninjured point on the muscle. This procedure reduces the repetitive stress of muscle contraction on the actual attachment. It prevents overstretching and potential re-injury of the healing tissue. The strap can be used not only during yoga practice but also during daily activities. To avoid pinching off blood circulation, it is important not to cinch the strap too tightly or to be used for too long a period of time.

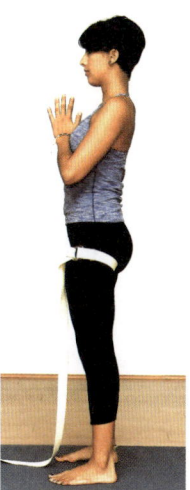

Restorative hamstring rehabilitation is effective, particularly for hamstring muscle-belly injuries. It requires an assortment of props and maintaining the posture for 5-15 minutes. The strategy is to apply external muscle compression onto the femur bone with *lengthwise contraction* through the leg. Compression is a valuable therapeutic tool for rehabilitating injured muscle and myofascia. Compression flattens the myofascia, widens the muscle fibers, and creates a neurologically calming effect similar to 'hugging" the muscles to the bone.

To set-up this therapy, sit in **Janu Sirsasana** (Knee Head Pose). Loop a yoga strap behind the hips at the level of the hip socket and around the heel, in line with the ankle joint. This step alone can be used as a complete, effective therapy. To go further, place a weight on the top of the thigh to compress the muscles into the femur bone and the leg to the floor. The amount of weight will vary, from one or two yoga sandbags to weightlifting plates of one hundred pounds or more. Be sure to cushion the flesh of the thigh from any hard edges of the weights being used.

An option is to sit against a wall for support and on blankets to better form the lumbar curve. If the straight leg does not touch the floor or if the knee is vulnerable to hyperextension injury, place blankets under the leg to provide firm contact from below.

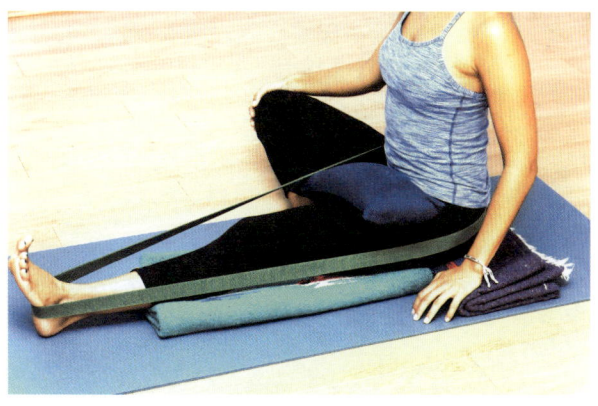

21 Knee Alignment Principles

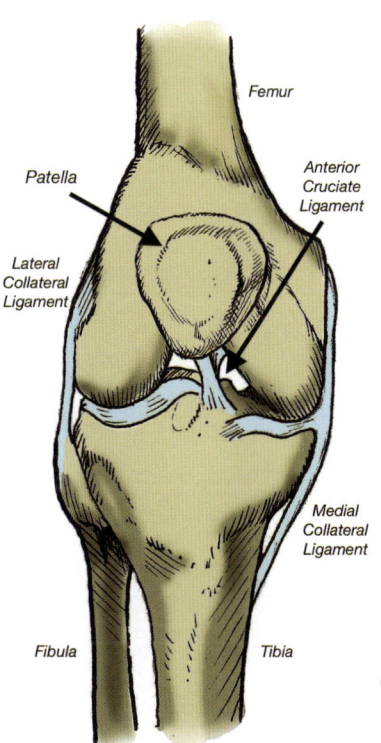

Hang around any gym or yoga studio and you will hear aging athletes lament their intractable knees. The knees are an almost universal area of complaint among those who have lived a physically full life. This chapter explores the anatomy and alignment principles of the knees. A greater understanding of their function can prevent knee injuries and offer therapeutic options for knees already injured.

The knee is the largest joint in the body. It is also one of the most complex. The knee faces a number of anatomical challenges. It must lock into position when stability and support are needed, yet be able to release quickly and manage rapid motion delivered by the force the body's most powerful muscles. To handle these mechanical demands, the knee has evolved an intricate design. In order to interlock securely, the knee's joint surfaces and cartilage (menisci) are irregular and asymmetrical in shape and size. Its ligaments wrap extensively around the joint. Although these irregularities stabilize the joint during extension, they predispose the knee to sprains, tears, and dislocations.

The knee is primarily a hinge joint with limited ability to pivot while bent. Knee flexion, the movement that brings the heel toward the buttock, is the knee's primary action and an important component of gait. Knee movement coordinates with the hip and the ankle during walking and running to allow the foot to land safely on irregular surfaces. When the leg is straight (extended), the knee joint itself is not extended. Rather, a straight leg is the neutral position of the knee. The knee joint is not designed to extend or move beyond this neutral position. From a position of flexion, the knee does extend *to return to neutral, using the powerful quadriceps muscles* to straighten the leg for support.

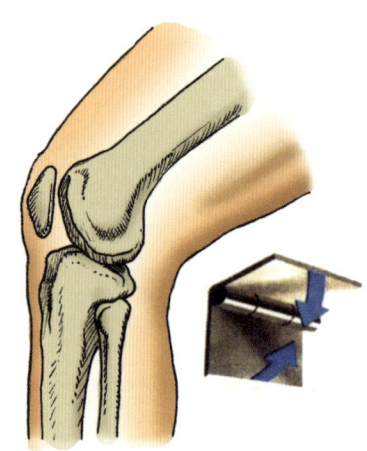

The knee is capable of internal and external rotation but only in flexion (bent). When the knee is fully extended (straight leg), no rotation is possible. The ability of the knee to rotate increases proportionally to the increase in the degree of flexion.

The muscles of the knees

The hamstring muscles, the three-muscle group located on the back of the thigh, are the primary knee flexors. As detailed in Chapter 20, the hamstring muscles originate at the pelvis on the ischial tuberosity and insert below the knee on the tibia and fibula.

Other muscles that participate in knee flexion include the *sartorius*, a long, thin muscle that crosses the front of the thigh and the *gracilis*, located at the inner thigh. The popliteus, a short muscle located behind the knee, plays an important role in knee flexion. When the leg is straight, the hamstring muscles require the assistance of the short, powerful *popliteus* to bend the knee. Along with the short head of the biceps femoris, the hamstring's built-in *key* muscle, the popliteus unlocks the knee from the straight-legged, fully-extended position.

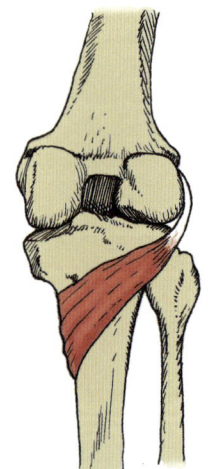

Popliteus

Extension

The four quadriceps muscles are located at the front of the thigh. They are the primary muscles that extend the knee. The quadriceps is comprised of the three vastus muscles – *vastus lateralis*, *medialis*, and *intermedius*. They originate on the femur and are dedicated to knee extension. The rectus femoris, the fourth and centrally positioned muscle of the group, originates on the ilium and both flexes the knee and the hip.

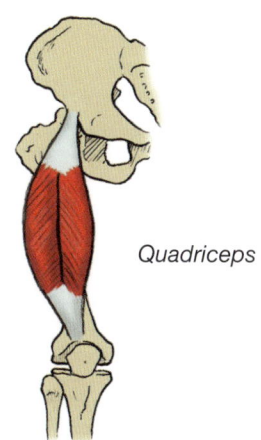

Quadriceps

Rotation

Rotation of the knee is only possible when the knee is bent. The internal rotator muscles are the *sartorius*, *gracilis*, *popliteus*, and two muscles of the hamstring, the *semitendinosus* and the *semimembranosus*. The external rotators are the *biceps femoris* (part of the hamstring muscle group) and the *tensor fascia lata* (upper thigh).[1]

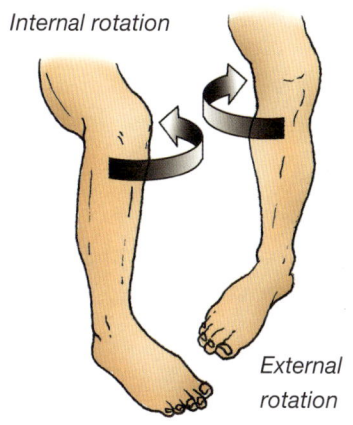

Internal rotation

External rotation

Knee injury statistics

In 2003, there were approximately 19.4 million visits to physicians' offices due to knee problems. Knee problems were reported to be the most common reason for visiting an orthopedic surgeon.[2]

Vulnerable knee positions

The knee is most stable when in full extension or full flexion. It also responds best to yoga therapy when fully extended or fully flexed. In between these extreme positions, the knee is most unstable and vulnerable to injury.

As the degree of internal rotation increases, the knee is more prone to damage. Forced or sudden extension from a position of internal rotation can easily torque and tear the meniscus cartilage. This is a common sports injury, one that occurs especially when kicking a ball.

Concussive forces on the knee that come from the outside (lateral to medial) are particularly damaging. Such a force is common in football tackles, martial arts, and side-impacting skiing injuries.

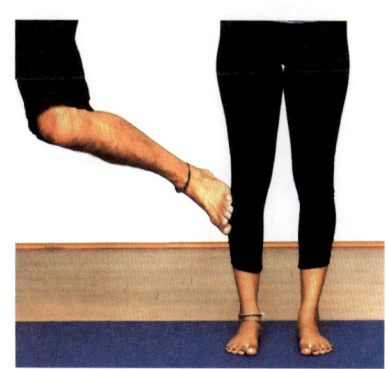

Meniscus – the cartilage of the knee

The *menisci* (plural) are irregularly shaped discs made of fibro-cartilage. The menisci attach to the tibial surface of the knee, following the contour of the inner surfaces of the tibial condyles. *Condyles* are the round prominences that form the ends of most long bones, often exaggerated in cartoon depictions of bones. The menisci cushion the forces of the femur bone as they impact the joint. The menisci attach only to the anterior portion of the tibia, allowing them to float and move with the knee. This configuration, however, makes knee cartilage susceptible to tearing.[3]

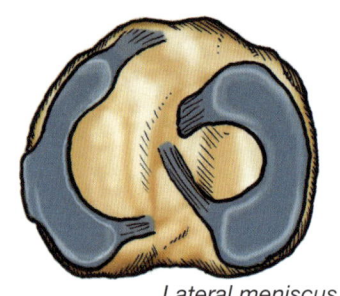

Medial meniscus

Lateral meniscus

Roll and glide

The knee joint moves like a mortar and pestle. As the knee flexes, the femoral condyles roll and glide from back to front over the menisci of the tibia. During this process, the unattached, posterior flap of the menisci can lift and become torn by the femur as it glides across the joint.

Knee flexion compresses the menisci, forcing them to shift within the joint to the outer edges. When the knee extends, the menisci reverse directions, moving medially to their original position.

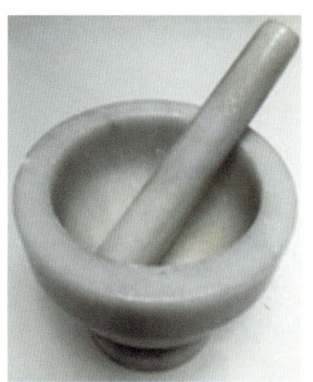

The medial meniscus is the one most easily injured. This is because of limited space medially within the joint, causing the medial meniscus to shift to the side. In fact, the medial meniscus is capable of displacing only half the distance of the lateral meniscus.

Inflammation of the knees resulting from injury is very common. S*ynovial fluid* is the viscous fluid that lubricates most joints. When the knee joint becomes inflamed, the synovial fluid stagnates and adheres to the surfaces of the menisci, making them more susceptible to being torn.

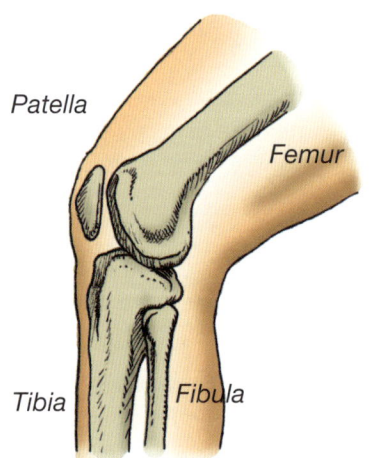

Patella

Femur

Tibia   *Fibula*

Ligaments of the knee – strips and crosses

Two sets of ligaments connect the femur with the tibia and fibula: the *collateral* ligaments, located on the sides of the knee, and the *cruciate* ligaments, located in the knee's interior. These ligaments are the primary stabilizers of the knee.[4]

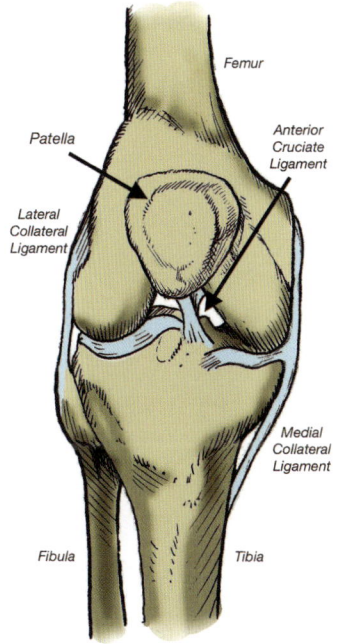

The medial collateral and lateral collateral ligaments run vertically down the inner and outer surfaces of the knee, respectively. These thick bands stabilize the knee by restricting the side-to-side movement of the knee joint. By interlinking with embedded fibers from the surrounding muscles, their ability to stabilize the joint is enhanced.[5]

The anterior and posterior cruciate ligaments are deeply recessed in the joint. The anterior cruciate ligament (ACL) criss-crosses toward the front of the knee and the posterior cruciate ligaments criss-cross toward the back. The cruciate ligaments provide stability to the front and rear of the joint.

Injury to the anterior cruciate ligament (ACL) is the most frequent ligament injury of the knee. The following are common causes of ACL injury:
- Direct trauma (e.g., injuries sustained in athletics)
- Quick change in direction or speed
- An abrupt jump into a squat
- Landing from a jump with body weight surging forward

Studies have shown that in certain sports female athletes have a higher incidence of ACL injury than males. Possible explanations may be women's increased Q-angle, differences in strength, or hormonal effects on ligament flexibility.

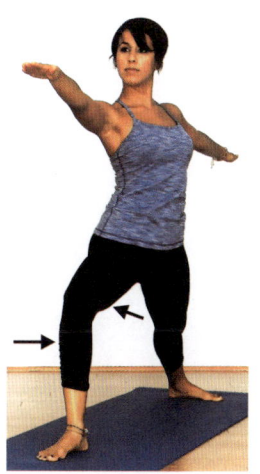

Shins in – thighs apart

> Embedded muscle fibers in ligaments create the ability to control the stability of the knees. Actions like *shins in-thighs apart* strengthen the knee during asana and can be used as yoga therapy to support weakened or damaged cartilage or ligaments.

Hyperextension and the posterior cruciate ligaments

As explained earlier, the knee joint does not extend. In the straight-legged position, the knee is in a neutral position. Extension would require the knee to go beyond neutral, what is referred to as *hyperextension* and is not desirable or mechanically safe. Habitually standing with the knees pressed beyond the neutral, straight-legged position causes the major posterior knee stabilizers, the posterior cruciate ligaments, to become overstretched. Overstretched, they fail to support the back of the knee.

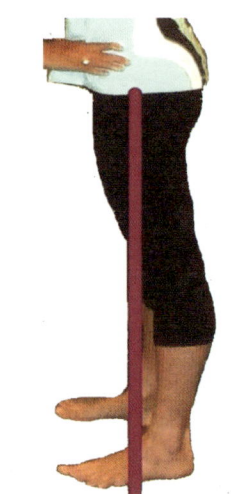

The following actions can reduce habitual hyperextension. The first two are particularly helpful:
- Micro-bend the knee when straightening the leg.
- Squeeze into the knee from its sides to engage the embedded accessory muscles of the knee. This helps keep the collateral ligaments strong and healthy.
- Squeeze the mid calf around its circumference to contract the soleus muscle, a foot extensor muscle responsible for plantar flexion.
- Press the shin forward while grounding the foot.
- Engage the peroneus brevis muscle, located on the side of the shin. This muscle is shaped like a racing stripe and flattens against the lateral shin.

Into the fold

The collateral and cruciate ligaments of the knee are the least elastic ligaments in the body, a design that fosters stability. To provide flexibility, these ligaments use their micro-pleating and wrap-around-the-bone properties to modulate their tension and relaxation. Using knee ligaments correctly creates strong yoga postures and prevents injuries.

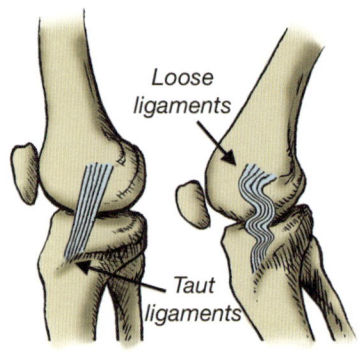

To perform **Virabhadrasana Two** (Warrior Two Pose), the front knee must be in flexion. Flexion, however, is a position that loosens the ligaments and reduces stability. To keep the knee stable, two other actions are available. Contract the muscles around the knee to isometrically create external rotation. Align the outer edge of the knee with the outer edge of the foot below and the outer surface of the hip. This alignment isometrically engages abduction, which tightens the ligaments and stabilizes the knee.

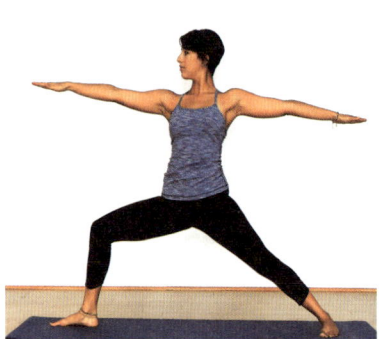

Detailed instructions for knee alignment in asana

Poor alignment produces faulty mechanics that places strain on the ligaments, cartilage and tendons of the knee. Over time, poor alignment causes degenerative damage. Knee injuries frequently occur as a result of yoga practice, however, many are preventable when integrative alignment is implemented in every asana. When adopting any alignment protocol, it is best to experiment with each action, remaining aware of which protocol offers a positive outcome, i.e. reduced pain, greater strength, or greater stability. The knee should not be forced directly into a specific position. Instead, engaging the alignment principles will bring the knee where is most appropriate. The following list presents the specific actions that bring the knees into alignment:

- Move the shins forward and the thighs back (*shins forward-thighs back*).
- Draw the shins in and the thighs apart (*shins in-thighs apart*).
- If the tendency is to hyperextend, follow the procedure outlined for hyperextension.
- Squeeze both sides of the knee to the center of the joint.
- Hug the quadriceps muscle to the femur bone and lift the kneecap toward the hip.
- Energetically draw the hamstring muscles down the back of the thighs and into the knee creases.
- Lift up the calf muscles toward the knee from below.
- Viewing from the side, align the femur and tibia vertically with each other. The difference in muscle mass between the thigh and the shin should be accounted for when making this observation.
- Viewing from the front and side, position the knee along a vertical line formed between the center of the hip and the center of the ankle, terminating through the second toe.

The Squat

The *half-squat,* a form of squatting common in Western culture, causes the femur to glide forward on the tibia with excessive force. This driving force on the knee causes the cartilage to compress and the anterior cruciate ligaments to strain.

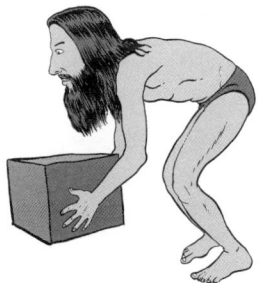

In deep squats, the form of squat practiced by yogis and people of many indigenous cultures, the femur does not compress the joint. Instead, as the hips drop below the knee, the femur draws away from the joint, leaving the tibia and menisci free of downward pressure.

In **Anjaneyasana** (Deep Knee-bending Lunge), the hips drop lower than the knee. This allows the front knee to move forward of the ankle safely with no risk of injury. Deep knee bends are therapeutic for knee injuries. **Utkatasana** (Chair Pose) is a half-squat posture. To avoid injury, the knees remain directly over the ankles and not beyond.

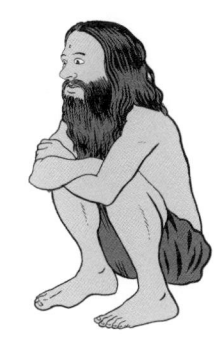

Meniscus therapy

The knee menisci function most safely when space is created behind the knee and the femur is lifted away from the tibia. After menisci injuries, knee cartilage will heal best when this space is maintained and compression of the menisci is avoided. Place a soft dowel (a rolled towel or section of a yoga mat) behind the knee. This procedure lifts the femur off of the cartilage and can be used in all postures where the knees are flexed. Before positioning the dowel, spread apart the calf muscles on the back shin. As yoga therapy, the soft dowel can be placed behind the deeply flexed knee and a secured with a yoga strap. If the yogi has an unresolved, torn anterior cruciate ligament this procedure may be contra-indicated.

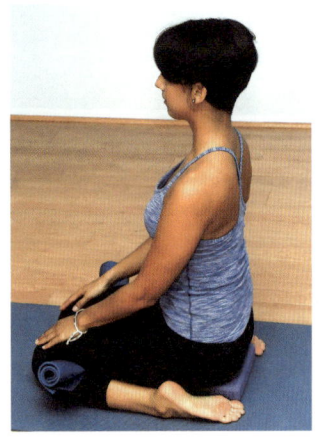
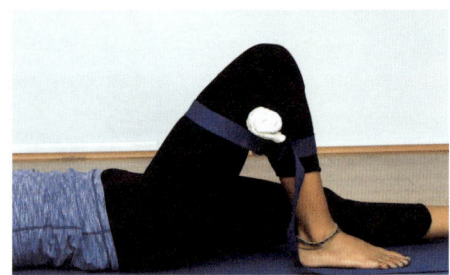

"X" and "O"

There are two common misalignments of the legs that affect knee alignment: *valgus* and *varus*. These misalignments are sometimes referred to as X and O. The term valgus comes from the Latin word for knock-kneed. With a valgus knee configuration, the legs resemble the shape of an "X". The valgus knee misalignment increases the Q-angle in the leg and can also contribute to bunion formation. Varus misalignments, in contrast, cause the knees to bow away from the midline, creating an "O" appearance to the legs. Hip disorders often accompany the presence of varus knee misalignment.

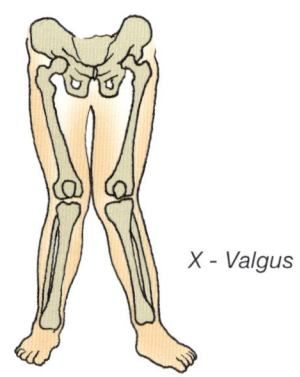

X - Valgus

The causes of both misalignments are various. Among them are leg muscle imbalances, faulty foot mechanics, hip disorders, and knee trauma. Varus/valgus misalignments damage the collateral ligaments and cause the menisci to degenerate.

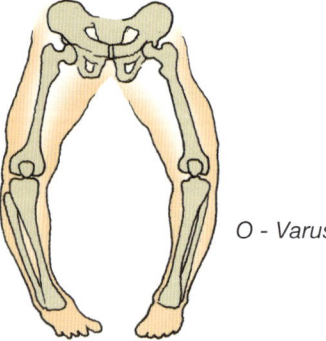

O - Varus

Valgus/Varus therapy

Yoga therapy can help reduce knee misalignments. These procedures for re-aligning the knees can be performed in either a standing or supine position with the help of yoga straps and blocks. For valgus knees (X), place a block between the knees and a strap across the shins. This creates *shins in,* drawing the lower legs to the midline and reducing the lateral displacement of the tibia. If the ankles come together when the knee block is positioned, a second block can be wedged between the ankles.

For varus knees (O), place a block between the inner ankles and tighten a strap around the shins. This will bring the legs inline.

When possible in the course of asana practice, place a block either between the knees or the ankles, depending on which misalignment is being addressed. In place of a strap, muscularly engage the action of shins-in.

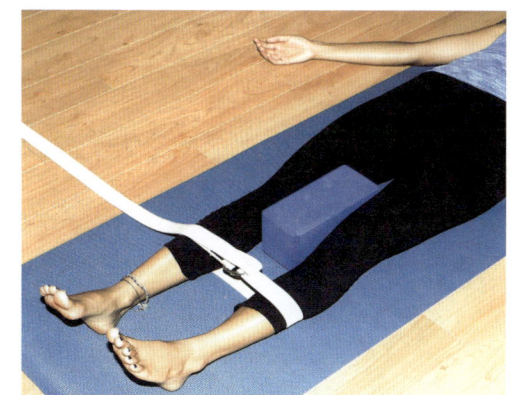

Valgus correction

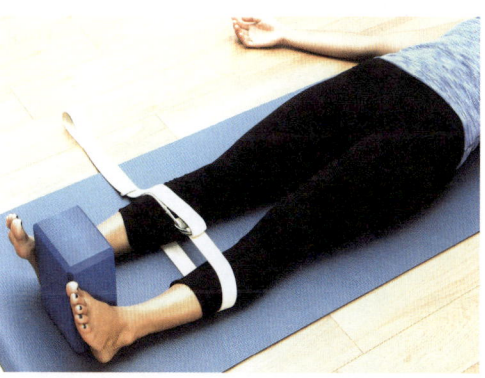

Varus correction

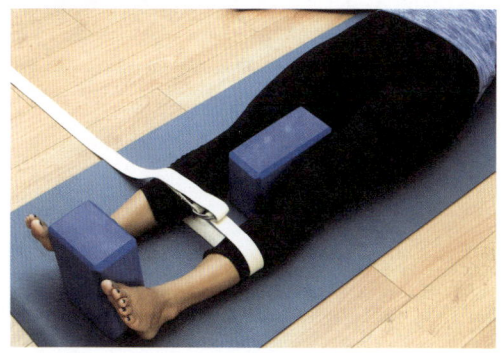

Valgus correction with ankle block

Tibial torsion

Tibial torsion is a rotational misalignment in which the tibia twists either inward or outward while the femur remains facing forward. It is a term usually associated with infant leg development, but is also used with adults when rotation of the tibia is greater than 25°.[6] Tibial torsion creates excessive stress on the knee and can cause serious damage to the knee. To protect the knee from torsion, press through the inner heel. The Achilles' tendon, behind the ankle, will be straight, unbent and unwrinkled.

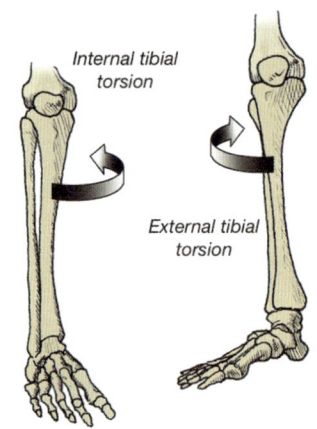

To therapeutically address tibial torsion, stand with the feet parallel and press their inner edges into a block placed between them. Slightly bend the knees and align them over the center of the ankle and in line with the second toe. Maintain the alignment as the knees are firmly straightened but not hyperextended.

Eka Pada Rajakapotasana (Pigeon Prep)

Pigeon Prep is an excellent pose for stretching many of the hip rotator muscles as well as the iliopsoas. Pigeon Prep, however, has hidden dangers for the knee. The outer shin of the front leg is placed parallel to the front of the mat and held in position by its contact with the floor. As the hips square to the front of the mat, the front thigh internally rotates. This produces tibial torsion and counter-strain on the menisci of the knee. Potential injury can be avoided by increasing hip flexibility. *Inward hip release*, engaged in both hips, will increase hip range of motion and allow the front shin to be parallel with less strain on the front knee. The knee and hip should not be forced to the floor. Rather, support the front hip with a block or blanket to position the knee without any rotation. Pressing through the inner heel will protect the knee from torsion.

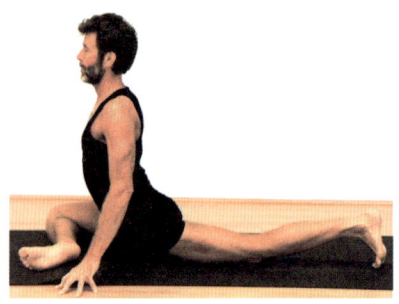

A remedial modification of Pigeon Prep pose is to deepen the bend in the front knee and rest the front of the shin on the floor instead of the outer shin. This position produces less tibial torque and keeps the knee positioned as a simple hinge, one of its safest positions.

The patella

The patella, or kneecap, is a small, boney plate located at the front of the knee. It is generally considered a protective shield for the knee. The patella sits in the special groove between the femoral condyles, riding above and slightly lateral of the center of the knee joint. The patella bears no weight and is held to the tibia by the patellar ligament. The patella is embedded in the quadriceps tendon where, acting as a pulley, it increases the efficiency of the quadriceps muscle.

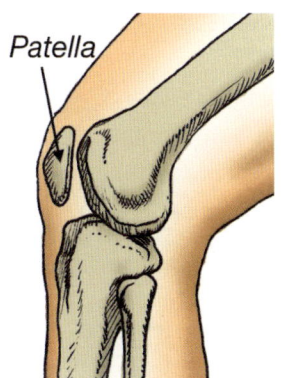

Baker's cyst

A Baker's cyst is a swelling behind the knee that is often painful and limits knee flexion. It results from aggressive muscle activity and can be mistaken for a hamstring tendon tear. Named after its discoverer, a Baker's cyst occurs when a portion of the joint lining, the *synovium*, gets trapped and bulges into the popliteal fossa, the space behind the knee. Baker's cysts often occur together with inflammation of the bursa on the semimembranosus tendon (on the hamstring) where it overlaps with the gastrocnemius (the calf muscle).[7]

Knee hyperextension is one cause of Baker's cysts. If the femoral condyles glide excessively posterior, the synovium becomes compressed and irritated and a cyst can form. Reducing hyperextension can prevent this condition or reduce the size of the cyst and the pain that results from it.

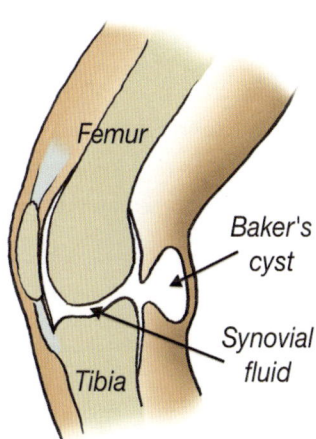

"**Don't it always seem to go, that you don't know what you've got 'til its gone...**"

Joni Mitchell's insight is true not only for parking lots but also for healthy knees. Our knees are taken for granted, abused, and forced to meet all sorts of unrealistic demands. If they become injured, the effect on our ease and confidence is immediate. Yoga and most daily tasks are compromised or stopped entirely.

By using precise alignment in asana practice and employing yoga therapy, students have reported significant improvement in knee conditions, from acute strains to meniscus tears to degenerative arthritis.

Meniscus tears are very common and surgery is a popular option. Although surgical procedures continually improve, long-term studies have shown that a positive outcome for patients receiving surgery is not guaranteed.[8] Furthermore, no studies have researched the effects of yoga therapy on meniscus tears. The use of yoga therapy for knee injuries, however, is not an either/or situation. Yoga can complement medical and surgical procedures and serve as excellent rehabilitation. Of course, in these circumstances, *precise alignment must be utilized!*

As with all advice in this book, the health care choices a student makes are personal. Hopefully they are done with a yogic mind. Conscious awareness, intelligence, and wisdom are ingredients for any successful outcome. *Pain* and *injury* can be our greatest teachers. If we respect their presence and listen to what they tell us, our yoga practice will serve us.

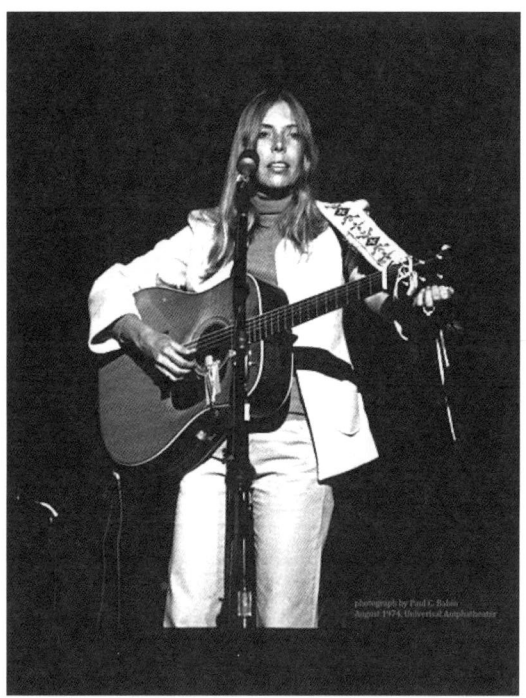

Joni Mitchell

22 The Ankle

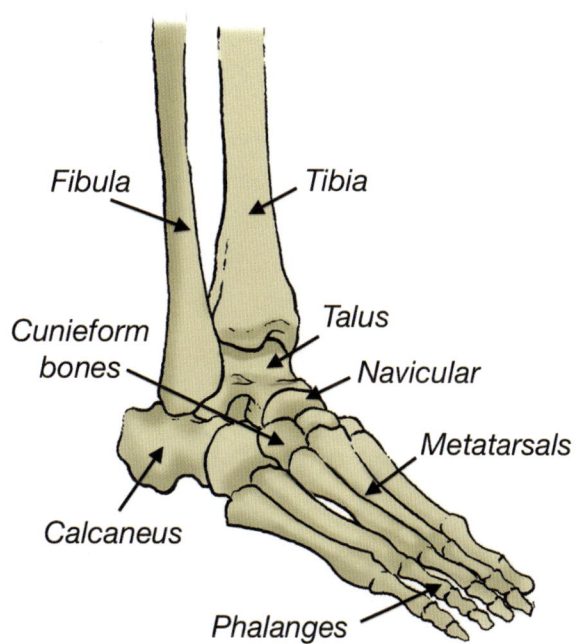

Hardly an athlete is without a story about spraining their ankle. Many sports careers have been compromised by a sprain or break to this complex joint. Yoga asana and yoga therapy can be effective in stabilizing the ankle and assisting its healing process.

Movement of the ankle is fully integrated into the body mechanics of the lower extremities. The finesse and grace expressed in the simple act of foot placement cannot occur without coordinated action from the hip and knee and ankle. Alignment of the ankle, as with all joints, is vital to its effectiveness and its safety.

The talus joint

The ankle, also called the *talus joint*, consists of three bones: the *tibia*, *fibula* and *talus*. It is a large hinge joint capable only of flexion and extension. Technically, the ankle is a rolling mortise joint, gliding and rolling in a fashion similar to the knee. The ankle's design allows it to absorb up-and-down shock with 70% of those forces being handled by the tibia and the remaining 30% by the fibula.[1] The inside "bump" of the ankle is the distal end of the tibia, called the *medial malleolus*. The outer ankle protrusion is the outer end of the lower fibula, called the *lateral malleolus*. The lateral malleolus is larger than the medial malleolus and is set more posterior.

Below the talus joint are two sub-talar joints that contribute to the function of the ankle, the *talar-calcaneus* and *talar-navicular* joints. These joints restrict excessive side-to-side motion as the forces of foot strike shift the anklebones to accommodate ground irregularities.

Inverted "T"

The alignment of the ankle with the foot forms the shape of a capital T. The T is inverted when looking down at your own feet and it is right side up when looking across at the feet of someone else. The top of the T cuts across the crease of the ankle, the talus joint. The stem of the T runs through two bones of the foot, the calcaneus and the cuboid, continuing through the 2nd metatarsal and second toe (phalanges).

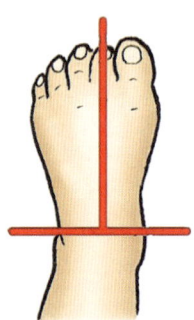

Details of ankle alignment while standing

- Keep the Achilles' tendon straight and smooth with no inward sickling (turning in).
- Lift the talus bone, moving it laterally to position it horizontal to the floor.
- Keep the ankle crease (the talus joint) perpendicular to the calcaneus.
- If the foot sickles, press the outer heel down and back.
- Deepen the ankle crease.
- Contract the calf muscles to lift the Achilles' tendon.

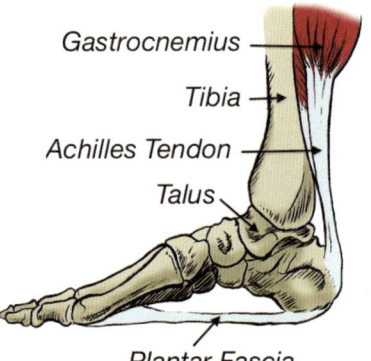

Here is a simple stretching procedure that helps Achilles' tendon injuries: Lift the heel; then contract the calf muscles. Keep the muscles contracted and squeezed onto the shinbones while returning the heel to the floor.

No wrinkles!

In **Padmottanasana** (Lotus Pose) and **Ardha Baddha Padmottanasana** (Half-bound Lotus Pose), maintain a straight, smooth Achilles' tendon with no visible wrinkles in its surrounding skin. Draw the inner talus bone toward the knee. Press out through the inner heel to keep the ankle neutral and balanced.

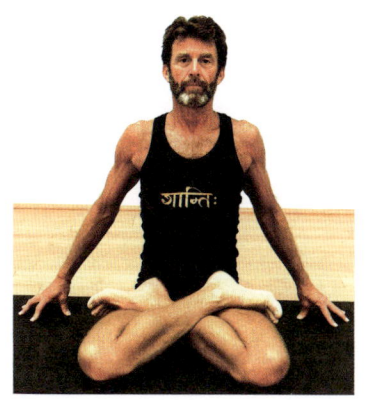

The powerful calf muscles

The calf consists of the *gastrocnemius* muscle, which, with its two unevenly sized heads, forms the bulge of the calf, and the underlying single-headed *soleus* muscle. Together they are often referred to as the *triceps surae*. The gastrocnemius is a powerful muscle but progressively weakens as the knee flexes. Rising from a position with the knees fully bent, requires the power of the soleus.

Because of the asymmetry of the calf muscles, the ankle tends to sickle inward (inversion) when non-weight bearing or with forceful contraction. Along with the ankle, the foot will also invert and supinate (details and definition of these terms follows in chapter 23).

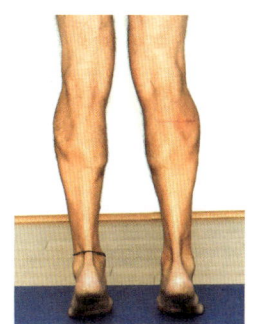

Using accessory muscles to reduce foot sickling

Foot sickling, in general, is undesirable in yoga postures. Feet are best kept in their neutral position in what is often referred to as *active feet*. (See Chapter 23 for details).

In order to limit foot inversion, calf muscles are kept more passive and the accessory, or secondary muscles of the joint are engaged. This reduces foot deviation and allows purer flexion and extension at the ankle.
The accessory muscles of the ankle are:
- Peroneus longus and brevis
- Tibialis anterior and tibialis posterior
- Flexor digitalis longus [3]

In **Paschimottanasana** (Seated Forward Bend), the yogi keeps the feet active by engaging *shins in*. This produces neutral, balanced alignment through the ankles.

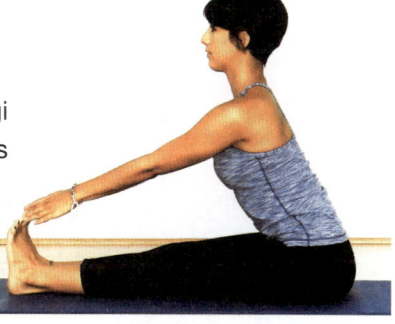

Motions of the ankle:

- Flexion   dorsi-flexion (top of foot flexes up)
- Extension   plantar-flexion (bottom of foot presses down)
- Adduction   same as medial rotation
- Abduction   same as lateral rotation
- Supination   the sole of the foot opens medially (inward)
- Pronation   the sole of the foot turns laterally (outward)

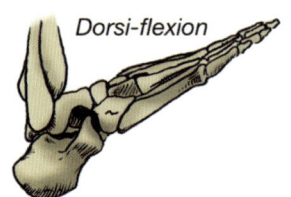
Dorsi-flexion

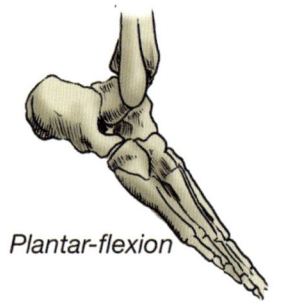
Plantar-flexion

Ankle ligaments

Transferring power and weight-bearing forces across the ankles requires an extensive system of thick and minimally elastic ligaments to support the joint structure. The major ligaments of the ankle are called the *collateral ligaments*. They provide side-to-side ankle stability. The medial collateral ligament of the ankle is called the *deltoid* ligament.[4]

Sprain has sprung

Imagine a cool, spring morning. A runner steps out of his front door, ready to finally get back into shape. But as he reaches the curb, he steps unknowingly on an uneven crack in the cement and turns his ankle. The foot gives way and the runner immediately collapses to the ground. In a matter of moments, the ankle is swollen and signs of blood appear under the skin, especially below the joint.

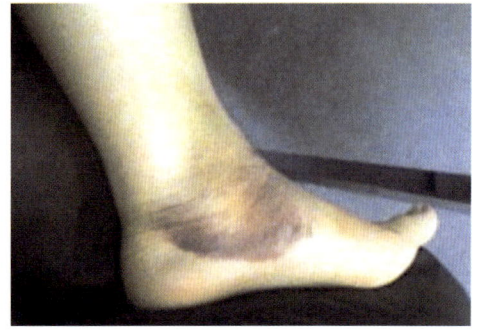

Across North America, sprained ankles occur at a frequency of 25,000 each day.[5] Once sprained, the overstretched ankle ligaments lead to chronic and usually permanent instability in the ankle joint.

Sprains are graded on a scale of one to four. Grade-1 is minor ligament damage. Grade-4 is a complete tear in the ligament's collagen fibers.

> Any severe injury should be professionally evaluated as soon as possible to be graded and to rule out fractures or other possible complications.

RICE, plus

The most accepted approach to soft tissue injury is known by the acronym RICE: Rest, Ice, Compress, and Elevate. How long these procedures should be applied depends on the severity of the injury. In most situations 24 to 48 hours is recommended, with ice being applied for 15-20 minutes out of each hour when possible.

In the rehabilitation process, alignment is critical. It allows the tissues to heal most effectively and with the least amount of scar tissue. When re-use and weight bearing is first attempted, neglecting alignment can re-injure the tissues and cause a return of pain and instability. Carefully aligned asana can provide excellent rehabilitation. Establishing precise alignment not only in the ankle but also in the lower limbs and pelvis will be immediately indicated by a decrease in pain and more stability in the ankle. Pain becomes a masterful teacher!

> Alignment is a powerful tool for rehabilitation. It speeds recovery time, reduces pain and creates the potential for high-quality healing.

General guidelines for soft tissue healing response

The list below, based on research and clinical experience, presents the approximate soft-tissue recovery times to reach minimal pain and reduced risk of re-injury. Of course, extraneous conditions cause variances in these estimates.

- Muscle injury   4-6 days
- Myofascia   2-4 weeks
- Ligaments   3-6 months
- Cartilage   6-12 months

Ankle support

The crease of the ankle draws back (posterior) when it is in correct alignment. If the ankle is injured, its ligaments cannot comfortably maintain the posterior position. **Virasana** (Hero Pose) requires the foot to bend back (plantar-flexion), which can force an unstable ankle anterior. Place a dowel, a rolled-up cloth, or the edge of a blanket in front of the ankle crease to support the ankle and keep it from collapsing anterior.

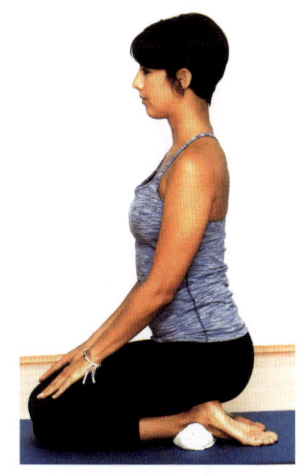

Virasana is an excellent posture for developing the strength of the arches of the feet. Engage the peroneus muscles located along the sides of the shins with *shins in* and press through the inner heels. Discussion of the arches of the feet is presented in Chapter 23.

Collapsed talus joint and foot pronation

The following set-up can help a variety of foot and ankle misalignments. Primarily, it strengthens all the shin muscles while the foot is in neutral position. This is excellent therapy for medially dropped talus bones and excessive pronation.

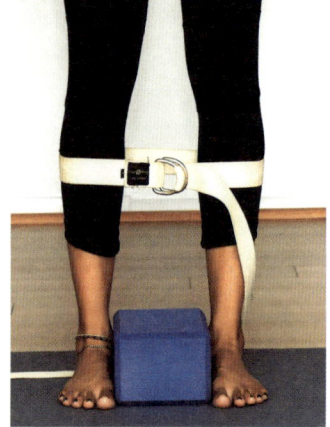

To apply, engage all four corners of the feet. Place a block firmly between the ankles. Lift the arches to bring them as close to neutral as possible. The pose can be performed with or without a strap. The strap placed around the shins (as shown) provides counter-resistance and allow the pose to be passive. Without the strap, engage *shins in*.

Should the knees rotate or collapse medially, an additional block can be placed between the knees. (not shown)

23 The Feet

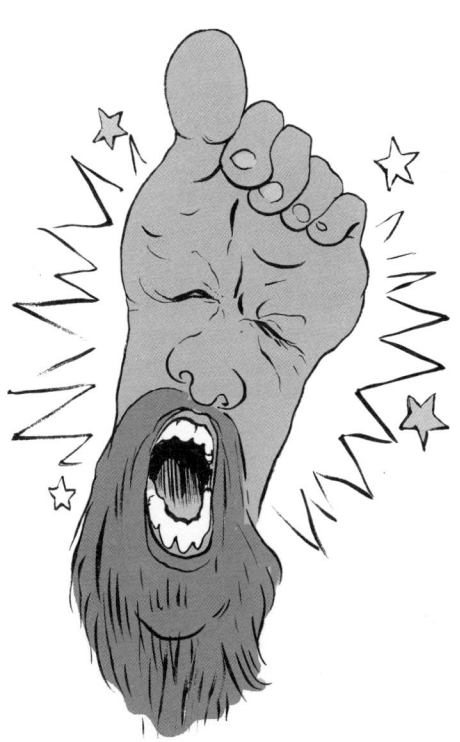

Many yoga students begin their morning practice standing at the front of their mat, staring down at those curious appendages below. They know that their feet are important because they form the foundation of the upcoming sun salutation series. But how do the feet engage? Do the toes spread apart or extend out? What alignment principles for the feet will best support and balance the weight of the body? The importance of the feet and their relationship to the rest of the body is often an afterthought, but to be sure, the feet work very hard in asana practice.

No wheelies, please!

Ideally, the foot distributes weight evenly on its four corners, balancing like an automobile on four tires. Additionally, each foot aligns with the other foot in the manner of two toy cars riding side-by-side on a track without colliding into each other or diverting to the side of the road.

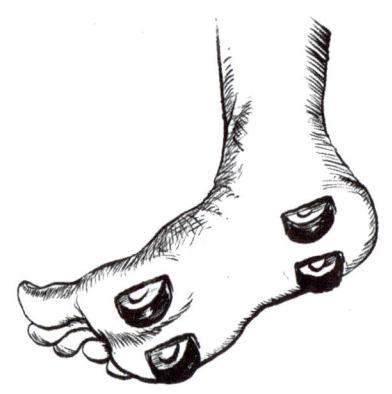

> In standing poses, such as Triangle, Warrior One, and Warrior Two, the four corners of both feet, and especially the rear foot, securely maintain equal pressure on the floor.

Integrative alignment of the foot

When jumping up and down, heel strike forces can reach nearly ten times body weight. The trampoline-like design of the feet provides spring and shock absorption to manage the concussive forces of foot strike. This is accomplished with three arches that cross the plantar (bottom) surface of the foot. The arches vault and the plantar fascia lifts to increase the spring tension of the tissues and to best absorb the shock. The arches of the feet also regulate side-to-side motion. This arch design safeguards the ankles that operate as simple forward-and-back hinge joints and are easily sprained.

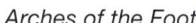
Arches of the Foot

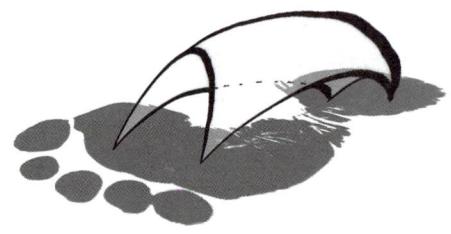

Follow this step-by-step procedure to most effectively engage the arches of the feet:

1. Press into the big toe ball mound (knuckle).
2. Press into the inner heel.
3. Diagonally cross the top of the foot and press into the outer toe ball mound.
4. Draw back from the small toe and press into the outer heel.

Muscles of the arches

The strength of the arches comes primarily from the ligaments and small muscles of the feet. The larger *peroneus* and *tibialis* muscles, located on the inner and outer shin, respectively, also help form and maintain the arches. The tendon of the peroneus longus, which crosses under the foot from behind the lateral malleolus (the outside ankle protuberance) and inserts into the first metatarsal (the most medial of the five long bones of the mid-foot), helps maintain all three arches.

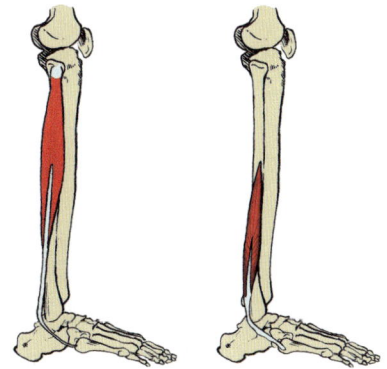
Peroneus longus and brevis

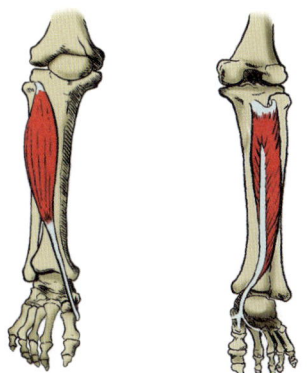
Tibialis anterior and posterior

How the feet remotely control posture

Some yoga teachers amaze their classes by looking at their students' feet and then advising them on seemingly unrelated, whole-body alignment issues. These teachers are aware of the alignment clues found in the distribution of pressure through the feet. If the foot is not balanced on its four corners, it will upset body alignment consistently in specific places.

Pressing into the foot from its corners changes body alignment as outlined below:

- Inner foot   Inner foot pressure increases internal rotation and adduction in the leg. It increases *inward hip release* in the hip and pelvis.
- Outer foot   Outer foot pressure externally rotates and abducts the leg. It encourages *forward tailbone scoop*.
- Front-of-foot   Pressing into the front of the foot most directly affects the ankle and knee.
- Rear-of-foot   Pressing into the back of the foot most directly affects hip and pelvis.

These concepts may seem difficult to picture at first. One yoga posture that helps explore the effects of foot pressure is **Virabhadrasana Two** (Warrior Two Pose).

Rear foot - Press fully into the inner heel of the rear foot to engage *inward hip release,* which increases mobility in the rear hip joint and releases the sacroiliac joint. Inner heel engagement internally rotates and draws the hip joint back, allowing the ligaments to release and the hamstring muscles to align for maximum efficiency.

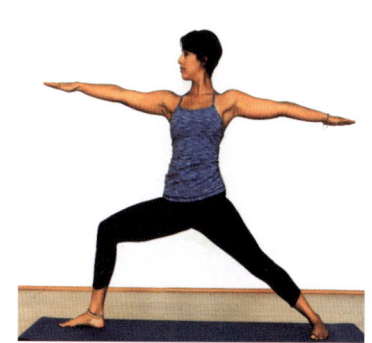

Front foot - Press into the outer, front portion of the front foot to externally rotate and abduct the knee and ankle of the front leg, bringing the knee to align with the outer hip and the outer border of the foot. Pressure on the outer heel is also recommended to additionally stabilize the hip and pelvis.

Additional details on foot mechanics

It is difficult to differentiate the mechanical actions of the ankle from those occurring in the twenty-six bones of the feet. The feet have limited large ranging movements but the subtle movements that control their vaulting and flattening are extensive.

Alignment of the numerous small joints of the foot can be engaged with the following actions:

- Spread the *metatarsal* (transverse) arch side-to-side across the front of the foot.
- Extend the toes straight out from the arch. The toes act as outriggers that improve balance by providing additional surface contact.
- Press the toe pads down evenly.
- Lift the *inter-phalangeal joints* (the joints between the outer sections of the toes) with a soft, claw-like gripping action).

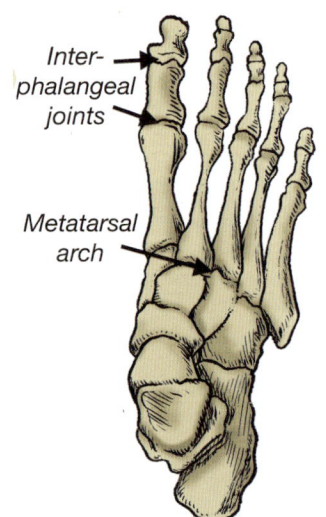

"Don't stand so close to me"   The Police

As discussed in previous chapters, the hips and knees also play a role in foot placement. While walking or running, the backward swing of the heel follows an arc that, at its upper limit, contacts the ischial tuberosity of the pelvis. This mechanical relationship offers a rationale for the distance between the ischial tuberosities (4-6 inches) being the natural distance of the feet in standing poses. Some yoga traditions teach Mountain Pose using a stance that has the feet completely touching. Keeping the feet together may seem like a minor teaching preference and a subtle action but it can produce a cascade of consequences, especially for yogis with naturally wide hips. Standing with the feet together increases the angle between the hip and knee, the Q-angle (see Chapter 19 for details on the Q-angle). Additionally, because the front of the foot is usually wider than the back, bringing the heels together can externally rotate the legs and force the thighs anterior. This will reduce *inward hip-release*, tighten the sacroiliac joints, and tense the lower back musculature.

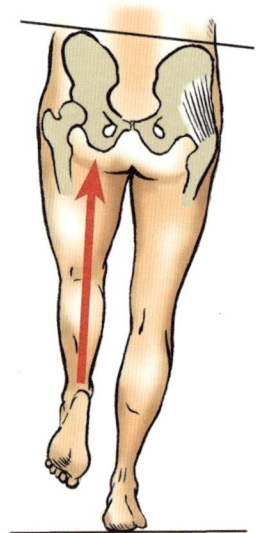

Eversion and inversion

Eversion is movement of the inner foot dropping medially (inward), causing the sole to turn to lift laterally (outward). Eversion greater than 25° is called *pronation*. The feet are designed to pronate when standing or in other weight-bearing positions. Pronation causes the arches to flatten and the talus bone to drop to the midline. The foot also pronates during the heel strike phase of walking. The inner heel is fleshier than the outer heel to maximize shock absorption.

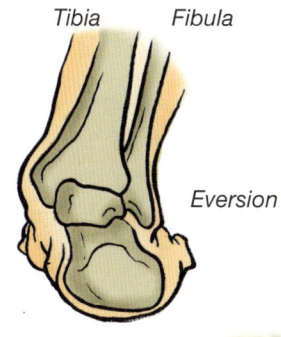

Inversion lifts the inner foot, turning the sole inward to face medially. The foot is considered to be in *supination* when it is inverted approximately 50°. When the feet are non-weight bearing, as in **Dandasana** (Staff Pose), they invert because of the asymmetrical tone of the calf muscles (see Chapter 22 for details).

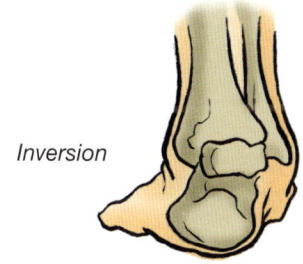

A weighty subject

Individuals with large body mass and those whose occupations require constant weight bearing place high levels of force on the arches of the feet. This causes the arches to collapse and flatten. When the arches collapse, the talus bone drops toward the midline, distorting leg alignment by rolling the knee and hip inward. Long-term weight bearing is a common cause of knee cartilage damage and joint degeneration of the knee and hip.

Plantar fasciitis

Plantar fascia, referred to as the *plantar aponeurosis*, is a thick band of fascia that runs along the bottom of the foot from the front of the calcaneus to the metatarsal arch. The plantar fascia consists of a dense strip of collagen fibers that orient lengthwise from the heel to the toes. It supports the arch of the foot by increasing muscular tension in the arch like the string of an archer's bow. The arches of the feet are not designed to hold the full static weight of the body but to support the body with a springy, diaphragmatic, pulse-like action.

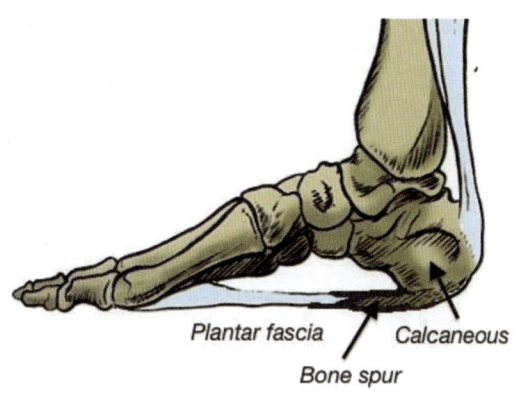

Plantar fasciitis is a painful inflammatory condition that affects the bottom of the foot. Pain is the primary indicator of plantar fasciitis. Diagnostically, lifting the toes (dorsi flexion) when standing will exacerbate the pain.

Plantar fasciitis is caused by excessive stretch or strain of the fascia, often the result of weight bearing. If the strain on the fascia becomes repetitive and chronic, the plantar fascial fibers tear and the protective fat tissue that cushions the fascia and bone from heel strike forces deteriorates. Plantar fasciitis is a common cause of heel pain that can lead eventually to heel spurs.

Plantar fasciitis rehabilitation

- It is important to reduce inflammation. Ice massage, which can reach deep between the torn fascial fibers, effectively reduces inflammation.
- Precise alignment of the feet and well-toned arches help the feet carry body weight and absorb the forces of heel strike.
- *Shins-in-thighs-apart* engages the peroneus muscles on the inside shin and improves the arches.
- Flexibility in the calf muscles, the Achilles' tendon, and the plantar fascia increases blood circulation and reduces inflammation. If the bottom of the foot is initially too painful to stretch, acute symptoms can be reduced by first stretching the calf and Achilles' tendon alone.
- Plantar fasciitis and the heel spurs that result from persistent fasciitis respond therapeutically to hugging the shin muscles firmly to the bone while moving into a deep squat.

Bunions

Hallux valgus is the anatomical term for bunion. Bunions occur when the two bones (phalanges) of the big toe are diverted toward the small-toe side of the foot (valgus). Bunions are often accompanied by shortening of the ligaments that encapsulate the joints between the metatarsals and phalanges and by weakness and imbalance in the foot's interosseous muscles, the small muscles between the bones of the feet.

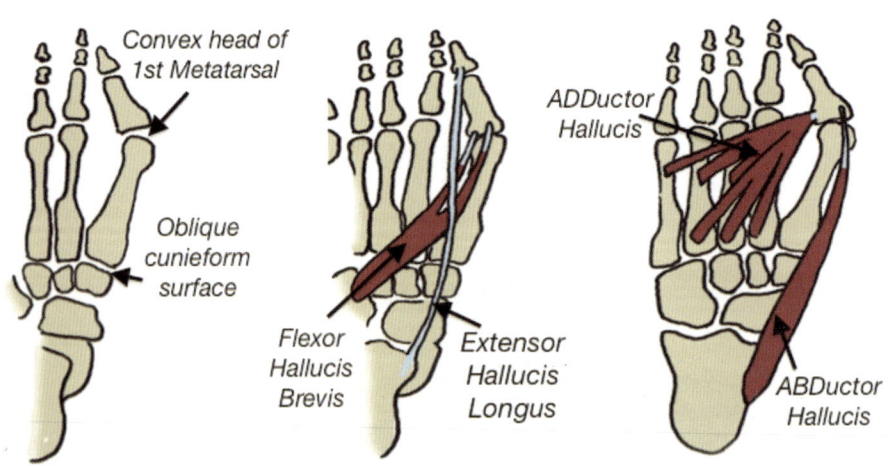

Bunions often occur in conjunction with *pes planus* (flat feet or severe pronation). Pes Planus drops the heel medially, increasing pressure on the big toe. This abnormal pressure causes the tibialis anterior and peroneus muscles to weaken. As a result, posture often distorts, causing external rotation of the hip, weak gluteus muscles, and medial rotation of the knee. Over time, degenerative damage will develop in the soft tissues and joints.

Yoga and yoga therapy can offer the best rehabilitation for bunions when the cause is muscular in nature, particularly when there is imbalance between the AdH and AbH (fig. C). To therapeutically address muscular-based bunion issues during asana practice, use the following procedures in all standing poses:

- Engage all four corners of the foot. This encourages a general release of tension in all of the hyper-contracted muscles of the foot.
- Stretch the metatarsal (transverse) arch, lengthening from the big toe to the little toe. This reduces hyper-contraction of the adductor hallucis muscle.
- Contract the muscles of the medial longitudinal arch that runs from the big toe to the inner heel. This strengthens the weakened abductor hallucis muscle.

Technically Speaking - Structural causes of bunions

Although the blame for bunions is often placed on shoes that are pointy or have high heels and small toe-boxes, there are structural conditions that are known to be involved.

- Misshapen bone. The distal head of the first metatarsal can be overly convex. Alternatively, the distal surface of the 1st cuneiform (medial tarsal bone) can be abnormally oblique. Both conditions can cause the proximal metatarsal to slide varus. (fig. A)

- Muscular balance. The flexor hallucis longus (FHL) and extensor hallucis longus (EHL) lift and bow the foot laterally (fig. B). If the adductor hallucis (AdH) is hyper-contracted, it can overpower the abductor hallucis (AbH), pulling the metatarsals towards the midline of the foot. (fig. C)

- Adductor hallucis. The adductor hallucis (AdH) plays an important role in creating the transverse arch. If hyper-contracted, it can cause the arch to malform. Adductor hallucis (AdH) contracture can also increase pronation and increase pressure on the 1st metatarsal. An indication of pressure is callous formation on the 1st metatarsal mound.

Twist walking

Twist walking is an excellent technique for addressing many conditions of the foot. It strengthens the arches, reduces plantar fasciitis, and can prevent or improve bunions.

How to twist walk:

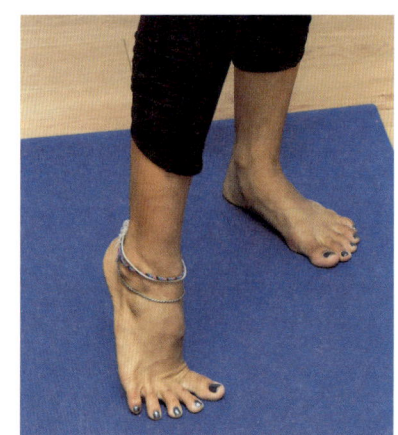

Standing on a sticky mat, turn one the foot inward and step forward, first pressing the pad of the big toe into the mat as if to extinguish a cigarette butt. Hold the big toe pad down while twisting the foot inward until the ball of the big toe presses into the floor. This action straightens the angled toe. Continue twisting inward, bringing the heel to the floor in line with the big toe and squaring the foot to the front of the mat. Engage the same actions with the opposite foot. Repeat with both feet as a walking therapy for at least the length of the yoga mat.

The high arch

Pes cavus (high arches or hyper-supination) is another challenge for the feet. One cause of this condition is weakness of the small, intrinsic muscles of the feet that attach from bone to bone. This allows the larger antagonist muscles, the *tibialis posterior* and *peroneus longus*, to over-contract and lift the arches. In more chronic cases of high arches, the tibialis posterior or the peroneus brevis may reach a state of fixed contraction (contracture).

* * * * * *

This chapter presented many anatomical and alignment details regarding the feet. Although the feet are a "distant" part of the body, their precise alignment offers many benefits to the performance of yoga asana. Skillful engagement of these movable foundations allows us to engage in the dance of awareness that we call yoga.

24 Anatomy of the Spine

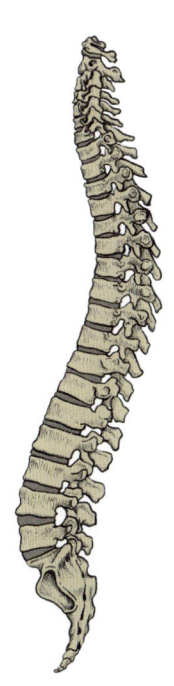

If the spine were free from the demands imposed by the upper and lower extremities, it would be able to maintain its neutral, **Tadasana** alignment with relative ease. The intention of asana practice is to maintain spinal alignment while the yogi moves through a series of increasingly complex postures that primarily challenge the strength and flexibility of the extremities. Specific alignment and anatomical considerations also apply directly to the spine. Students who understand the anatomy and mechanics of the spine will find alignment easier to apply to their practices.

The adult spinal column consists of 24 movable vertebrae. The five fused vertebrae of the sacrum and four fused vertebrae of the coccyx are considered pelvic structures.

Being the point of attachment for the ribs, the spine is the torso's structural center and is referred to as the "keel" of the body. Core musculature attaches to the many processes that protrude from the posterior portion of the spine. Its front surface is smooth to avoid puncturing the internal organs. In addition to its mechanical duties providing locomotion and weight bearing, the spinal column provides protection against outside trauma for the delicate nervous system housed inside the spinal canal.

Physiologists regard the spine as a curved column consisting of three functional curves: the cervical, thoracic and lumbar curves. The curved design provides shock absorption and allows the spine's central vertical axis to resist forces (axial compression) up to ten times that of a straight column.[1]

Architecture of a vertebra

Vertebrae have two sections. The anterior portion is called the *vertebral body*, and the posterior portion, the *vertebral ring*.

The vertebral body is a thick, kidney-shaped block of bone, designed to carry the central vector of the force of body weight. Many of the internal organs abut or suspend from the smooth and rounded anterior surface of the vertebral body.

The vertebral ring is the "business end" of the vertebra. It is referred to as the *motor unit* because most mechanical movements of the spine occur here. Seven boney processes on the vertebral ring serve as attachment sites for the ligaments that stabilize the spinal segments and the muscles that move entire regions of the spine and torso. There are four spinal *facets*, the hinges that are positioned at the top and bottom of each side of each vertebra (except for the top of the first cervical vertebrae). The facets are the primary sites of spinal movement with surfaces flat and smooth to optimize gliding motion.

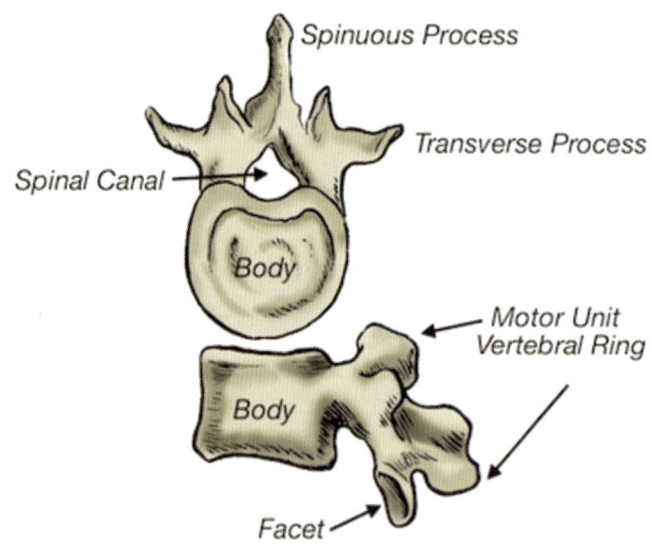

The disc

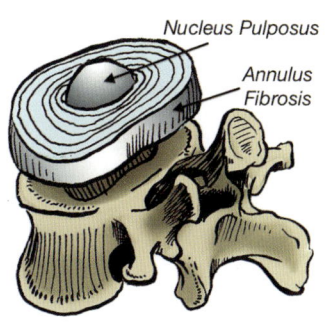

Spinal discs are located between vertebrae, beginning with the second and third cervical vertebrae. Spinal discs absorb shock and create space for the spinal nerves to exit the spinal column. The discs are equal in height, front and back. They do not naturally wedge or angle, even where the spinal curve deepens. A disc has two distinct parts. The outer portion, the *annulus fibrosis*, comprises concentric rings of fibro-cartilage and absorbs 75% of the forces applied to the disc. The disc's center, the *nucleus pulposus*, is a round, gel-filled sac of protein that absorbs the remaining 25%.

Rupture, herniation, bulge, protrusion, prolapse, slipped disc and tears

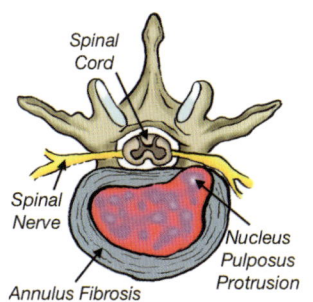

Many words are used to describe vertebral disc injuries. Following are two terms that best and most simply cover the full extent of the subject:

A *disc protrusion* stretches and causes minor tears in the fibro-cartilage rings of the outer disc. This causes the disc to bulge like a bubble in a bicycle tire. A disc can protrude medially or laterally to the opening where the nerve exits from the spine. A "disc bulge" is considered a protruded disc.

In a *prolapsed disc*, the "bubble" breaks and the protein gel of the nucleus pulposus leaks though the outer rings of the disc, coming into contact with the surrounding tissues. A disc prolapse is referred to as a ruptured or herniated disc.

The American Academy of Orthopedic Surgeons estimates that between 60 and 80% of North Americans will experience low back pain at some point in their lives. A prolapsed disc will be present in a high percentage of these cases.

> ### Technically Speaking - Tolerances before disc prolapse
>
> Spinal discs are designed to manage high amounts of axial loading (vertical force). Discs in the young adult spine can support 800 kilograms per square inch before prolapse, yet discs in the aged adult spine can handle only 450 kilograms per square inch. Carrying or lifting weight exponentially increases pressure on spinal discs. A 10-kilogram weight, when lifted with knees bent and the spine upright, produces approximately 100 kilograms of pressure on discs. When 10 kilograms is lifted while bending forward, with the arms and legs straight, a force of up to 700 kilograms per square inch is generated, more than enough force to damage a disc.
>
> Twists and torques produce shearing forces on the disc. Torsional forces on a disc that exceed 15° rotation can tear the annular fibers in the disc's outer rings.

Shear madness

In side-bending poses, teachers often instruct students to begin by shifting their hips to the opposite side of the one toward which they are bending. Horizontally displacing the hips causes the lumbar vertebrae to shear across the discs, increasing the likelihood of tearing. To safely perform these poses, lift and lengthen the body on the side that is being bent toward (the concavity). This elongates the concave side of the pose and initiates a smooth, curved movement instead of a sharp and angular one that causes the discs to wedge and compress.

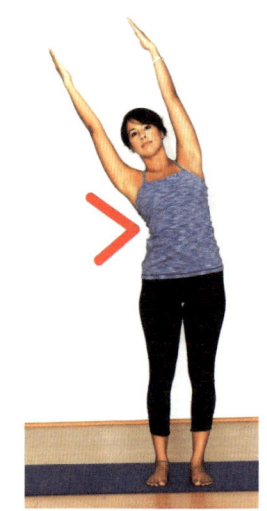

Back pain- mechanical or chemical?

The human body has a sophisticated strategy for distinguishing "I" from "other". The immune system responds to invaders, whether they are viruses, bacteria, or biological venoms. It amasses a detailed memory of the materials to which it has been exposed throughout a lifetime. It is particularly responsive to proteins.

A prolapsed disc will leak proteins from the disc's nucleus into nearby tissues, proteins that, until the moment of rupture, had been walled off from the rest of the body.

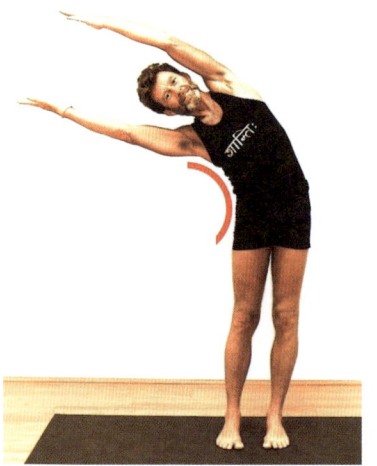

If the immune system does not recognize the newly exposed disc material as "self", it will attack the disc protein and initiate an inflammatory process in the region, a common auto-immune reaction. Adding to an environment already constricted by a swollen disc, inflammation further reduces the small opening between the vertebrae (foramen) through which the nerve root glides.[2] This leads to nerve compression and pain.

Esoteric qualities can heal disc injuries

An MRI is an imaging tool that can diagnose potential causes of back pain. It provides a detailed view of the spine, the discs, and the surrounding soft tissues. An MRI can show not only current conditions, but also offer insight into past injuries. A patient is often told by a doctor that a disc prolapse has been identified on an MRI to be the cause of the current pain and that older disc injuries are also visible, ones that occurred many years prior. Bewildered, the patient exclaims, "But I never had any back pain before this happened!" How could someone be aware of one injury and not others when they are so similar? The answer is found in how an individual's immune system responds to stress. If a disc prolapse occurs during a state of panic or protracted stress, the immune system, unable to pinpoint the source of the "foreign" protein, can overreact. The system goes on alert and creates massive inflammation.

If a person is managing stress in a calm manner during the incident, the immune system may react minimally, causing a more subdued inflammatory process, or none at all.

Breathless in yogasana

Breath has a direct effect on spinal disc pressure. When used effectively, breath can provide great stability and protect discs from damage. Improper breathing, however, can increase disc pressure to dangerous levels. Many yoga traditions incorporate *Kumbhaka* (breath retention) and *Bandha* (breath lock). These two procedures are practices of *Kriya* (cleansing) yoga and *Pranayama* (energy flow), but they also play an important role in asana. More details on bandhas and breath practices are presented in Chapter 29.

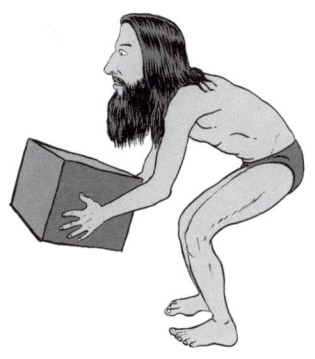

As mentioned, disc pressure increases in forward bending positions, especially when the spine is loaded with weight or when the breath is held. If the breath is held while forward bending, pressure inside the discs can rise to levels where lifting a 20-pound weight can prolapse a disc.

Two physiological phenomena protect discs from what may seem like inevitable damage. The first is that the majority of the vertical force hitting the discs naturally shifts from the gel-like nucleus to the outer rings of cartilage. Of course, for this to occur, maintaining correct spinal alignment is vital.

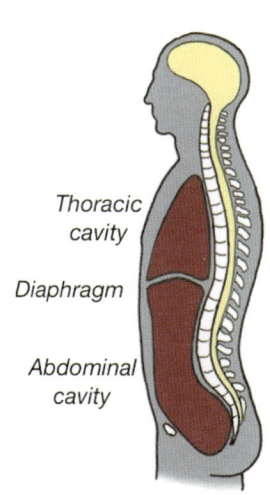

The second protective mechanism is called the *Valsalva effect*. The Valsalva effect happens when air is compressed in the thoracic and abdominal cavities. The trapped air increases intra-abdominal pressure and significantly reduces pressure on the discs. The sequestered air acts as a rigid, inflated beam that transfers forces to the abdomen that would otherwise be placed on the spine. The effect is short-acting and designed primarily to protect the discs when a heavy object is first lifted. The Valsalva effect reduces axial compression by 50% on the T_{12}-L_1 disc and by 30% on the L_5-S_1 disc.[3,4]

Applying the bandhas engages the Valsalva effect, trapping air in the abdominal and thoracic cavities to carry the forces weighing on the spine. There is a definite, critical difference between holding the breath, which increases disc pressure, and trapping air in the cavities, which reduces disc pressure. When practicing asana, breathe fully and evenly. Apply the bandhas without holding the breath. This keeps disc pressure normalized. As will be explored in Chapter 29, full breathing and bandha engagement can take place simultaneously.

How many movements can the spine make?

When asked this question, yoga students are often perplexed, not knowing where to begin to find the answer. They are aware that the spine is fluid and mobile, but determining the number of separate spinal movements is not something they previously considered. The purpose of this accounting is more than mere curiosity. When yoga students understand what movements are possible, it is easier to make them happen. What is clear to all is that the more fully the spine can be mobilized, the greater the overall flexibility and the deeper the yoga practice.

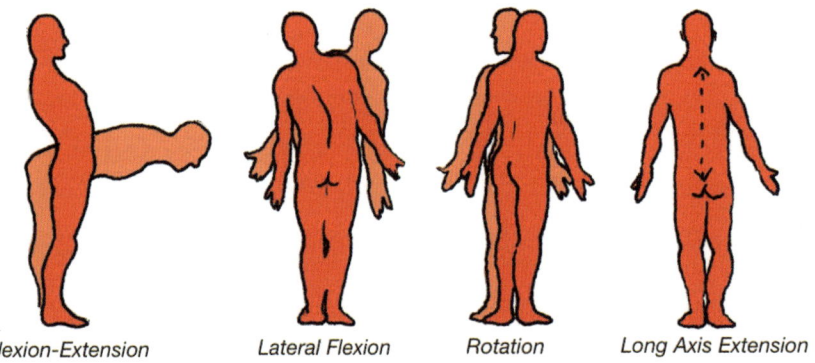

Flexion-Extension *Lateral Flexion* *Rotation* *Long Axis Extension*

The total spinal movement question can be explored as follows:

- Each vertebra moves in seven different directions. Each vertebra can: *flex* and *extend*; *laterally flex* (side bending) left and right; and *rotate* left and right. Additionally, like a coiled spring elongating, each vertebra can extend through the vertical axis of the spine, what is called *long axis extension*.[5]

- Each facet joint is capable of moving independently in all seven directions, even where the facet's orientation favors one direction of movement over the others.

- With 24 moveable vertebrae in the adult spine, each moving in 7 directions, there is a sub-total of 168 movements in the spine. But this is not the final count. Movement occurs at each facet joint, gliding between the vertebra above and below. From the sacrum to the atlas (the top vertebra), the number of facet joints is 48. This brings the total to 336 independent, spinal movements, more than enough to create the snake-like, undulating movements we associate with a healthy spine.[6]

Most of us, including many of the most accomplished yogis, have never learned to engage the spine's full capabilities. Poor postural habits and injuries also limit the ability to utilize many of the spine's subtle movements. The thoracic spine, in conjunction with the rib cage, has 216 movements; yet the thoracic cage is often moved as a solid piece. Perhaps belly dancers fare better than yogis in accessing this extensive mobility!

> Breath is full and even in asana practice, neither restricted nor retained.
> Engaging the bandhas is a protective practice that creates core stability.

Independent facet movement

Facet joints glide independently of each other. Even on the same vertebra, some joints can move freely while others are *fixated* (locked in place). When movement in a facet joint is reduced, other joints compensate to take up the slack. The facet joints with the most mobility are compelled to move beyond their normal range. Unfortunately, these subtle compensations rarely reach a yogi's awareness until the joints are weak and unstable. Hypermobile joints become strained and inflamed. Fixated joints, due to lack of motion, become adhered. Over time, degenerative changes occur, including calcium deposits, spur formation and, eventually, spinal fusion. Although this is the "typical" aging process, restoring mobility and practicing yoga with correct alignment can curtail its occurrence.

Hypermobility, clicks and cracks

Some yoga students are familiar with the creaking and cracking that occurs in the spine when twisting and turning to engage postures. When the back cracks, substances are released called *endorphins*. Endorphins are neurotransmitters that are chemically similar to morphine. They produce sensations of pleasure and relief that some students, and teachers alike, pursue by constantly cracking their backs. Most cracking that recurs when moving through postures has little therapeutic value. These generalized cracks and pops do not release "stuck" joints, as chiropractic procedures may do, but instead move already unstable ones. Repetitive movement of unstable joints stretches soft tissue and leads to chronic hypermobility in that joint. Moving hypermobile joints can feel empowering at first, with some movements seeming easier than before. This "benefit" rapidly diminishes, however, when the hypermobile regions become inflamed and painful. If hypermobility continues to be exploited, the slow process of degeneration will begin in the spine and discs.

Yoga – the cause or the cure

Certain regions of the body may seem flexible or freely moveable in comparison to others that are more recalcitrant. Breath and awareness can detect areas of restricted spinal mobility and bring attention to other areas that respond with strain and hypermobility. *Moving from the least mobile areas first* and maintaining precise postural alignment reduces the potential for damage from imbalanced joint mobility.

Rag Doll Forward Bend is a deceptively complex pose that offers more than a simple stretch of the back body. In Rag Doll Pose, the body can experience the energetic contrast between *ease* and *tension*. Areas of tension are less mobile and feel stuck, unable to find ease. When in Rag Doll Pose, release deeply into the joints and tissues of the tense regions by focusing the breath on these specific areas. With each exhalation, lengthen and release the tension. Be aware of adjacent areas of the spine that are free moving and attempt to compensate by overstretching.

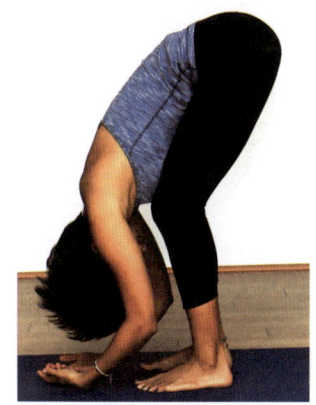

The Cat-Cow series can be modified to produce undulating movement along the spine that engages all seven directions of movement in each vertebra. To begin, move the spine with an effortless, wave-like motion. Notice areas not joining the movement and regions that are being exploited for their greater ease and freedom of movement. Once a pattern is clear, use successive waves of Cat-Cow to increase motion where it is limited and reduce motion where the spine over-engages. Eventually, a more fluid and balanced flow through the spine is attained.

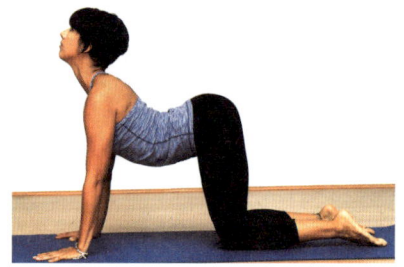

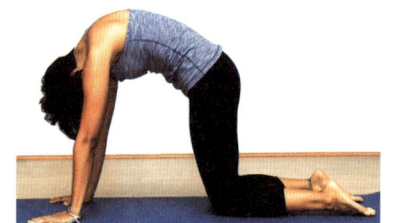

The "Dead Zone"

Twisting poses, such as Revolved Triangle or Revolved Lunge, can be used to evaluate the spine and detect regions that are relatively immobile in comparison to fully mobile areas. This procedure is best performed with assistance. The student assumes either pose. The evaluator gently palpates the spine, looking for tight or immobile sections by pressing into each vertebra just off the center of the spinous process. The sections where the spine feels stiff and hard, as opposed to springy, are called, affectionately, *dead zones*. With practice, the evaluator can identify subtle variations in the stiff areas of the spine. He can distinguish muscular tension, which offers back a slight springiness when deeply pressed, from that of joint immobility, which presents firm resistance, what is referred to as a *hard end feel*. The evaluator can also detect the presence of hyper-mobile segments, which are often interspersed between immobile ones. If no evaluator or assistant is available, the student can perform gentle undulations while in one of these revolved postures. If carried out with focus and attention, the student can get a sense of their own pattern of spinal movement.

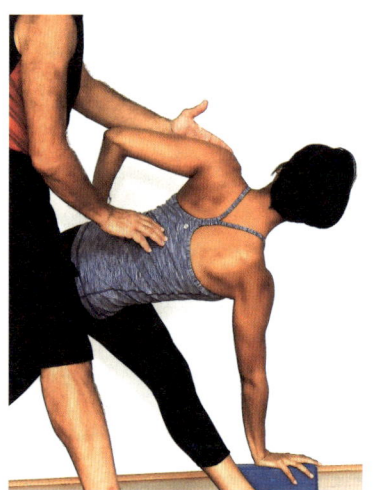

Changes in spinal curves throughout life

If we were looking from a distance at a group of people and could make out only their general outlines, we would instinctively have a sense of their age and level of vitality. The uprightness of their spines and the rhythm of their gaits send visual cues hard-wired into our basic consciousness.

At birth, the curve of the human spine retains its fetal form: a rounded C-shape. The concavity of the fetal curve faces anterior, what is referred to as a *kyphosis*. When the infant begins to lift its head in search of food from the breast or bottle, the neck muscles strengthen, and, over time, the cervical spine reverses its curve to exhibit a posterior concavity, or *lordosis*.

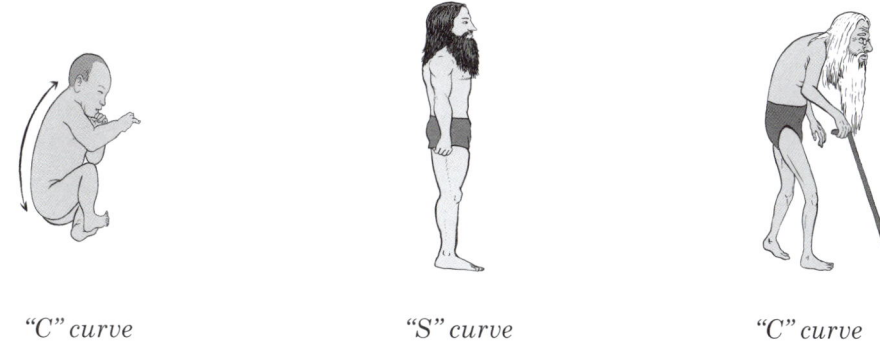

"C" curve   "S" curve   "C" curve

When a baby begins to crawl, the hipbones recess into the acetabulum, stimulating deep hip sockets to form. Crawling and, eventually walking, cause the lumbar spine, like the cervical spine, to reverse into a *lordotic* curve. Because of the space needed for the lungs and heart, the thoracic spine retains its original *kyphotic* curve.

The three curves of the adult spinal - cervical, thoracic, and lumbar- form an overall S-shape. Like springs, the S-shape design best manages the shocks and forces transferred through the body's central axis.

Finally, as we advance in years, the overall curve of the spine often returns whence it came. The effects of a long lifetime of wear and tear and the loss of muscular strength result in degenerative changes that cause the spine to collapse and return to a C-shaped curve.

Scoliosis – dangerous curves ahead

A lateral (side-to-side) spinal curvature is called *scoliosis*. Although not normal, the spine is pre-disposed to scoliosis and is a common occurrence. The heart in the initial stages of human embryonic development is large and positioned at the center of the growing fetus. In some cases, the developing spine deviates to the right to accommodate for the heart, and the deviation may persist into adulthood. Spinal rotation is also commonly found in regions where scoliosis forms, although not in every case. As the degree of curvature increases, the scoliosis becomes progressively problematic. At extreme degrees of curve, scoliosis can compromise the function of the heart, lungs, and diaphragm, as well as other internal organs.

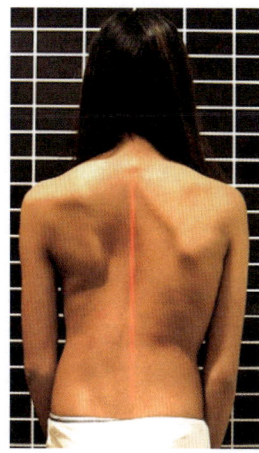

Besides the heart-development catalyst, a few other known causes are:
- Uneven hips or uneven leg lengths
- A wedge-shaped vertebra (in place of a square one)
- Muscular asymmetry or underdevelopment
- A hyper-flexible spine stabilizing itself by generating the additional curves of a scoliosis.

The cause of scoliosis is often unknown and given the name *idiopathic*, from the Greek, "one's own suffering".

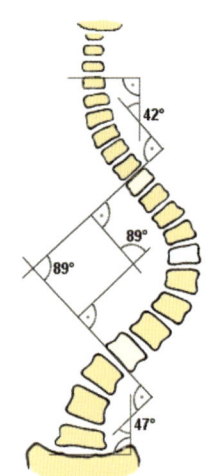

Scoliosis and mobility

As it is vital in a healthy spine, mobility is especially important when scoliosis is present. Mobility, however, is not just indiscriminate movements, but balanced and well-dispersed motion throughout the spine. The degree to which scoliosis causes compensations and eventually degenerative damage depends on fluid spinal mobility. The more that the spine can engage its 336 subtle, inter-segmental movements in their normal ranges of motion, the less likely damage will occur.

Scoliosis is observed most often in students who are hyper-flexible and who have unstable spines. Their anterior and posterior spinal curves are usually straighter and flatter than the normal spine. Scoliosis formation may be a secondary response to a flat, unstable spine, the body creating curves wherever it can in order to bolster stability.

Vital yogic principles for scoliosis

Samasthiti: the asana quality where every muscle and body tissue is physically and energetically balanced along each surface of each bone and each joint. This fundamental principle is especially important to apply when scoliosis is present. Even if a student is unaware of the causes of imbalance in their spine and torso, Samasthiti will significantly reduce the effects of scoliosis.

Move from the least mobile regions first. Initiating movement from the least mobile joints will produce fluid and graceful action, even when imbalances are present. When a yoga student habitually moves the least mobile regions first, the spine can re-pattern its mechanical activity. These pattern-changes make asana practice therapeutic and reduce the tendency of scoliosis to accelerate spinal degeneration.

Lengthen along the vertical axis of the spine (long axis extension). With scoliosis, the spine tends to compress and shorten. Over many years, the spine in affected regions may collapse, resulting in an observable loss of height. Extending the spine at the deepest portions of the curve lengthens the spinal muscles, which, in time, become more balanced and help keep the spine straighter.

> Regardless of whether or not scoliosis is present, yoga students should learn about their spines, identifying where movement is excessive or absent or normal. This information is fundamental to a safe and therapeutic asana practice.

Scoliosis and yoga therapy

Yoga therapy provides many approaches for reducing the effects of scoliosis. This is an extensive topic that a number of masterful teachers and books address comprehensively. This book does not intend to cover the topics of yoga therapy and scoliosis fully; however, here is one example of how restorative asana and props can effectively address scoliosis.

With the student in a restorative side posture, place a bolster at the convexity of the lateral curve. The student lengthens the spine and uses breath to expand the spine and rib cage.

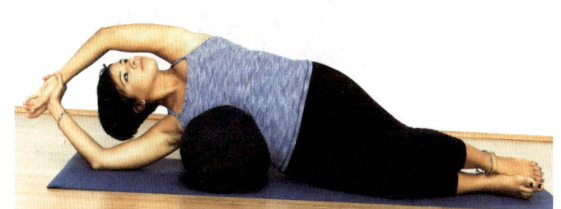

Mapping out the spine

Whether scoliosis is present or not, understanding our habits and postural tendencies is necessary for making asana a safe and therapeutic experience. If someone were to ask, "Which of your shoulders is higher?" or "Which hip is more forward?", could you answer with certainty? This information is important and unique to each person. It is best learned by direct observation.

The best approach is to "map out" our bodies. When our baseline posture and personal habits are known, a greater opportunity exists to reduce the negative health effects of poor alignment on and off the yoga mat.

With the help of a teacher, an assistant, or professional, assess the appearance of these anatomical markers, looking for levelness and balance:
- Are the collarbones square and level?
- Is the head and neck centered over the breastbone?
- Are the bottom tips of the shoulder blades level?
- Is one shoulder blade farther back or does one rotate forward and off the spine?
- Are the lower ribs symmetrical and level with each other?
- Does the rib cage jut forward on either side?
- Do the crests of the hips appear level?
- Is one hip forward of the other?
- Is the soft tissue and muscle over the hips evenly toned or does one side bound up?
- Are the knees in line horizontally with each other?
- Can scoliosis be visually observed when looking at the back?
- When bending forward to a half forward fold, does the spine straighten or are there areas that remain curved or that bound up? This observation indicates whether a scoliosis is *functional* (a consequence of movement patterns) or *structural* (resulting from bone and muscle development).

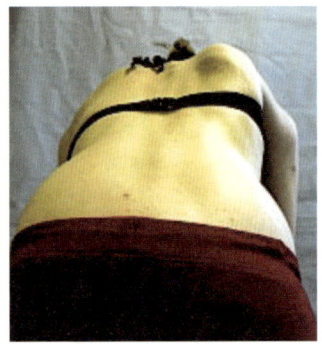
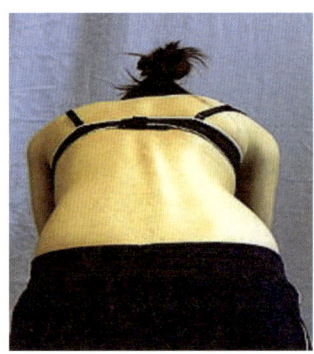

Severe scoliosis *Mild Scoliosis*

Once we understand spinal movement and locate our imbalances, we can bring this knowledge and these vital statistics to yoga practice. In each asana, we can make subtle adjustments to balance the postural tendencies discovered through personal evaluation.

Imbalanced spinal mobility

Every vertebra of the spine is designed to move individually, without strain or excessive wear-and-tear. Every vertebra's movement is also interdependent with all others, especially the ones in the same region. If one vertebra becomes "stuck", nearby vertebrae compensate by becoming hypermobile, increasing their ranges of motion. Over many years of compensation, the spine will show signs of degenerative damage. Spinal discs wear thin and the surfaces of hypermobile vertebral bodies become rough and irregular, producing boney extensions called *spurs*, indicative of the spine's attempt to create stability. This wear-and tear degeneration is called *osteoarthritis*. In its more advanced stages, two or more vertebrae may fuse together, what is called boney *ankylosis*.

Students with less a flexible body type must be careful not to force their asana. Joints that are immobile will not simply release; instead freely moveable segments will overwork and eventually become hypermobile and unstable. It is best to move slowly into immobile regions, using the awareness of breath to increase mobility.

Over time, once flexible, hypermobile regions of the spine become immobilized as degenerative changes reduce the ability of spinal joints to move. To avoid this outcome, especially for the highly flexible students amongst us, resist exploiting the regions of instability and hypermobility. Instead, focus on detecting and initiating movements from the regions of limited spinal motion. The yoga alignment principles for the pelvis and hips and yoga therapy and yoga props are essential tools for changing spinal movement patterns. Manipulative therapeutic approaches, such as chiropractic, can help identify and restore lost movement and help in reversing the destructive outcome of imbalanced spinal mobility.

25 The Lumbar Spine

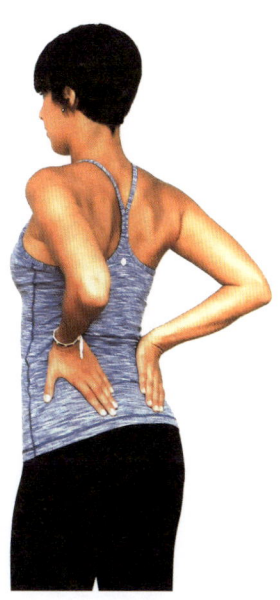

Lower back pain incidence has reached epidemic levels, becoming the nemesis of western civilization. With a lifestyle that has devolved to riding in automobiles, sinking into soft couches, and never developing the ability to comfortably squat, the human frame has become vulnerable to lumbar spine injury.

In a recent study of lower back pain trends, it was reported that 25% of Americans, 76.2 million people, experienced lower back pain during a recent, three-month period. Over a one-year period, that number increased to nearly 50%.[1] Over a lifetime, an estimated 80% of Americans will experience back pain.[2] Most low back pain results from mechanical dysfunctions of the spine. Fewer back complaints originate from organic conditions, such as inflammatory arthritis, infection or cancer.

There are no magical cure-alls for low back pain and yoga certainly cannot be considered one. Yoga, however, offers an excellent approach to managing lower back issues. Alignment-based asana practice can identify muscular weakness, poor posture and unhealthy mechanical patterns that cause spinal joint damage. And, of course, yoga can deliver alignment to the spine that will prove therapeutic and regenerative.

Motion of the lumbar spine

Isolating the nearly 70 movements within the segments of the lumbar spine can be, at best, a difficult task. Traditional orthopedic testing combines lumbar and thoracic spinal movement into a single measurement, referred to as the *thoraco-lumbar* ranges of motion. The lumbar facets orientate front-to-back (sagittal plane), making flexion and extension the easiest movements for the lumbar spine to engage. Lateral flexion and rotation are more limited.

Lumbar Ranges of Motion:
- Flexion   40°
- Extension   30°
- Lateral flexion 20 -30°
- Rotation   10°   (2° at each segment or 1° each direction)

The ilio-lumbar ligaments

The pelvis is the foundation of the spine. To remain stable, the pelvis is anchored to the pelvis by the *ilio-lumbar ligaments*. The ilio-lumbar ligaments are large bands of tissue that are dense and highly collagenous. They attach on the lowest two lumbar vertebrae (L4, L5) and the iliac portions of the pelvis. The ilio-lumbar ligaments also help to stabilize the sacroiliac joints by preventing movement that would exceed their modest range.

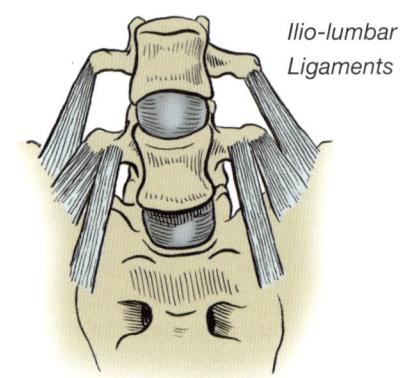

Ilio-lumbar Ligaments

Happy baby, indeed!

Have you ever wondered how happy, little babies effortlessly round their backs and put their toes in their mouth? They tauntingly look up at their mothers with an expression that says "Go ahead, try this, Big Strange Creature!"

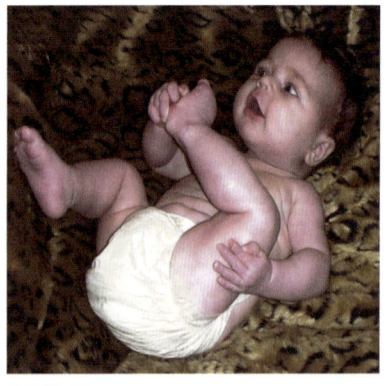

At childbirth, the ilio-lumbar ligaments are rudimentary. They form during childhood and become fully developed in the early teen years. If children have poor posture during these critical years of development, the ligaments develop elongated and over-stretched.

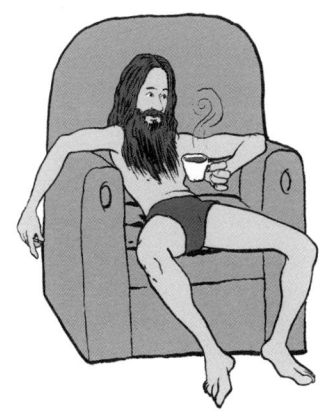

The elongated ligaments lose their ability to provide support, which results in permanent instability of the L4 and L5 vertebrae. Poor postural habits that continue as an adult and lower back injuries that accumulate during a lifetime lead to permanent structural weakness in the lower spine. An unstable spine resulting from weak ilio-lumbar ligaments could well be the primary reason for the high incidence of lower back issues.

Stiff, or not stiff? That is the question!

Lower back pain and stiffness are often the reasons students attend their first yoga class. New students often complain that their lower backs are stiff and inflexible. Stiff-backed students usually believe inflexibility to be the cause of their troubles. To support this assumption, they bend forward, displaying a rounded lower back and a finger-reach at a great distance from their distant appendages. It is true that these students may never make the final cut for Cirque du Soleil®. Yet, when on all-fours, they have no difficulty curving their lumbar spine toward the floor. If a student's "stiffness" were caused by inflexibility, the spine would remain rounded in a Cow Pose, exhibiting limited ability to change shape and form a concavity. Rather than inflexibility, the issue turns out to be instability. In forward-bending postures, weak, overstretched ligaments are neither able to stabilize the lumbar curve nor prevent the spine from rounding farther than is safe. In response, muscles become tense and strained, and tissues become inflamed. It is tense muscles and inflamed tissues that cause stiffness and the misperception of inflexibility.

Yoga practice can be a valuable part of the solution for improving the unstable, but stiff lower back. Yoga asana develops good posture and healthy spinal curves when practiced with precise alignment. By maintaining a proper curve, the lumbar spine is not only stable but able to move more freely than if the spine was rounded.

Spinal stenosis

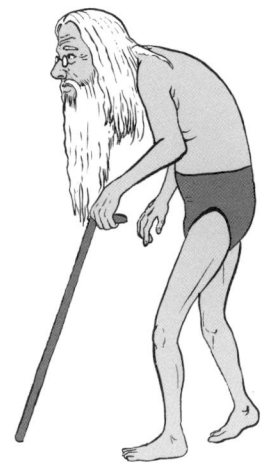

If you spend time at a senior community, you begin to notice characteristics shared by the wonderful residents living there. Beyond the obvious slow-shuffling gates and rounded upper backs, a discerning eye is aware of another senior feature: straight lumbar spines and flattened buttocks. This state is often the result of a condition known as *spinal stenosis*. Spinal stenosis is an increasingly common condition, often initiated by weak ilio-lumbar ligaments and a lifetime of spinal instability.

Spinal stenosis is a narrowing of the spinal canal. Stenosis is usually the result of a thickening of the posterior rings of the vertebrae. Normally, body weight is carried by the massive front body of the vertebrae. If the center of gravity shifts posterior, the weight is transferred to the more slender posterior rings. Over time, the rings thicken and in the process, the canal that it forms narrows. The space for the spinal cord and its multi-fibril tail becomes compromised, causing severe discomfort in and dysfunction of the back and lower extremities. Spinal stenosis can occur in other regions, frequently in the cervical spine.

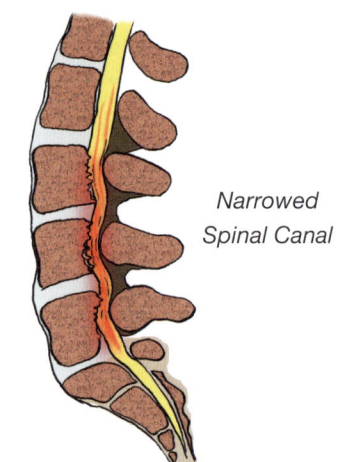

Narrowed Spinal Canal

When to surrender

For lumbar stability, the normal curve of the lumbar spine (lordosis) must be maintained in essentially every position the body assumes. As mentioned in previous chapters, in the final position of **Paschimottanasana** (Seated Forward Fold), after muscular tension releases, the lumbar spine will often round. Allowing the lumbar spine to round while surrendering into Forward Fold Pose is of little negative consequence for someone with a healthy, flexible spine. But this deep position is not beneficial for students who have lumbar instability or stenosis. For those students, it is better to remain more erect, maintaining an egg-sized lumbar curve in the final position. This will keep the pose therapeutic for lumbar instability and spinal stenosis. Modifications using yoga props, such as sitting on blankets or a bolster, often help keep the lumbar curve intact while in a seated forward fold.

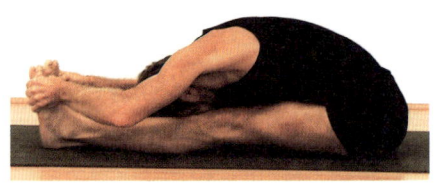

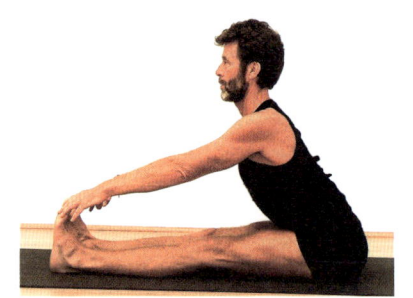

Rounded Postures

Most lifestyles are filled with situations that require the back to round. Yoga practice does not need to reinforce this undesirable posture. If a sequence of asana omits the rounding of the spine altogether, students would be better for it!

Tip of the pelvis, wag of the spine

Spinal curves are directly affected by the tilt of the pelvis. The top surface of the sacrum is actually the *sacral base* and forms the foundation of the spine. *Pelvic tilt* shifts the sacral base in relation to the horizontal plane. An anterior pelvis tilts the sacrum forward and increases the sacral base angle. As a result, the foundation of the spine tips forward, causing the lumbar curve to increase. A posterior pelvis tilts the sacrum backward, bringing the sacral base more horizontal. This reduces the sacral base angle and causes the lumbar curve to flatten. With a posterior pelvis, the thighs tend to shift forward unconsciously. In this position, the body is not correctly aligned and hip joints can weaken and become damaged. Initiating pelvic tilt from the Mula (Muladhara) moderates pelvic tilt's otherwise overpowering effect on the legs and hips. *Moving from the Mula* is the safest and most effective way to move the pelvis and preserve integrative alignment in the entire region.

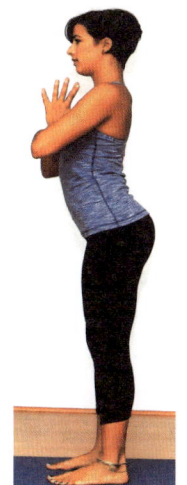
Anterior tilt

Many students have been told that performing sit-ups and other abdominal exercises keep the lower back strong. This is true, but only to an extent. Of course, if one's abdominal muscles are weak, a modest abdominal exercise regimen will have noticeable results. The abdominal muscles, however, are only part of the story. Complete structural health and alignment of the lumbar spine is only possible when the three primary, lower core muscle groups are balanced: the *abdominal muscles*, the *psoas major*, and the *lumbar paraspinal muscles*.

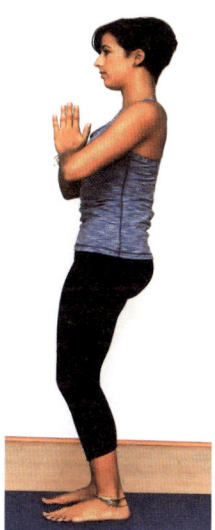
Posterior tilt

At first, the amount of strategizing needed to balance the lumbar spine may seem overwhelming and confusing. The good news is that the same pelvic integrative alignment principles used in all other asana regulate and balance the lumbar spine's musculature. *Inward hip release* increases the lumbar curve, while *forward tailbone scoop* flattens the curve (Review Chapter 14 for details). The point between these two actions where an egg-sized lumbar curve is formed is also the point of balance between the three core muscle groups. And that, as Goldilocks would say, is "just right."

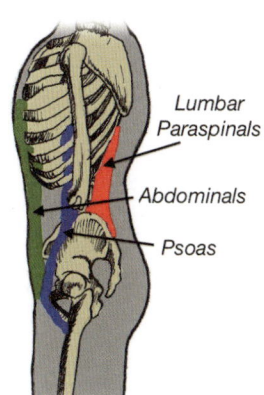

Don't crush the egg!

Which comes first, the egg-sized lumbar curve or balanced core muscles? As in the chicken and egg riddle, the answer is *both* or, maybe, *either*.

The lumbar curve is ideally formed when an egg could be nestled snuggly between the two long bands of paraspinal muscles in the small of the back (L2-L5). If supine, the egg would fit under the back and would neither roll out nor get crushed.

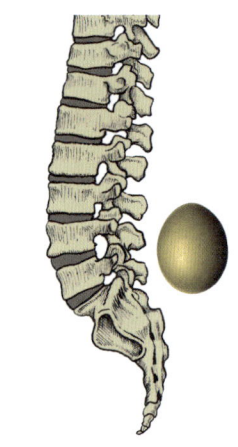

> A lumbar curve that provides both spinal stability and muscular balance is approximately the size of an egg.

When the hips flex deeply and the pelvis rolls posterior, as in **Ananda Balasana** (Happy Baby Pose), the lumbar spine usually flattens to the mat. Despite this tendency, Happy Baby Pose is correctly performed with the sacrum on the mat and an egg-sized curve retained in the lumbar spine. A happy baby does not crush the egg!

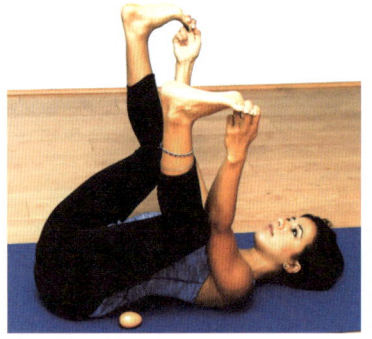

When lying supine and lowering a straightened leg, the lumbar spine tends to lift and increase its curve. Engage the core musculature and *forward tailbone scoop* to keep the curve to the size of one egg, not a half dozen.

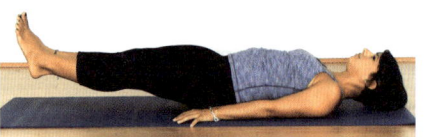

The abdominal obliques

The abdominal obliques (*internal*, *external*, and *transverse*) play a role in strengthening and stabilizing the lumbar spine. They attach above on the lower seven ribs, and below anchored to the pelvis, in part, by the *inguinal ligament*, a common location for hernias. The obliques are a diamond-shaped group of muscles that encircle the lower torso like a girdle. The function of the abdominal obliques is to twist the lower torso, including lumbar rotation. The abdominal obliques contract with a characteristic "parabolic" action that is responsible for forming the hollowed shape of the waist.

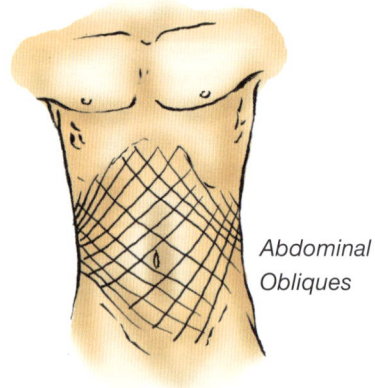

Abdominal Obliques

This parabolic action can be best understood by picturing closely packed strings suspended between two rings with the upper ring representing the lower rib cage and the lower ring representing the pelvic brim. For a twist to occur, one of the rings must remain stable while the other turns, or both rings can turn in opposite directions. If both the lower rib cage and the pelvis turn in the same direction, neither significant twisting nor the waist-narrowing engagement of the muscles occurs.

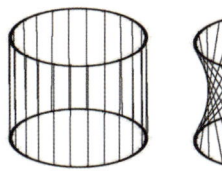

Twist Engaged   *Not engaged*

In Revolved Lunge Pose, stabilize the pelvis (the lower ring) by squaring it to the front of the mat while the lower rib cage (the upper ring) twists. This action strongly engages the abdominal obliques and provides a therapeutic "squeezing" of the internal organs.

In Supine Twist Pose, keep the lower ribs (upper ring) stable and rotate the pelvis (lower ring). Lumbar spinal twists have therapeutic value for the lower back. They are most effective and safe when the abdominal obliques are engaged in this fashion.

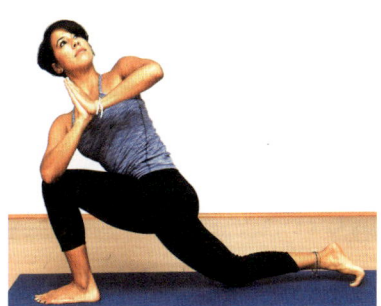

Keep the spine straight when twisting

In a supine twist, the knees are bent and stacked one over the other. When the knees drop to one side, the spine will deviate from its central axis the distance of half the width of the pelvis. To keep the spine in line, shift the entire pelvis 10-14 inches to the opposite side before dropping the knees.

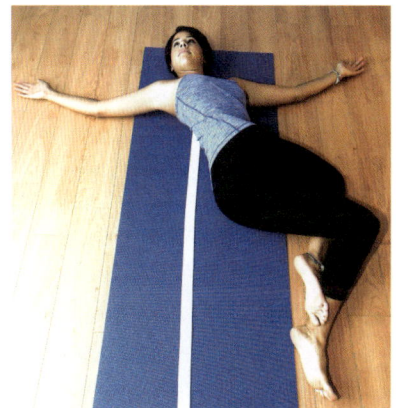

The "black hole" of the belly

For building a six-pack abdomen, yoga is not the first choice as a physical activity. Most yoga postures do not isolate the abdominal muscles or engage them with the firmness required to develop a six-pack. Nothing is wrong with developing "washboard abs" as long as doing so does not develop the abdominals to the point where they overpower the psoas and lumbar paraspinal muscles.

Using a subtle, yet definite degree of effort, draw the abdominal musculature inward from every direction toward the navel. The navel is like a *black hole* in the universe, drawing all surrounding matter and energy into its center. The abdominals remain engaged throughout the entire yoga practice without releasing their subtle contraction, a process similar to the method of engaging the bandhas.

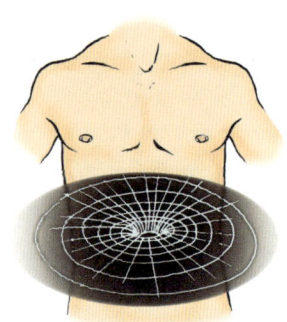

Spondylolisthesis

Approximately 5% of the general population has a structural defect in one or more vertebrae called *spondylolisthesis*. Spondylolisthesis is a break in or a non-fusion of the posterior vertebral ring, creating a persistent instability and tendency for the impaired vertebra to slip forward. With spondylolisthesis, managing the force of gravity becomes problematic. Weight-bearing activities and back-bending postures must be performed with caution to not aggravate the condition.

Spondylo, as this condition is called, may cause the lumbar spine to appear deeply curved, collapsed or compressed. Typically, however, the pelvis of someone with spondylo is not tilted forward, as would be expected in the presence of deep lumbar curves, but retains a neutral position.

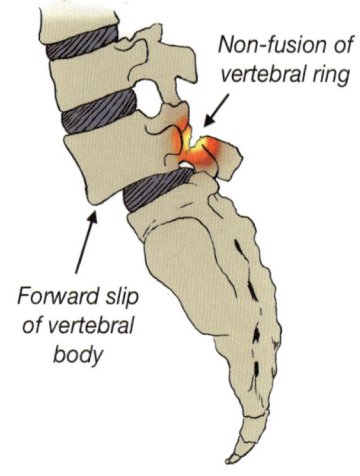

Non-fusion of vertebral ring

Forward slip of vertebral body

No special yoga postures or physical therapies can "fix" a spondylolisthesis. The integrative alignment instructions presented in this book, however, are a preventative to help keep an affected lumbar vertebra from drifting forward. Alignment can play a significant role in reducing the pain and limitations experienced with this condition. Precise alignment can keep yoga practice safe and therapeutic even in the presence of spondylolisthesis.

These previously-presented alignment principles can help manage a spondylolisthesis safely:

- *Move from the Mula.* This action prevents the center of gravity from shifting forward and placing stress on the spondylo.
- *Scoop the tailbone, Scoop the breastbone, Draw-in-the-Navel* (Chapter 11). This group of actions is the most effective way to reduce compression of the lumbar vertebrae.
- Engage the abdominal "black hole" continuously.

Supported bridge for spondylolisthesis

Supported bridge pose is an excellent restorative posture for spondylolisthesis. When lifted and suspended from the block, the lumbar spine is put into traction (mechanically lengthened in long axis extension).

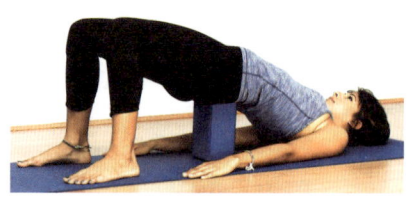

With the assistance of gravity, the vertebra with spondylolisthesis drops posterior, reducing its pre-disposition to shift forward. Reducing the anterior stress on the weakened vertebra can offer great pain relief and stabilization.

Place the block at any height or width, as long as it rests on the sacrum and not the lumbar spine. Use this modified Bridge Pose daily as an effective therapeutic approach to spondylolisthesis.

Sciatica

The sciatic nerve travels down the back of the leg. It is the largest and longest nerve in the body. It comprises a network of nerve root fibers that exit the spine from the L3 to S2 segments. *Sciatic neuritis*, the proper term for sciatica, results from inflammation of one or more of the sciatic nerve's roots. It can produce deep buttock pain that can radiate down the leg to as far as the foot. Sciatic neuritis is most often caused by disc protrusion.

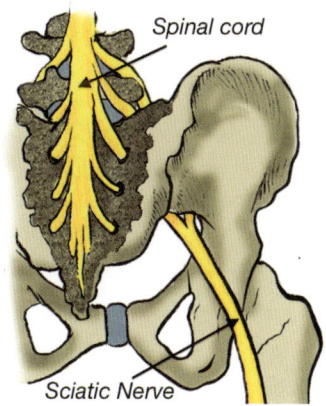

The sciatic nerve roots exiting between the vertebrae normally slide a distance of approximately 12 millimeters. In the orthopedic test for sciatica, the Lasegue's test, a leg is lifted while straight. The limit of 12 millimeters is reached at the point where the leg flexes to approximately 60° of lift.

A healthy sciatic nerve can continue to stretch beyond this point without producing tension or irritation. If a disc is protruded or swollen, the nerve may be trapped or have to travel an extra distance beyond 12 millimeters to go around the bulge. The increase in nerve tension produces pain well before 60° of leg lift is reached. Leg pain that begins after 60° is usually not the caused by sciatica but the result of other conditions, such as sacroiliac dysfunction, hip issues, or problems originating in the musculature, particularly in the piriformis or hamstring muscles.[3]

The straight-leg-raise test is not conclusive for a disc protrusion, however, it does provide a yoga teacher with information that can be used to responsibly advise students about how to modify their practice or to see a healthcare professional.

The **piriformis muscle** externally rotates the hip. Its path courses directly over the sciatic nerve. In some individuals, the sciatic nerve travels through the center of the muscle. If the piriformis muscle is weak it may collapse onto the nerve, producing pressure. If the muscle spasms, it can create a vise-like grip around the nerve. Either of these piriformis conditions can produce sciatic pain, although the pain is usually confined to the buttock region and rarely travels down the leg.

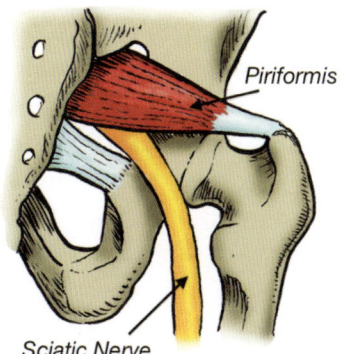

A tear in the **hamstring muscle** attachment at the ischial tuberosity can be equally uncomfortable and mimic the pain of sciatic nerve inflammation. It is a common cause of the painful variety of "yoga butt". A tight, but not torn hamstring muscle can also produce leg pain that runs down the back of the thigh and behind the knee. This pain is not usually confused with sciatica because it tends to be localized within the muscle itself.

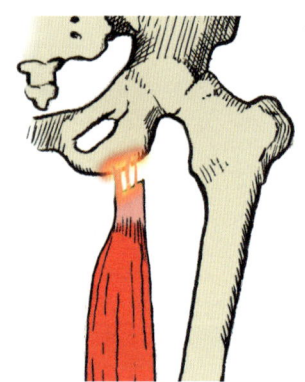

Muscle-related back pain

Although spinal disc injuries occur frequently, the most common cause of back pain is localized muscle strain. An overly diligent yoga student may strain a muscle and cause it to become irritated or slightly torn. Pain from muscle strain is relatively short lived, lasting two to five days. Chronic muscle pain, however, is often a sign of underlying mechanical dysfunction. Chronic muscle pain indicates that muscles are attempting to compensate for structural weakness elsewhere and straining beyond their limits. As an example, muscles will overwork when a joint becomes unstable and when its ligaments are unable to provide support. Conversely, when joints lose mobility, muscles weaken as a result of a lack of mechanical stimulation. In either case, if the cause of the pain is mechanical and structural, improving body alignment helps resolve the issue.

It is also important to remain conscious of the larger health picture. Any pain that persists and does not improve through rest, rehabilitative exercise, or greater precision of alignment can have other organic or metabolic causes. The conscious yogi never ignores unresolved pain.

Move gently out of backbends

Immediate or rapid reversal of the lumbar curve is not safe practice. After deep back-bending poses such as **Urdvha Dhanurasana** (Reversed Bow Pose), a neutral-spine pose such as Downward Facing Dog is a safer counter-balancing pose than immediately hugging the knees to the chest or attempting a full forward bend such as **Uttanasana**.

The safest way to perform all backbend postures is to treat them as chest openers. This encourages the less mobile region, the thoracic spine, to be more involved in the pose and reduces the dependency on the lower back to do most of the work in the pose. Engage the alignment principle of *Scoop the tailbone, Scoop the breastbone, Draw-In-The-Navel* with all back-bending postures to prevent hyperextension of the lumbar spine.

26 Yoga Butt

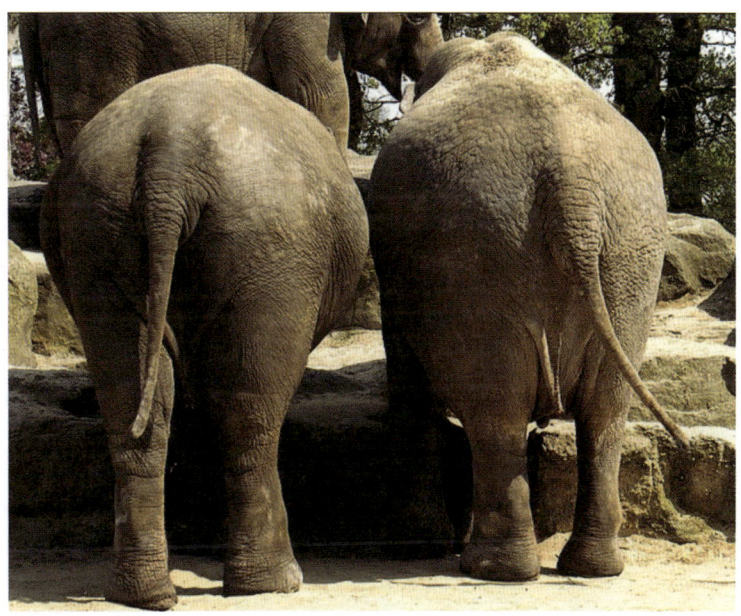

In any crowded yoga studio, it is not uncommon to observe what is sometimes affectionately referred to as *yoga butt*. Usually, this is the natural physique of a yogi, not the consequence of practicing a specific style of yoga. Some students and teachers see the development of yoga butt as a desirable trait and encourage it. Natural or not, yoga butt can predispose those who possess it to injury, shifting from compliment to curse.

Yoga butt is recognizable by a number of features, most obviously an exaggerated anterior tilt of the pelvis. Accompanying the anterior pelvis is a marked lift of the buttock muscles. The knees are usually hyper-extended, creating the potential for knee cartilage compression and weakening of the posterior ligaments. The hamstring muscle tendons, especially at the buttocks, are often chronically overstretched as a result of being lengthened by a flexed, anterior pelvis. It is also common for students with yoga butt to have a flat thoracic curve and jutted-forward lower rib cage.

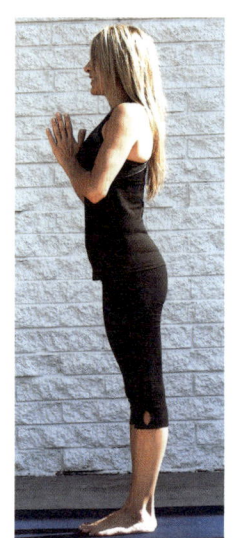

Springing into action

The curves of the spine function similarly to coils of a spring. Like a spring, mobility of the spine increases as the spine elongates. When the curves deepen, the spine (and spring) can better absorb shock and provide stability. Also like a spring, as the forces of gravity and weight-bearing load onto the spine, the curves deepen, compress and round.

When the entire spine is straight and flat-curved, making it unstable, stability can most easily be achieved by deepening the lumbar curve. To create a deeper lumbar curve, the pelvis must tilt anteriorly to angle the base of the sacrum forward. To counter the forward-shifting of the body's center of gravity, the muscles that anchor the pelvis to the legs, the gluteal and hamstring muscle groups, must become stronger. Over time, these muscles increase in mass and size. This will cause the buttocks to lift and protrude. Large thighs can also result from a pronounced yoga butt.

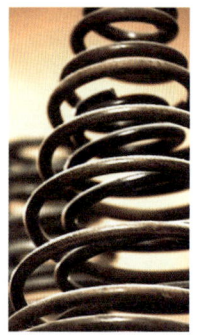

Pain in the yoga butt

Pain from yoga butt can occur at the hamstring attachment. Anterior pelvic tilt resulting from yoga butt lengthens the hamstring muscles. Elongated hamstring muscles increase flexibility but they also significantly increase tension in their tendons, becoming highly susceptible to injury. The hamstring muscle attachment at the ischial tuberosity can tear, which produces deep buttock pain. If the muscle tears free from the bone, it is called an *avulsion*.

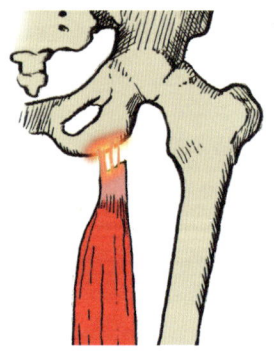

Pain from hamstring tendon tears is easily confused with the nerve pain of sciatica. Piriformis muscle strain is another injury commonly confused with hamstring attachment tears.

Problematic postural habits develop early as a result of yoga butt and a straight upper spine. The shoulders tend to round forward with the head too far forward, causing the upper back muscles to become tense. The knees may also become hyperextended.

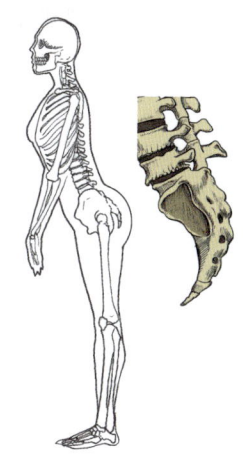

Yoga butt may also cause injury to the spine. Yoga butt increases the lumbar curve, compressing and increasing pressure on the spinal discs. The shifting forward of the center of gravity produces shearing forces across the spinal discs that cause damage. Degenerative wear and tear develops over time, causing the vertebral discs to narrow and the vertebral bodies to become rough and irregular.

In a small percentage of people, as discussed in Chapter 24, the vertebral defect known as *spondylolisthesis* may produce a postural appearance similar to yoga butt. With spondylolisthesis, however, anterior pelvic tilt is often absent

The righting reflex

The nervous system has a mechanism called the *righting reflex* that perpetually adjusts our center of gravity. The purpose of the righting reflex is to keep the head balanced in relation to the horizon so that the eyes and ears receive stimulus symmetrically. To attain this balance, the body may develop complex postural distortions. One example occurs when, due to an injury or postural defect, the neck slants to one side. In this situation, the shoulders will tilt down on the opposite side in order to re-establish the horizontal orientation of the head. Another example is when a visual or auditory imbalance, such as astigmatism of the eyes, causes the body to contort itself in order to bring about visual symmetry.

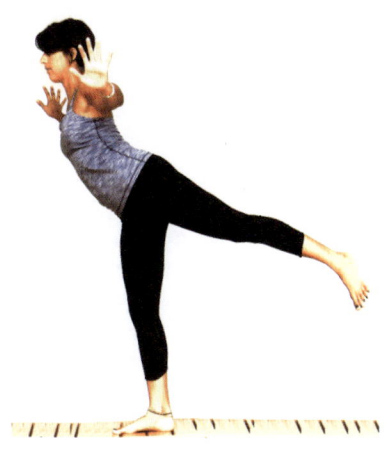

You may be asking yourself, how does this relate to yoga butt? The righting reflex can also produce undesirable effects. Yoga butt can begin with the pelvis tilting anteriorly, not only as compensation for a flattened spine. If the buttocks protrude, the righting reflex activates to restore structural balance by elongating the thoracic and cervical curves, two undesirable consequences.

On the positive note, the righting reflex plays an important role in rehabilitation. Newly developed postural patterns become instinctual more quickly and easier to learn when the body can use sensory cues to find balance.

Steps to reduce yoga butt posture

- First, establish a stable foundation with each foot balanced on its four corners.
- Engage *shins-forward* and *thighs-back,* even if only isometrically. This action prevents the knees from hyper-extending.
- Align the center of the hips vertically over the ankles.
- Engage *inward hip release* and *forward tailbone scoop* to balance the pelvis in a neutral position. The key indicator of a neutral pelvis is having an egg-sized curve in the lumbar spine.
- Draw the lower rib cage back.
- Increase the volume of the upper thoracic region by engaging *chest integration*. This is achieved by breathing 360° around the upper chest, at the level just below the collarbones. Remember that the lungs are not only in the front of the body and that the rib cage can expand in all directions. Even though this action may be challenging at first, expand the sides of the lungs at the inner armpits and across the upper back. Chest integration creates a fuller, rounder thoracic spine and a broader foundation for the neck, which allows the cervical curve to deepen. More details regarding chest integration are provided in Chapter 29.

In my professional experience, following the steps outlined above is highly effective in reducing trauma from excessive anterior tilt, or yoga butt. These procedures change the very nature of how the body is inhabited, not just physically, but mentally and emotionally as well.

Precise alignment requires an amount of detail that may seem overwhelming. The yogi's mental resistance may override the patience needed to carefully learn, imagine, and implement the actions as described.

Throughout this book, there are reminders that alignment principles are the same for all asana and do not vary pose to pose. There is only one set of principles to learn and they apply to everything in yoga practice, including assists, adjustments and therapy.

With patience, the yogi can develop finely tuned observation skills. This heightened awareness helps unlock the true potential of yoga.

27 The Psoas Muscle

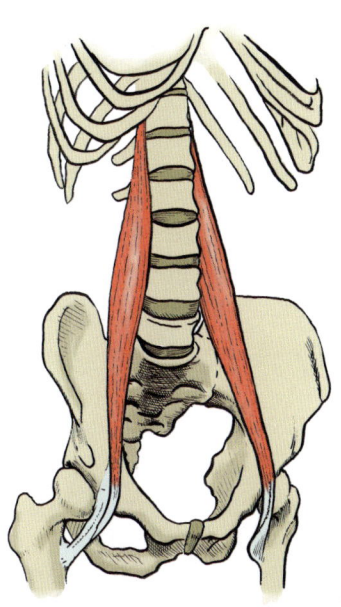

"So as the psoas, so as the core"

True, and fun to say!

The psoas muscle, pronounced "so-as," has emerged from relative obscurity to being a subject of strong curiosity, but not without considerable differences of opinion about how it actually works. Despite ongoing debate regarding the significance of the psoas, this core muscle plays a central role in yoga alignment.

The psoas muscle has two parts, the major and minor psoas. The psoas major is long and tapered at both ends (fusiform). Between 40% and 50% of the human population also have a psoas minor. The smaller psoas minor has no separate role but contributes to the function of the psoas major. General convention refers to both muscles together as, simply, the psoas. For those who find it interesting, the psoas muscle of cattle is highly coveted in the beef industry. With its extensive blood supply and rich red color, the psoas is the filet mignon and tenderloin cuts of steak.

The psoas muscle is located deep within the lower torso and pelvis. It courses anterior to the large quadratus lumborum and forms part of the supportive wall behind the internal organs of the abdomen. The psoas originates from the transverse processes and vertebral bodies of the twelfth thoracic vertebra and each of the five vertebrae of the lumbar spine. Its extensive attachments send fibers directly into the vertebral discs and the spinal (annular) ligaments. The psoas interweaves its fibers into the thoracic diaphragm and the quadratus lumborum.

The psoas is a core muscle that plays a key role in integrating the intricate relationships of the lower spine, pelvis and hips. The psoas runs an oblique course, crossing but not attaching to any portion of the pelvis. Having no attachment to the pelvis gives the psoas great mechanical advantage by allowing it to execute long, unobstructed, and efficient pulls on the spine. The psoas insertion is on the lesser trochanter, a small protrusion on the upper, inner neck of the femur. Chapter 25, introduced the psoas muscle as part of a three-muscle group, that along with the abdominal and lumbar paraspinal muscles, balances and stabilizes the lower back.

The traditionally-accepted actions of the psoas are flexion (thigh to torso) and external rotation of the hip. Some anatomists contend that the psoas muscle does not concentrically contract (shorten) during hip flexion and therefore cannot be considered a flexor muscle.[1] As this chapter will present, psoas function is a complex a topic, but knowing how to correctly use the psoas in asana is relatively easy.

Iliopsoas

Combined, the psoas and iliacus muscles form the *iliopsoas* muscle. The iliopsoas is the primary muscle that flexes the thigh to the torso and externally rotates the hip. The two muscles, the psoas and iliacus, share a common tendon that terminates at the lesser trochanter. The nerve supply to each muscle, however, is separate and distinct.

The iliacus originates on the inner bowl of the pelvis and has no contact with or influence on the spine. Its function is to provide hip flexion. The iliacus does not have adequate efficiency to flex the hip beyond 90° without the assistance of the psoas. Along with the gluteal muscles and the long head of the biceps femoris, the iliacus is used to engage *forward tailbone scoop*.

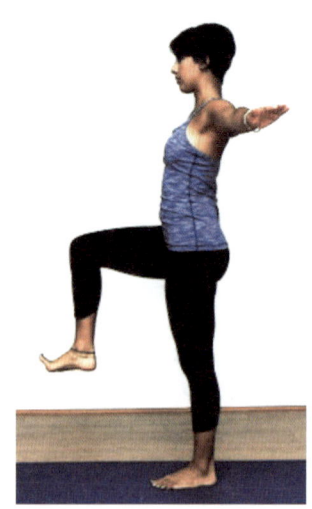

The elusive psoas

Psoas function is difficult to observe because of the muscle's deep location. The psoas cannot be directly palpated or massaged from the body's outer surface, nor can its action be isolated from that of surrounding muscles. Additionally, when the position of the spine, hips, or legs is significantly altered, the psoas can reverse the direction of its contraction. Instead of contracting to deepen the lumbar curve, that contraction can flatten it. Each of the following conditions alters the normal action of the psoas muscle:

- Tight hamstrings
- Misalignment of the pelvis
- Limited hip mobility
- Limited lumbar spine mobility
- Conditions that restrict the shape of the lumbar curve, such as stenosis

The dual nature of the psoas

Yoga asana usually focuses on either strength or flexibility. For example, a standing pose may concentrate more on the flexibility of the hamstring muscles and less on its strength. For the psoas, however, focus on strength and flexibility will always coincide. The following chart lists the actions that are caused or will be caused by the psoas, either during stretching or contraction.

Psoas Stretch
- Femur heads draw back
- Engaging *inward hip release*
- Anterior pelvic tilt
- Open the sacroiliac joints
- Increased lumbar curve

Psoas Contraction
- Femur heads press forward
- Engaging *forward tailbone scoop*
- Posterior pelvic tilt
- Sacroiliac joints close
- Lumbar curve flattens

Technically Speaking: Psoas stretching vs. contraction

Stretching
Psoas stretch pulls on the spine from segments T-12 to L-5, drawing the lumbar spine posterior of its central axis. This causes the lumbar curve to protrude forward and deepen. Psoas stretch produces an anterior tilt of the pelvis, increasing the sacral base angle and with that, the lumbar curve.

Contraction
Psoas contraction pulls the lumbar spine anterior of its central axis, causing it to straighten. Psoas contraction tilts the pelvis posteriorly, causing the sacral base to become more horizontal and flatten the lumbar curve.

Stretching lengthens a muscle, increasing flexibility and mobility.
Contraction shortens a muscle, producing force that provides strength and power.

Psoas strength in asana

In **Paripurna Navasana** (Boat Pose) the abdominal muscles hold the lower torso straight and stable. The iliopsoas is important in Boat Pose because of its strength as the primary muscle to flex the hip and hold the legs to the trunk. A lengthened, yet strong psoas muscle maintains the lumbar curve and keeps the back from rounding in the pose. Tight hamstring muscles limit the ability of the pelvis to tilt forward in the pose, making the lumbar curve difficult to establish and maintain.

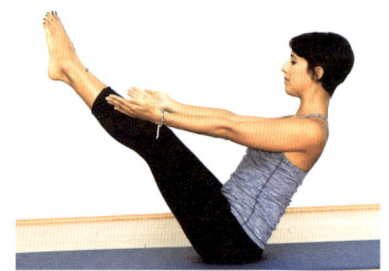

When the legs are on the ground as in the Pilates Roll Up, the psoas assists the abdominals in pulling the trunk toward the thighs. Performing this action is not recommended if the lumbar spine is unstable.

Single-sided (unilateral) psoas engagement laterally flexes the lower trunk. This occurs in standing side-bending poses.

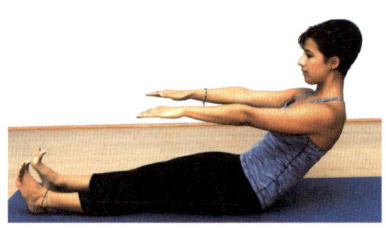

In one-legged standing balancing poses, psoas contraction on the same side as the standing leg stabilizes the torso in a straight and vertical position.

On the raised leg side, the psoas helps to lift the leg but also rotates the trunk in the opposite direction (contra-lateral rotation), as in **Parivrtta Hasta Padangusthasana One** (Revolved Hand-to-Big Toe Pose).

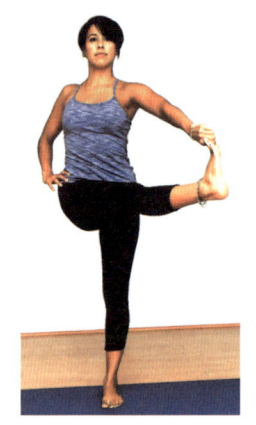

Anterior pelvic tilt, *inward hip release* and psoas stretching

When the pelvis tilts forward, *inward hip release* is activated, drawing back and inwardly rotating the femurs from the lesser trochanters. This rotation stretches the psoas an additional 20% of its resting length, the point where it achieves optimal efficiency. If the pelvis is unable to tilt forward, the sacral base angle cannot increase and the lumbar curve remains flat, leaving the psoas unable to stretch to its full capacity.

> The psoas is involved in *inward hip release*, while the iliacus participates in *forward tailbone scoop*.

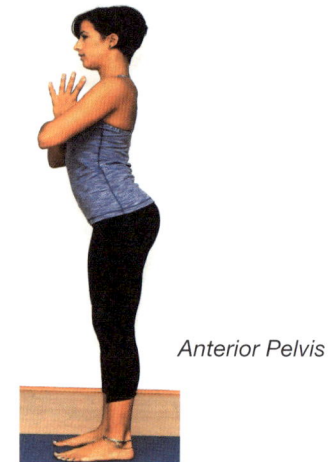

Anterior Pelvis

Hamstring muscles and the psoas

Tight hamstring muscles cause the psoas to become short and tight. The hamstring muscles anchor to the pelvis at the ischial tuberosities and, if the muscles are tight, anterior pelvic tilt becomes restricted. If severely tight, the pelvis can move opposite of the desired direction, tilting posteriorly. Posterior pelvic tilt presses the hip joints forward, prevents *inward hip release* and inhibits psoas stretching.

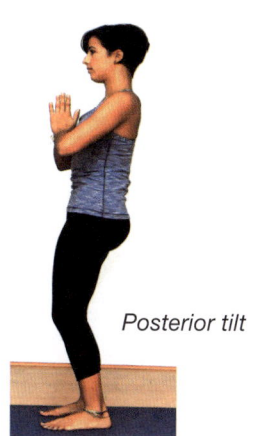
Posterior tilt

A short, tight psoas muscle

Any muscle forced to stretch more than 10% beyond its maximum length is at risk of being overstretched, inflamed or torn. This rarely occurs with the psoas because of limitations in hip extension that keep the psoas from exceeding dangerous lengths. A short, tight psoas, however, is more frequent and more likely to predispose yoga students to injury. Performing asana with a short, tight psoas muscle can quickly turn a relatively conservative stretch into one that crosses the lines of safe practice.

The common cause of most musculo-skeletal injuries is poor structural alignment. The role of the psoas in the mechanics of the lower spine and pelvis is significant. Utilizing the integrative alignment principles of *inward hip release* and *forward tailbone scoop* is essential for the psoas to lengthen and function safely. The egg-sized lumbar curve that results from correct alignment is the hallmark of a well-toned psoas.

Some causes of short, tight psoas muscles are:

- Sitting in car seats or sofas that cause the hips to drop lower than the thighs.
- Practicing old-style sit-ups that position the pelvis in a posterior tilt.
- Cycling with a too-low seat height that causes the knees over bend and splay outward.

A psoas that is tight on a single side can laterally distort the trunk. This type of psoas imbalance shortens the length of the torso and spine on the affected side. Psoas side-to-side imbalances are associated with scoliosis.

Urdvha Hastasana (Raised Hands Pose) provides a general but useful evaluation of side-to-side psoas length. When the arms are raised overhead, one arm appearing shorter than the other may indicate that the psoas is short and contracted on that side. Of course, factors unrelated to the psoas should also be considered but this test has shown to be reliable.

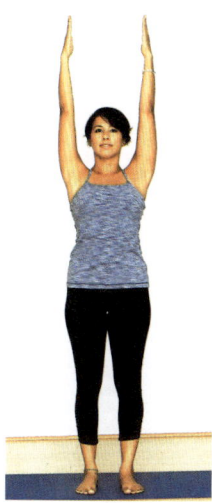

> The hallmark of a well-toned psoas is a single egg-sized lumbar curve.

Psoas stretch increases sacroiliac joint mobility

The psoas has no direct muscular interaction with the sacroiliac joints. The psoas and sacroiliac joints, however, have great impact on each other. A healthy, functioning psoas, lengthens to facilitate *inward hip release*, which opens the sacroiliac joints and enables their mobility. When the sacroiliac joints are unstable, the psoas muscle may be forced to overexert in an attempt to provide the missing support. Kinesiological muscle testing performed by health professionals may discover that the psoas has become weak from performing extra duties for an unstable sacroiliac joint.

Asana for psoas stretching

Setu Bandha Sarvangasana (Bridge Pose)

Bridge Pose is an excellent pose for evaluating the psoas. If the knees in Bridge or in the more advanced **Urdvha Dhanurasana** (Wheel Pose) are unable to remain in line with the hips but bow outward, it often indicates that the psoas is short and tight. If this is the case, gently squeeze a block placed between the knees to prevent outward splaying of the knees and to encourage *inward hip release*. This will help to lengthen the psoas. As in all asana, the action of *forward tailbone scoop* always follows. In back-bending poses such as these, *forward tailbone scoop* is essential for protecting the sacroiliac joints and lumbar spine from injury.

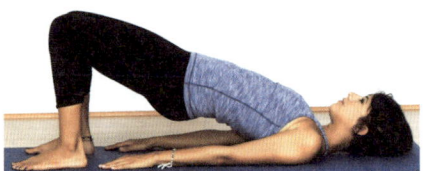

Lunge Pose, **Anjaneyasana** (Low Lunge), and **Hanumanasana** (Forward Split) are excellent postures to stretch the psoas. In these poses, the straight, rear leg receives the psoas stretch. *Inward hip release* is engaged in the rear leg to release the hips and hamstring muscles and to prevent injury. The effectiveness of the stretch depends on the rear thigh remaining integrated into the posture.

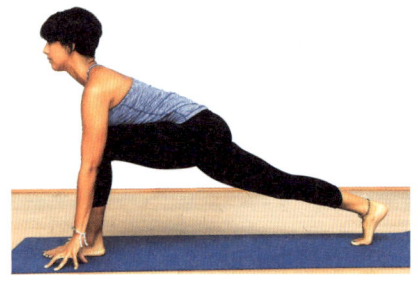

In **Supta Padangusthasana One** (Supine Single-Leg Lift), the leg on the mat remains flush with the floor. If the leg lifts from the floor and buckles or turns outward, it often indicates that the psoas on that side is short and tight.

In **Savasana** (Corpse Pose) with the legs straight out on the mat, a properly toned psoas creates a curve at the small of the back that is no more than egg-sized. With the knees bent and the feet on the floor, a well-toned psoas allows the lower back to flatten onto the floor.

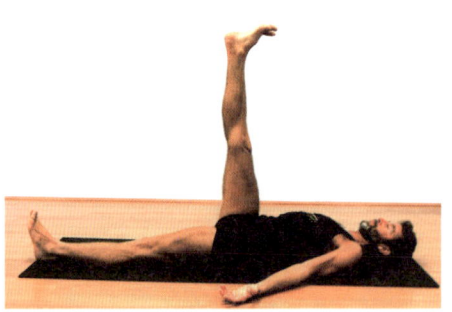

The psoas and the abdominal organs

Adverse health conditions have been associated with chronically shortened and tight psoas muscles. When the psoas muscles are habitually tight, the thighs protrude forward and the spine flattens. This results in limited space in the abdominal cavity. The lower abdominal organs, which rest against the psoas muscles from behind, actually roll forward, which can trigger dysfunction of the digestive track, bladder, or sexual organs. The kidneys are located in a pocket of connective tissue that attaches directly to the psoas muscle. Tension in the psoas muscle may have an impact on kidney function. Improving psoas function through yoga alignment may provide positive changes in some of these organic issues. Of course, psoas dysfunction is not the root cause of all organic ailments.

What is the sound of one hip snapping?

In **Supta Padangusthasana One** (Supine Single-Leg Lift), when lowering the straight leg, a loud "pluck" can sometimes be heard across the entire yoga studio. The snapping sound is the iliopsoas tendon, shifting lateral to medial and getting trapped against either the iliopectineal eminence on the front of the hipbone or the collar that surrounds the femur head. Most often the snap is produced when bringing the hip from a flexed position into either extension or abduction. If pain accompanies the sound, the tendon may be inflamed, indicating a tight psoas. To improve this condition, lengthen or press through the inner heel as the leg is being lowered and increase *inward hip release*. This will often eliminate the snap of the tendon.

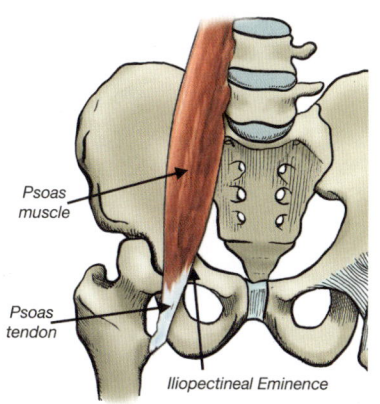

Iliopsoas muscle stretch

This stretch is also presented in Chapter 18 where it describes the iliopsoas muscle as the antagonist to the gluteal muscles. With hip extension being naturally limited, the iliopsoas has few opportunities to be fully stretched.

In a supine position, drop one leg over the edge of a table or a set of raised yoga blocks. The dropped leg extends the hip and its iliopsoas stretches. The torso must firmly maintain **Tadasana** alignment. To prevent lumbar hyperextension and sacroiliac strain, engage *Scoop the tailbone, Scoop the breastbone, Draw in the navel*. The leg that is dropped, considered the rear leg of the posture, actively engages *inward hip release* with the thigh rolled-in and drawn back.[2] This stretch can also be performed with a block under the sacrum and both legs stretched toward the floor.

28 The Thoracic Spine

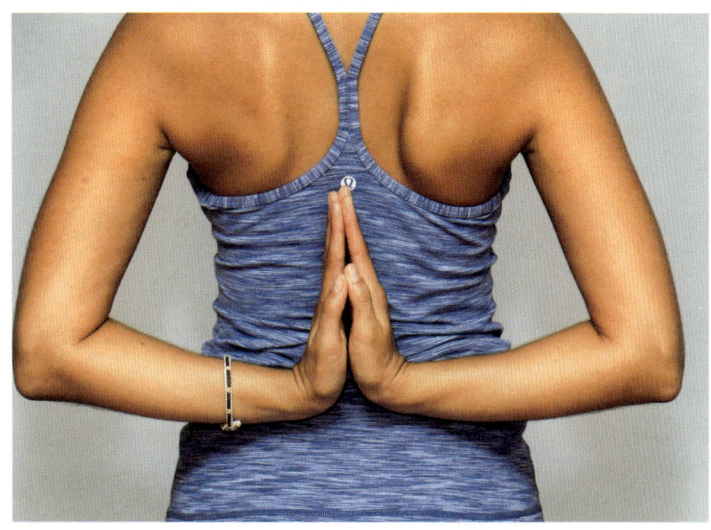

Imagine an early morning yoga class with the rising sun's soft light initiating the start of practice. The teacher instructs his students to draw the lower ribs back, extend the upper chest forward, and lift their arms overhead into **Urdvha Hastasana** (Upward Hands Pose). For many students, being instructed to move one section of the thoracic cage in one direction while moving another section in the opposite direction is quite perplexing. The very idea that individual regions of the spine and rib cage can move independently, not as one fixed unit, is new to many. Although the thoracic spine is not a region of broad, sweeping mobility, its subtle, intra-joint movements are extensive. The twelve thoracic vertebrae move in seven different directions at their facets, producing a surprising total of 182 individual movements! The essence of yoga practice is to develop awareness of this mobility potential and the skills to access it.

Spinal movement is best understood as having two components: broad *ranges of motion* that move entire regions of the spine; and *inter-segmental movement*, the small, subtle movements that occur at each facet joint. The thoracic spine has significantly less range of motion than the cervical and lumbar regions. Being the pillar that supports the rib cage, the thoracic spine is restricted, obviously, because of its attachments to the ribs. Additionally, with the thoracic-spine facets opening along the frontal plane, flexion and extension are limited. Extension is further restricted by the long, central spinous processes of each vertebra that spike downward, practically coming into contact with each other in the neutral-spine position even before any extension takes place.[1]

Range of motion in the thoracic spine

As mentioned in Chapter 25, it is difficult to isolate and measure the thoracic ranges of motion with reliability. Orthopedic testing resigns itself to using a single, combined, *thoraco-lumbar* measurement of the thoracic and lumbar regions.

As much as its movement can be isolated, the thoracic spine is predicted to have the following ranges of motion:[2]

- Lateral flexion   20° bilaterally
- Rotation   35° bilaterally
- Flexion   60°
- Extension   35°

The rib cage

The rib cage is an enclosure that protects the vital organs of the upper body. The rib cage must also move freely to expand and contract with the complex mechanisms of breathing. The thoracic spine is the central support for the framework of ribs that creates the rib cage.

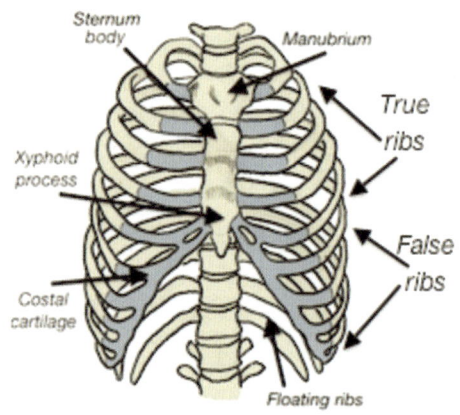

There are twelve pairs of ribs that form the rib cage. Not all ribs, however, are the same. The top seven are called *true ribs* because they attach in front, directly to the breastbone (sternum) at the center of the chest. Because of the boney attachment of these ribs to both the spine and sternum, the upper thoracic spine has the least mobility within the thoracic region.

The thoracic curve's apex, its least mobile section, is the seventh thoracic vertebra (T-7). The five lower sets of ribs are called *false ribs*. The first three sets do not attach directly to the sternum but to cartilage extending from the sternum to the ribs. The bottom two sets of ribs are called *floating ribs* because they are free of any type of anterior attachments.

In aging individuals, limited thoracic mobility is common. Over time, the upper back becomes rigid, immobile and rounded. This posture coincides with diminished health and vitality.

The upper back is subject to bone loss (osteoporosis) and compression fractures. Although hormonal and dietary components play a major role, poor posture and lack of mobility significantly reduce mechanical stimulation of these upper vertebrae, making them particularly susceptible to loss of density and eventually structural collapse.

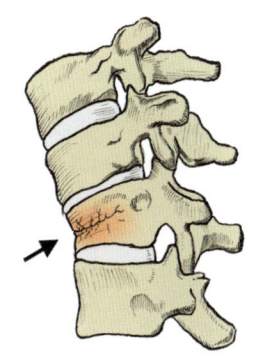

Compression Fracture

The 12th thoracic vertebra

Located at the transition point between the thoracic and lumbar curves, the 12th thoracic vertebra is a biomechanically unique vertebra. It is the primary swivel (rotation) point for the entire vertebral axis. To facilitate rotation, the vertebra's anterior body is uncharacteristically larger than its posterior ring. The deep muscles of the spine do not attach to the posterior ring of T-12, a distinctive design that reduces muscular hindrance to rotation. While having extensive rotation, the 12th thoracic vertebra, like the rest of the thoracic spine, is limited in flexion and extension.

The diaphragm, psoas, and trapezius muscles all attach to the 12th thoracic vertebra. This common point of connection at T-12 allows these important muscles to influence each other's action.

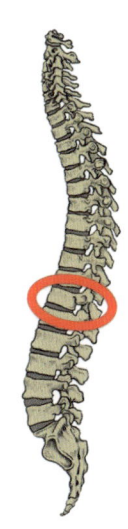

Moving the thoracic spine

For yogis and non-yogis alike, it is challenging to freely and independently engage the vertebrae of the thoracic spine. The best strategy for moving the thoracic spine is to begin movement from the least mobile vertebrae. Limited mobility may be the result of injury, habit or the presence of scoliosis. Use the breath to expand the thoracic region and help discover the most restricted areas. If there are no obvious restrictions, initiate movement from the level of the heart, the anatomically least mobile portion of the thoracic spine. Movement of the lower thoracic spine has additional conditions and alignment requirements, details of which are presented in Chapter 15.

Thoracic spinal mobility is also a prerequisite for safe, efficient function of the shoulder girdle. As will be presented in Chapter 31, the principles of shoulder integrative alignment initiate with the thoracic spine, before any shoulder positioning is addressed.

Learning to access the subtle movements of the thoracic spine is enhanced by two procedures that have been presented in previous chapters.

- First, practice undulating the spine, as discussed in Chapter 24, to develop the skill to isolate independent spinal movements, from vertebra to vertebra.
- Second, when attempting to move the thoracic spine in asana, take advantage of the *lock and load* principle (see Chapter 11) by first drawing the lower rib cage back and locking it into position. Once the lower thoracic spine is stabilized, successively move the vertebrae above, especially those of the upper thoracic region.

Kyphosis – the rounded back

The thoracic spinal curve is convex. It rounds posteriorly, creating space needed for the heart and expanding lungs. This curve is called a *kyphosis*, from the Greek term for hump, *kyphos*. Kyphosis refers to any posterior curve, including ones that are normal in depth. As mentioned in Chapter 24, the entire spinal curve of the fetus and newborn is a kyphosis (C-curve). Kyphosis is typically used to refer to a curve that demonstrates excessive rounding, although technically, the correct term is *hyper-kyphosis*.

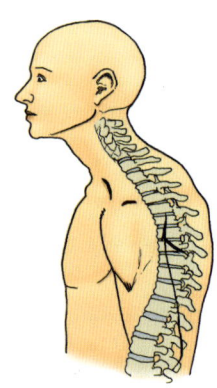

Because deeper curves are less mobile, the greater the degree of kyphosis, the more difficult it is for the spine to move. When the degree of kyphosis is extremely large, spine and rib cage mobility becomes severely limited, compromising healthy function of the cardio-pulmonary system.

Excessive kyphosis causes the spine to protrude on the back beyond the shoulder blades. This sets up a physical barrier that blocks the natural gliding of the shoulder blades toward the center of the back. Actions such as lifting the arms overhead become impaired because the spine cannot extend and the shoulders cannot shift fully onto the back. The yoga student with a thoracic hyper-kyphosis often compensates by rolling their shoulders and rib cage forward to raise the arms. The shoulders are extremely vulnerable to traumatic injury in this position. When the thoracic spine is rounded, it also becomes difficult to create the broad foundation across the shoulder girdle that the head and neck require to establish their alignment over the shoulders.

The flat thoracic curve

The thoracic curve can also become too flat. The term assigned to a flattened thoracic spine is *hypo-kyphosis*. Normally, the shoulder blades and the spinous processes of the upper thoracic spine form a gentle arch across the upper back. With hypo-kyphosis, a pronounced, recessed space is visible between the shoulder blades.

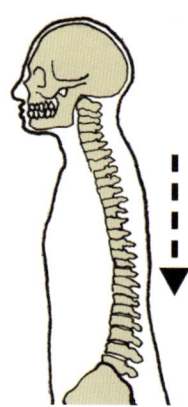

A flattened curve is elongated and generally over-flexible. Students with a "flat back" should use their breath to expand the thoracic cage. Fully inflating the upper lungs and maintaining their volume, even during exhalation, will help the thoracic spine increase its curve and develop more stability. The integrative alignment principle of *chest integration* that follows effectively improves a flattened thoracic spine.

Chest integration

Chest integration increases the volume of the upper thoracic region. This is achieved by breathing 360° around the upper chest, at a level just below the collarbones. To engage chest integration, breathe and expand fully, not only the chest, but the side-body ribs within the armpit and across the upper back. Keep the region inflated, even with exhalation. The action is similar to pumping a bicycle tire. The tire remains full and inflated, even between pumps when the handle releases and the pump is not injecting air into the tire. Chest integration will increase the kyphosis of the thoracic spine and create the broad foundation for the head and neck that is necessary for the cervical curve to form correctly. As will be presented in Chapter 31, chest integration is important for all types of spines.

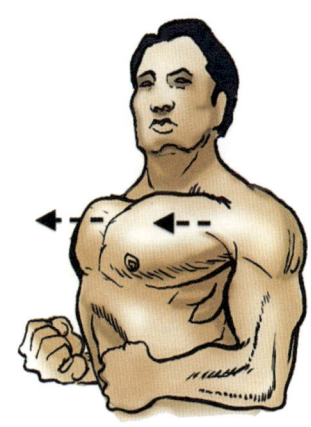

See-saw rib cage

As much as students attempt to move the thoracic vertebrae and ribs individually, it is still the almost natural tendency to move the thoracic cage as one block, rocking the rib cage and spine like a see-saw, from top and bottom. When safety in a posture depends on precise thoracic alignment, such as in Warrior One, students can take advantage of the see-saw principle by drawing the lower ribs back and rocking the chest forward.

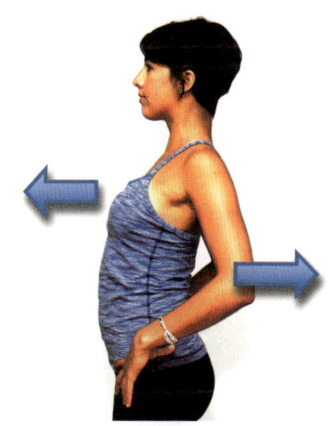

Rounding the upper back?   Not on my watch!

Yoga teachers sometimes offer students the verbal instruction to round their back when moving into a forward bend pose. This prompt may be given when sinking back into **Balasana** (Child's Pose) or when bending forward into **Upavistha Konasana** (Wide-Angle Forward Fold). The typical yoga student never needs to purposely round the upper back in any pose, or, in daily life, for that matter.

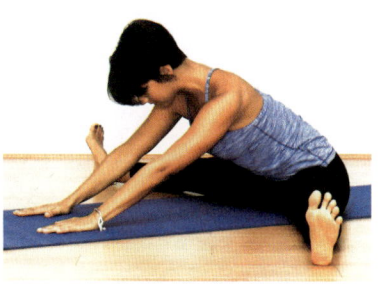

In some advanced, bound yoga postures, the student may need to initially round the spine in order to clasp and bind. However, once the clasp is made, the student lengthens the back, moving it toward being straight in the final position of the pose. The same concept applies to spinal twist poses.

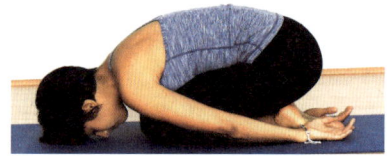

Child's Pose

In the posture **Paschimottanasana** (Seated Forward Fold), the "surrender" and release into the final stage of the pose can be performed without the shoulders rolling forward of the chest by keeping the elbows lifting and pointed outward.

Most yoga students are challenged to fully extend their thoracic spine. Being instructed to "round the back" takes them opposite the desired direction. Students will, in fact, have better aligned, safer poses by flattening the thoracic spine each time a teacher tells them to round it.

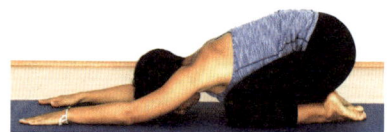

Extended Child's Pose

In the classic Child's Pose, the shoulders roll forward and the thoracic spine rounds and tightens, instead of releasing. Many yoga instructors replace Child's Pose with Extended Child's Pose. With the arms overhead, it is easier to keep the shoulders on the back body and the thoracic spine extended.

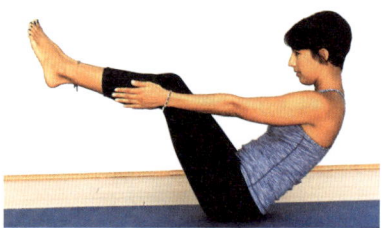

"Rounded" Navasana

"What is round will roll!"

This simple but insightful mantra is offered by Anusara yoga teacher Jaye Martin. It is most evident in **Navasana** (Boat Pose) where a rounded spine causes students to roll back but a straight and extended thoracic spine keeps the pose straight.

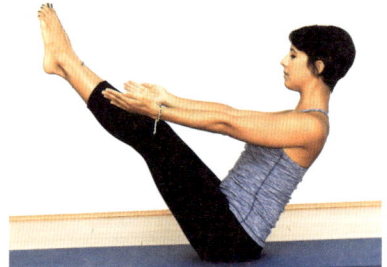

And, one more thing...

By the same reasoning as that for not rounding the spine, shrugging the shoulders is another unnecessary action for general yoga practice. In performing activities of daily life, most people spend an inordinate amount of time with their shoulders tucked up under their ears. There is no need to further develop this "skill" with our yoga practices.

> In every asana, the upper thoracic spine moves forward while the lower rib cage moves back.

29 The Breath and the Bandhas

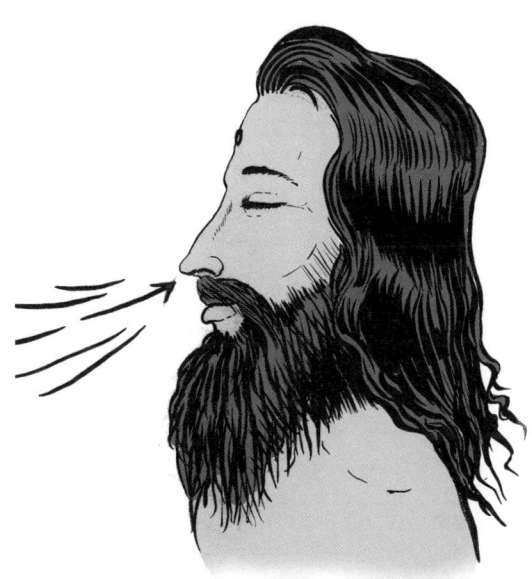

The coordination of movement and breath is a distinctive feature of yoga. In some traditions, breath control is essential to asana practice, its cycle synchronized with specific positions and postures. Other systems of yoga take a less stringent approach. A few traditions place the primary focus on the practice of *Pranayama*, harnessing the power of breath through a complex series of breathing patterns. Regardless of how formal the attention someone chooses to place on the breath, yoga practitioners all seem to agree that free flowing and unimpeded breath is necessary for asana practice.

Breathing is the act of *respiration*, the biological term that describes the lungs' exchange of oxygen from the environment with the body's discharge of carbon dioxide and water. It consists of two stages, *inspiration* (inhalation) and *expiration* (exhalation). The average adult experiences 18-20 cycles of respiration each minute. Trained yogis may reduce the cycle to as low as 1-2 per minute. The ability to control the fullness and rhythm of breath is an indication of the health and vitality of the heart and lungs. Yoga practice provides a great opportunity to influence this vital body system.

The diaphragm

The *diaphragm* is the primary muscle of respiration. It is a dome-shaped tissue that separates the thoracic cavity from the abdominal cavity, forming a barrier between the internal organs in each region. It is composed of large flat sections of muscle, interwoven with fascia that connects to a large central tendon. When breathing in, the diaphragm moves down as it contracts. Upon exhalation, the diaphragm lifts and relaxes.

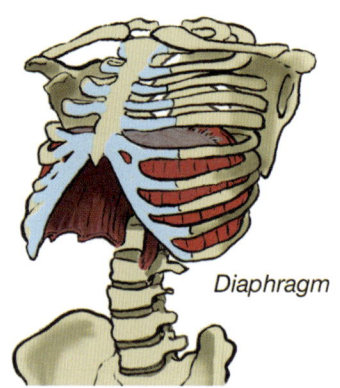
Diaphragm

The diaphragm's attachments to the skeleton are extensive. On the front of the body, the diaphragm embeds its fibers into the base of the two lowest ribs, the costal cartilage (cartilage that attaches the ribs to the sternum) and the tip of the breastbone (xiphoid process). The posterior insertion of the diaphragm is on the vertebral bodies of T12 to L2 where it interweaves its muscle and tendon fibers into the psoas and quadratus lumborum. These interconnections establish a mechanical relationship between the breath, the lower back and the pelvis.[1] The diaphragm's nerve supply is the *phrenic* nerve, emanating from the mid-cervical spine.

The diaphragm during respiration

At first glance, the diaphragm's movements seem counter-intuitive. When a typical muscle contracts, it shortens, reducing the space between the bones to which it attaches. Conversely, contraction of the diaphragm lengthens the muscle and increases space.

When a breath is taken in, the diaphragm contracts and is pulled down from its central tendon. The unique design of the central tendon allows contraction and relaxation of the diaphragm to change the shape of the thoracic cavity in all of its three diameters.[2]

When the diaphragm contracts, the thoracic cavity expands in the directions that follow:

- Vertically, dropping into the abdomen up to the neck, causing both the belly and chest to expand.[3]
- Transversely, (side-to-side and front-to-back) by using its attachment to the sternum as leverage to lift the lower ribs.

Diaphragm expiration

Expiration reverses the action of the diaphragm. When the diaphragm relaxes, its central tendon is drawn up into the thorax. The chest contracts and the belly flattens.

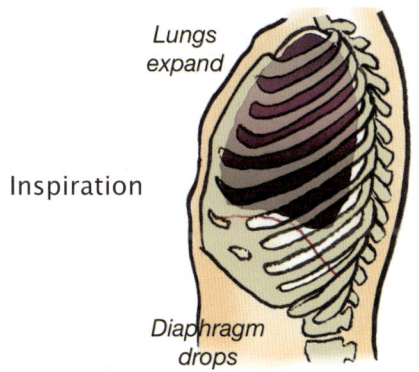
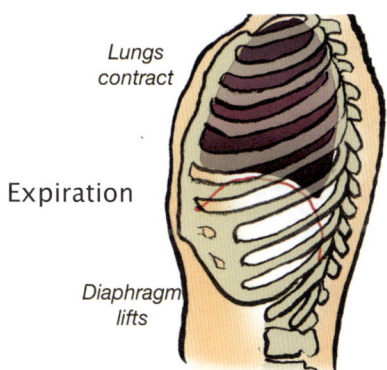

Protruding lower ribs

The efficiency of the diaphragm can increase up to 20% by lifting and jutting the lower rib cage forward. This action increases muscular tension on the diaphragm and allows the lungs and thorax to expand more effectively.[4] The increase in diaphragm efficiency may explain the natural tendency for the lower rib cage to jut forward, especially in backbending postures where the thoracic spine flattens and reduces the volume of the thoracic cavity.

The efficiency achieved by jutting the ribs forward, however, is reached within the first 1-3 inches of movement. Beyond that point, excessive forward protrusion of the lower ribs decreases the diaphragm's efficiency as it adversely effects the alignment of the spine.

The decrease in diaphragmatic efficiency that accompanies excessively protruded lower ribs can be experienced during deep backbend poses. As backbending postures lift the lower rib cage, the initial stretch on the diaphragm may "feel good" but once the ribs protrude too far, the pose becomes painful and breathing restricted. If the backbend continues beyond the point of relative comfort, the lumbar spinal discs compress and back pain often results. The ability to comfortably breathe in a backbend pose is a reliable sign that the asana is being executed safely.

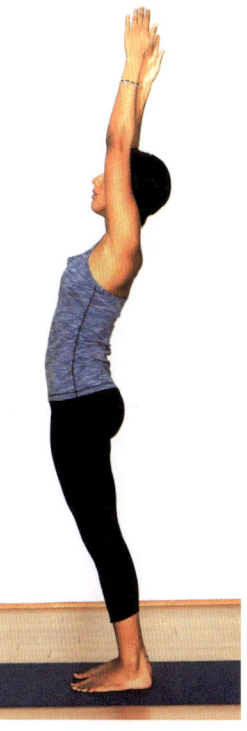

Effective diaphragm engagement

Backbending asana (extension postures) begin with the inhalation phase of respiration. To increase the efficiency of the breath, lengthen the side body rib cage to lift the diaphragm.

When runners are exhausted, they bend forward, drawing the belly in and the lower ribs back. This position relaxes an overstressed diaphragm, allowing it to recovery faster from fatigue. Propping up the chest and shoulders by pushing against the knees, another exhaustion response in runners, increases lung volume.

Other muscles that play an accessory role in inspiration are the sterno-cleido-mastoid, serratus anterior, pectoralis major and minor, and the latissimus dorsi. Allowing these minor muscles to excessively contribute to inspiration causes the shoulder girdle and neck to tighten, lift and shrug. This results in stress, strain and potential injury.

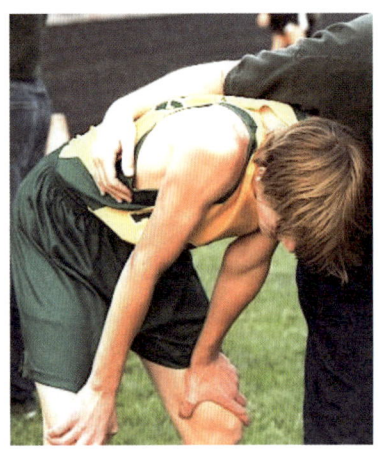

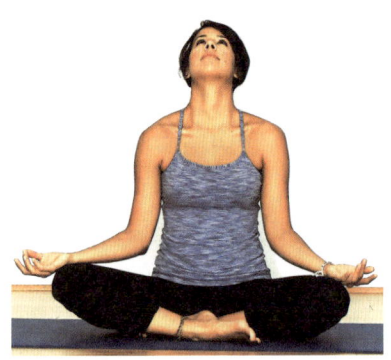

Overuse of accessory muscles tightens the neck, shoulders and upper back

The abdominals

The abdominal muscles are the antagonist muscles of the diaphragm. They play a role in both cycles of respiration, however, they are the primary muscles of expiration. During expiration, the abdominals draw the ribs and sternum inward, causing the diaphragm's central tendon to lift and all three diameters of the thoracic cavity to reduce. Both the abdominals and the diaphragm are always actively engaged in both cycles of respiration but the strength of their contraction varies inversely. Their reciprocal relationship is referred to as *floating equilibrium*.[4] Coordinated action between the diaphragm and abdominal muscles pumps air through the abdomen to help stabilize the spine. Because abdominal contraction engages the muscles that flex the torso, most yoga postures incorporate exhalation with forward folding movements.

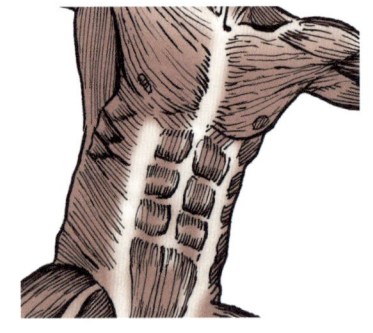

> Forward bends are performed on the exhalation.
> Backbends are performed on the inhalation.

Paradoxical respiration

Although breathing is a natural, unconscious action, many students have difficulty coordinating their breath cycles with diaphragm and abdominal contraction. In some cases, students reverse the contraction/relaxation cycle and contract the abdominal muscles when they inhale and relax them during exhalation. This is called *paradoxical respiration*. During paradoxical respiration, the abdominal cavity fails to expand, leaving the spinal discs vulnerable to injury during weight bearing activities. Details on the relationship between the abdominal cavity and the lumbar spinal discs can be reviewed in Chapter 24's discussion of the *Valsalva effect*.

Should breathing imbalances exist, yoga students can practice the following:
While exhaling, gently lift both the perineum and diaphragm and draw in the navel. This exercise and other yogic breath practices can help re-establish the natural breath cycle.

Nose breathing

There is a simple adage that is usually attributed to B.K.S. Iyengar, "the mouth is for eating and the nose for breathing."

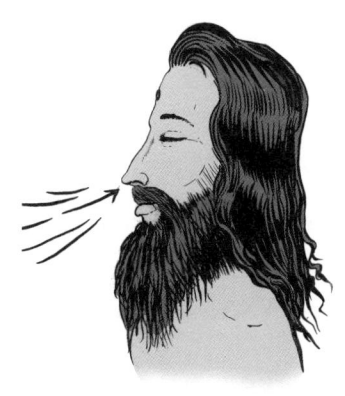

Nose breathing offers numerous physiological advantages over breathing through the mouth. Breathing through the nose filters bacteria and pollutants, preventing them from entering the body. Circulating breath through the nasal cavities and sinuses warms and humidifies the air before it reaches the inner tissues of the body. Breath entering the sinuses and porous, inner surfaces of the skull oxygenates the outer surfaces of the brain cavity. Nose breathing also retains moisture in the lungs, which helps hydrate the body.[5]

Other benefits of nose breathing are less obvious but also important, especially to the practice of yoga. Breathing exclusively through the nose has been shown to produce a positive shift in brain waves. Laboratory studies were performed at Maharishi University (MUM) in Fairfield, Iowa on the physiological effects of breathing. Test subjects used nose and mouth breathing combinations during various physical activities, such as running and weight lifting. When mouth breathing was used during either cycle of breath, test subjects produced mostly beta brain waves. Beta waves are cycles of electrical energy elicited when the mind is engaged in highly cognitive activities, such as thinking, talking, remaining alert, and concentrating. The studies further demonstrated that when nose breathing exclusively was used, on both inhalation and exhalation, the brain produced an increase in alpha, delta, and theta waves. These are the electrical wave patterns associated with states of deep relaxation, meditation and "higher" states of consciousness. These wave lengths have been associated with healing from illness, better-balanced hormone levels, and heightened states of spirituality.[6]

Nose breathing while exercising can maintain a heart rate below 60% of the maximum heart rate (MHR).[7] Yogic breathing techniques used by researchers at MUM kept the heart rates of athletes below 60% while performing sports that usually produce high spikes in the heart rate.

Athletes were tested in sports, ranging from long-distance running to power lifting, and lower heart rates were sustained without loss in performance. The benefits from this are inexhaustible! Nose breathing delays sports fatigue because lactic acid production is reduced as a result of the blood and muscles remaining oxygenated for longer periods.[8]

Nose breathing techniques stimulate the metabolism to burn fats. Exercising with a heart rate at 60% of MHR or lower stimulates the body to burn stored fat to fuel the muscles. Higher heart rates are interpreted by the body as a state of stress or survival and will reduce fat burning. Instead, the body shifts its energy source to carbohydrates and protein, muscle fuels that require less energy to metabolize.

Mouth breathing and stress

Ever notice that after a stressful situation, the first instinct it to let out a deep breathy "Whew"! This mouth exhalation is part of the body's stress response. Students who habitually exhale through the mouth over-produce and release stress hormones that can lead to deleterious health effects. Meditation and breathing techniques during asana that focus predominantly on nose breathing and discourage mouth breathing contribute to yoga's ability to reduce anxiety and daily stress.

The heart of the yogi

Non-yogic breathing patterns can create an abnormal overdevelopment of the heart muscle and its surrounding blood vessels, a condition know as *cardiac hypertrophy*. The heart and its large blood vessels function the same as other muscular tissues: they change in size because of the demand placed upon them. Chronic *high stroke volume* (the amount of blood pumped by the left ventricle of the heart) causes the heart and aorta to enlarge. A heart that has enlarged to meet the demands of explosive power sports creates a life-threatening situation once the level of exercise lessens. After tossing baseballs is replaced by tossing back beers, an ex-athlete's risk of heart attack increases. Once the hypertrophied heart is under-exercised, it becomes fatty and inefficient, producing an energetic drain on the body and making it prone to cardiac incidents.

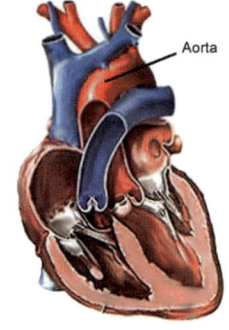

Normal heart tissue

Using nose breathing to lower heart rate reduces the volume of blood (per stroke, or beat) passing through the heart's walls and chambers. This lowers the demand on the heart and aorta and prevents them from enlarging. The heart can remain small, compact and highly efficient, which is more in line with yogic principles.

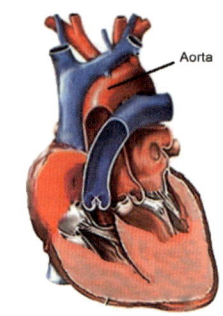

Thickened heart muscle

Blood pressure and yoga

This is a subject that produces strong and contradictory opinions. Medical advice is generally cautious about cardiovascular issues and what is a safe blood pressure for practicing vigorous exercise, including some forms of yoga. Concerns regarding the risks of **Sirsana** (Headstand Pose) and its effect on blood circulation in the brain are well established. At the same time, some authors with backgrounds in both medicine and yoga, regard vigorous practice and inversions as not only preventative but also restorative, even in cases of advanced cardiovascular disease.[9, 10]

There are no absolute answers to the many questions and considerations that arise regarding high blood pressure. Since a fundamental tenant of yoga is Ahimsa, *do no harm*, caution is the wisest approach to take for all students. The benefits derived from advanced postures can often be completely achieved in modified and remedial poses. This approach is best not only for cardiovascular issues, but orthopedic ones as well.

Bringing wisdom to all thought and concern about illness or disease is the very essence of yoga. Resisting the drive of the ego to attempt risky postures is the true practice of yoga. Managing any major health condition requires great personal responsibility. A student with heart issues must do diligent research and seek unbiased medical consultation. Then, with all the wisdom the student can muster, a skillful yoga practice can be designed.

> Serious yoga students eventually realize that wisdom is not necessarily in the answers, but in the deepest exploration of the questions themselves.

Advanced yogic breathing techniques

Yoga incorporates a sophisticated system of breath practice that is not asana, but is still considered Hatha. The methods used derive from the practices of *Kriya* yoga and *Pranayama*.[11] Kriya yoga refers to actions, deeds and efforts that are designed to remove obstructions in the relationship between the body and mind. Kriyas are a variety of practices for psychological and physiological cleansing. These include hygienic bodily cleanings as well as *mudras* (body and hand positions that increase prana), *mantras* and *meditations*.

Pranayama is primarily the yogic practice of breath control. Derived from Sanskrit, Pranayama refers to the practice of extending and drawing out the breath and life force. Yoga teacher Richard Freeman describes Pranayama as the "release of life energy from its bounds."[12]

Pranayama is considered an advanced, esoteric practice of yoga. As with other, non-yogic, spiritual pursuits, esoteric study is considered the realm of the more advanced practitioner. The sometimes, simple appearing breathing techniques require a level of awareness that often requires years of asana practice to fully develop. Breathing techniques, nonetheless, are presented to students at most levels of yoga practice. A few basic Pranayama techniques are explored here in this chapter that are appropriate for students of all levels of asana practice.

Basic three-part breath

Lie supine, relaxed, but *not* in full Corpse Pose. Inhale by first filling the abdomen; then hold the breath. While retaining the breath in the abdomen, further breathe to fill the chest. While retaining breath in these first two cavities, take a third breath into the throat. After a short retention of breath in all three regions, exhale, releasing the breath in the reversed order taken during inhalation. Practice this exercise with the hands placed over the belly to feel the abdomen expand. Alternatively, place one hand over the belly and the other on the chest to bring better focus to the breath. A rolled or folded blanket can be placed lengthwise under the spine to facilitate the practice.

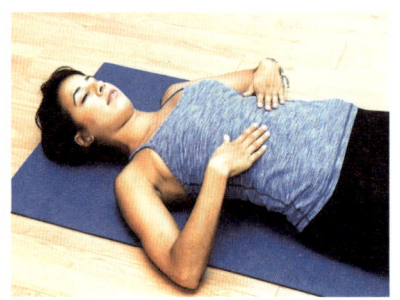

Alternate nostril breathing

Alternate nostril breathing is a rhythmic series of inhalation, breath retention, and exhalation. Known as **Nadi Shodhana** and **Anulom Viloma Pranayam**, these popular practices are found in many yoga classes. They are excellent methods for developing breath control and for balancing the neurological activities of the two brain hemispheres.

Here is a series that can be followed:

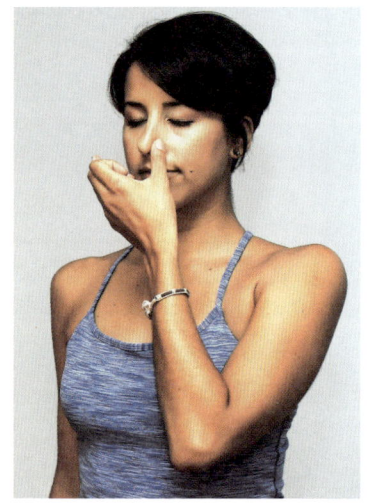

- Gently close one nostril, with or without finger pressure.
- Inhale for a count of four; retain the breath for a count of four; reverse whichever nostril is closed and exhale for a count of eight.
- Inhale through the now-unobstructed nostril, repeating the procedure starting from the other side.
- With each successive round of breathing, the count for each step can be lengthened proportionally.

There are many breath counting methods and variations of the finger configurations (mudras) used for alternate nostril breathing. Yoga students and teachers often create their own methods and most will be appropriate.

Of course, alignment of the body, particularly the shoulders, upper back, neck and head, is maintained throughout the practice. Students, often as they fatigue, may incorrectly point their elbow away from the body, causing the shoulder to round forward. This impedes breath flow by constricting the upper quadrants of the lungs. Nose-clasping by the fingers will be more stable if the arm is placed in a **Chatarunga-like** position with the collarbones lengthened wide and the upper arm held close the side body.

Holding the breath – Kumbhaka

Part of the alternate nostril breathing sequence is the practice of *Kumbhaka* (breath retention). Breath retention strengthens the muscles of respiration; however, it can also increase cardio-pulmonary pressure. If practiced in a safe, non-competitive manner, Kumbhaka can provide heart-health benefits similar to those received from cardiovascular exercises such as running.

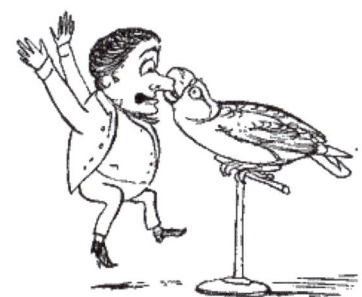

Kumbhaka derives from the Sanskrit word for "pot," in particular, a container that is sometimes full and sometimes empty. In breath retention, the chest is the pot that alternates between being full (chest filled with air) and being empty (air emptied out of chest). Kumbhaka is inherent in every breath cycle, occurring naturally at the end of each inhalation (*anatara*- breath inside) and each exhalation (*bahya* - breath outside). This routine action of Kumbhaka is skillfully harnessed in Pranayama and used as preparatory practice for meditation. The Kumbhaka procedure is applied to engaging the *bandhas*, or breath locks, a practice that can re-vitalize the tissue linings between the ribs and lungs. (bandha discussion to follow).

Kumbhaka must be performed with awareness, as it increases pressure in the spinal discs. It should not be performed while engaging extreme forward bending postures or when the spine is bearing weight. **Padmasana** (Lotus Pose) or **Siddhasanana** (Easy Sitting Pose) are appropriate postures for the practice of Kumbhaka, not during more active asana postures.

The Bandhas

The Sanskrit term *bandha* translates to lock, knot or bond. These words are associated with the actions of binding, restraining, or capturing. In yoga, a bandha is the restraint of breath for the purpose of regulating the flow of prana. As a Kriya practice, bandhas stimulate the internal organs.

Bandha locking is practiced either as an asana unto itself or as an underlying energetic action that accompanies all other asana. As an asana, bandhas are most often performed in a sitting or standing position and use a firm muscular action.

More often, bandhas are used to create an ever-present core tension that is both muscular and energetic. Some teachers in the *Astaṅga* tradition of *K. Pattabhi Jois* will instruct students to engage their bandhas "24/7".

Engaging bandha lock by squeezing the anus or performing a *Kegel-type* exercise is a misguided understanding of the action.[12] Bandha engagement is barely physical but is subtle and energetic, making its constant use possible.

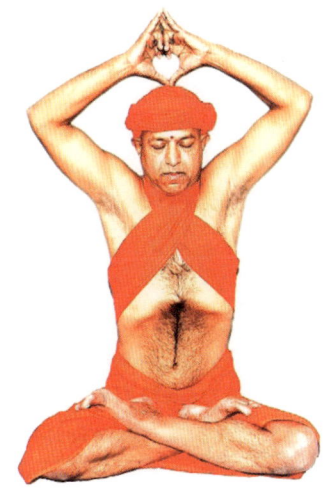

Uddiyana bandha

The three most commonly engaged bandhas are:

- Muladhara (Mula) bandha - engaged with a gentle lift from the center of the perineum.[14]
- Uddiyana bandha - engaged by the diaphragm retracting the abdomen toward the spine.
- Jalandhara bandha - engaged by closing the glottis and leveling the soft palate.

From an esoteric perspective, Mula bandha is the "root" lock that helps propel the upward flow of prana. Prana rises, molten-like, in a spiraling fashion through the *Sushumna*, the central channel of the core, and exits the body through the posterior fontanel of the skull. Pranic channels also run to the palms of the hands and the soles of the feet, which are also considered to be bandhas by some yogic traditions.

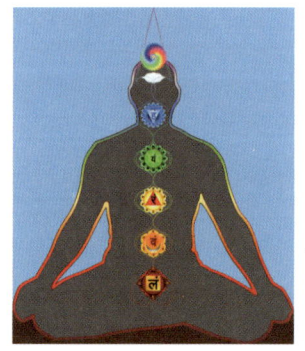

Bandhas, from an anatomical point of view

As first discussed in Chapter 14, bandha engagement can be used as a simple, but effective method of establishing postural alignment through the central axis of the body.

Essentially, bandha locks are contractions of the diaphragms. The diaphragms vault up in a dome-like fashion as the bandhas are engaged. The core contractions of the bandhas provide a deep sense of integration and safety. Lifting of the bandhas/diaphragms initiates at the Mula, through the thoracic diaphragm, up through the roof of the mouth, and continues with an energetic exit through the posterior fontanelle of the skull. *Forward tailbone scoop* engages the Mula bandha. This action stimulates the plexus of parasympathetic nerves on the pelvic floor, nestled under the inner surface of the tailbone (coccyx). The parasympathetic nervous system has a calming effect on the body, which the yogi may experience when engaging Mula bandha.

Ujjayi Pranayama – the victorious breath

If you walk past an Astaṅga yoga class in progress, you might hear a deep synchronized, hissing sound that causes you to quickly turn around with your light saber in full force, looking for Darth Vader.[13] *Ujjayi* breath creates this hissing sound by directing both inhalation and exhalation across the back of a partially closed glottis, the area of the throat that closes when swallowing. If partially closed, the air passing over the glottis will resonate, creating the deep sound from the throat and vocal chords. Ujjayi is performed with a closed mouth but is not a "sniff" from the nose. The sound emanates from the back of the throat, producing a deep, guttural reverberation. When performed correctly, more air enters the lungs than is possible from the nose or with simple mouth breathing. Ujjayi breathing is often a challenging practice for the beginner student.

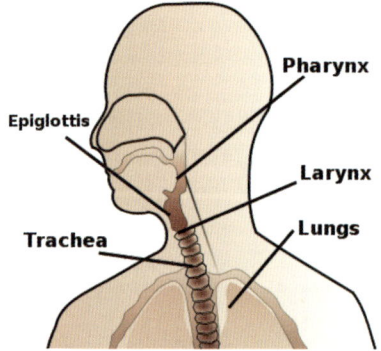

How loud is the Ujjayi call to victory?

The question of how audible Ujjayi breathing should be is met with differences of opinion by yoga traditions. Some schools of yoga insist that the Ujjayi breath be distinctly heard, and teachers will emphatically instruct to that effect. Other yogic schools of thought believe that constant, deep vibration of the vocal chords is irritating and dries out the delicate mucous membranes of the vocal chords, leading to sustained damage.

From a physiological point of view, Ujjayi is a valuable tool to calm the nervous system and maximize the exchange of airflow. It can easily be performed, practically in silence and present no risk of injuring the vocal chords. This wins out as the safest method.

The Valsalva Effect and breath

Introduced in Chapter 24, the Valsalva effect is a hydraulic-like action of the diaphragm and abdominals that traps air within the anterior cavities of the body. It provides structural support for the lumbar spine. Holding the breath is sometimes taught as the method to engage the bandhas, however, it is not recommended because it increases spinal disc pressure. Instead, apply the bandhas in a gentle yet deliberate fashion during *both* inhalation and exhalation.

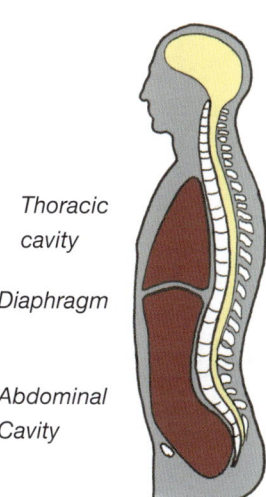

Thoracic cavity

Diaphragm

Abdominal Cavity

> Cycles of full-breath inspiration and expiration and the continuous, gentle application of the bandhas are the best way to align the core and keep the spine safe.

Back off the bandha!

The instruction to firmly squeeze the buttock to engage Mula bandha is often given by yoga teachers who have yet to fully explore the subject. A hard, forceful action causes students to miss the subtle effects of the action that are so calming to the nervous system.

The amount of lift required to engage Mula bandha has been suggested to be equivalent to the amount of effort used to lift a bubble from a soapy bowl.

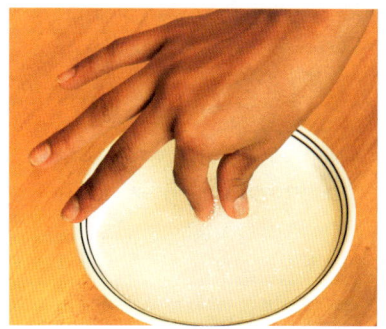

30 Shoulder Anatomy

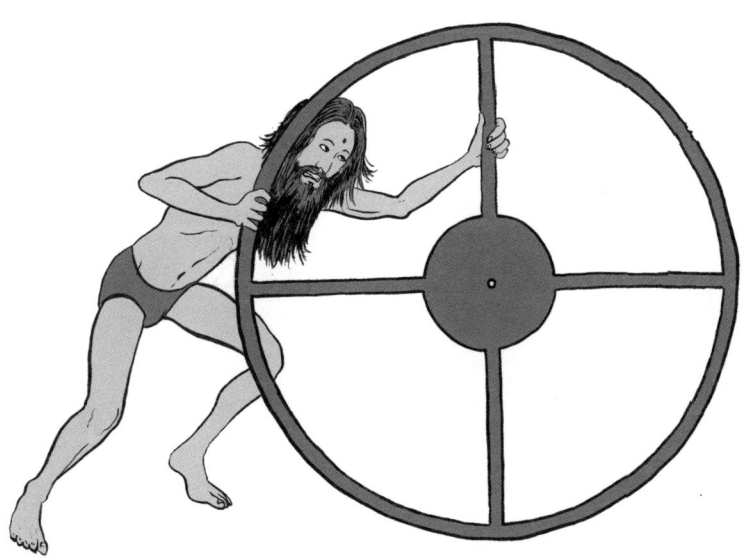

You will need to put your shoulder to the wheel in order to master the principles in this chapter, but it will be well worth the effort. Developing strong, well-functioning shoulders and preventing their injury is achievable when alignment is fully incorporated into yoga practice. And, as always, first learning the anatomy will help make applying the alignment easier.

The shoulders, along with the upper spine, are part of a functionally integrated system that includes the upper extremities and the head and neck. Precise alignment and integration of the shoulders is required in order to prevent injury not only to the shoulders, but also to these associated regions. The shoulders are capable of a multiplicity of actions. They have powerful muscular strength and, at the same time, the broadest joint range of motion found in the body.

Shoulder mobility

The term used to describe the general movement of the shoulder joint is *circumduction*. Circumduction combines all of the shoulder's possible actions in a single, cone-shaped movement that radiates outward from the shoulder. Shoulder movement arcs forward, intended to allow the eyes to easily follow the position of the hand. The shoulder's separate ranges of motion, sometimes called degrees of freedom, are as follows:

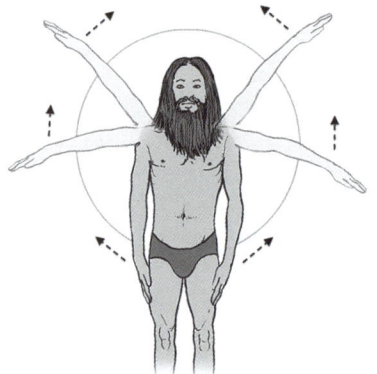

- Flexion   180°
- Extension   50°
- External rotation   80°
- Internal rotation   110° with arm behind trunk
- Abduction   180°
- Adduction   0° due to obstruction by the torso; adduction must be combined with flexion or extension

The full ranges of flexion and abduction bring the shoulder to the same final position overhead.

The three mechanical components of the shoulder

- Gleno-humeral joint
- Clavicular component
    - Acromio-clavicular joint
    - Sterno-clavicular joint
- Scapulo-thoracic "joint"

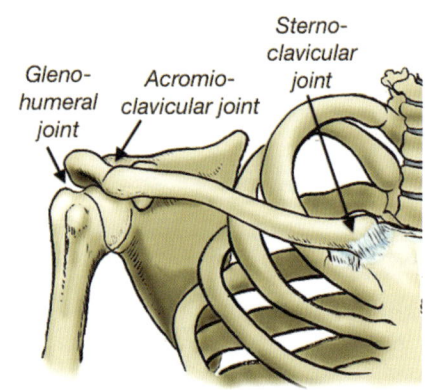

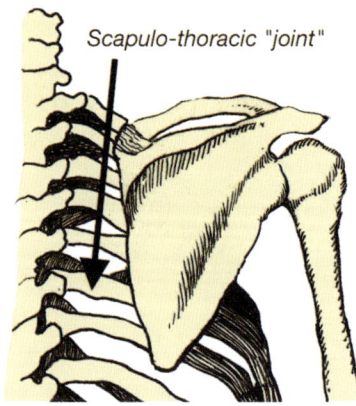

The gleno-humeral joint

The primary, most mobile joint of the shoulder forms between the *humerus* (upper arm bone) and the *scapula* (shoulder blade). It forms a ball-and-socket system called the *gleno-humeral joint*. The *glenoid fossa*, from the Greek *glene* for socket, is a pear-shaped cavity located on the lateral aspect of the scapula. It is small and shallow, technically not deep enough to be categorized a socket.

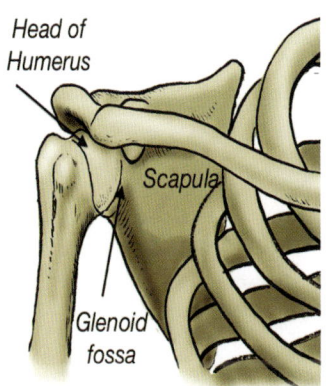

A cartilage collar called the *labrum* surrounds the glenoid fossa to create a snug fit for the large, spherical head of the humerus. The joint is loosely bound, held by a capsular ligament that surrounds the joint and contains lubricating synovial fluid. This capsule is loose on the bottom and taut along its top border.

Unlike the hip joint, which has a sharply defined central axis of rotation and limited *joint play*, the shoulder can shift its central axis as much as one to two inches. The floating central axis design allows the shoulder to achieve fluid circumduction and to rapidly change its direction or the angle of the joint. In the first 90° of circumduction, movement take place primarily in the gleno-humeral joint. The *deltoid* and *supraspinatus* muscles provide the majority of strength in this phase of circumduction that lifts the arm from the side.[1]

Comparing the hip and shoulder "sockets"

The hip: the *acetabulum* is deep and round. Its large rim holds the femur head snug inside the cup of its socket, preventing the hip from deviating off its central axis as it moves in all its directions.

The shoulder: the *glenoid fossa* is the shallow "socket" on the scapula that forms a joint with the head of the upper arm bone (humerus). It is a loose, lax, joint with a central axis that shifts between 1-2 inches during circumduction. This provides the shoulder joint with the widest range of motion of any joint in the body.

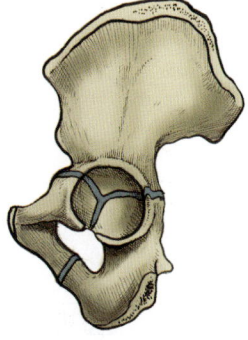   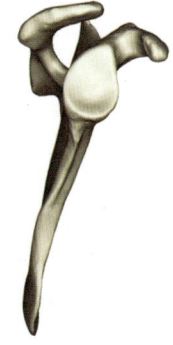

Hip and acetabulum   *Scapula and glenoid fossa*

Biceps tendon

The *biceps brachii* is a bi-articular muscle (crosses two joints) that flexes the elbow and shoulder. It also stabilizes the gleno-humeral joint. As the term *biceps* implies, it has two heads (muscle bundles), a long head and a short head. The long head tendon enters the joint over the top of the humeral head and attaches deep inside the capsule. It supports the joint, preventing dislocation of the humerus when the arm is pulled forcefully from any direction. The long head biceps tendon is vulnerable to injury, due its tenuous path through constricted and mechanically demanding areas of the shoulder. Extreme forces will tear the tendon.

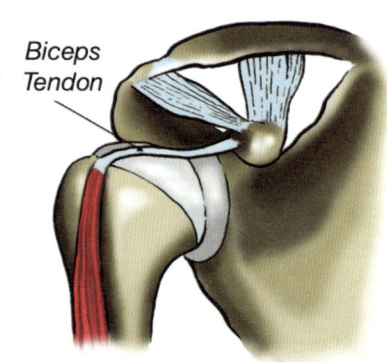

To keep the biceps tendon safe when it is engaged:
- Draw the head of the humerus back into the joint.
- Keep the collarbones lengthened horizontally.

Clearance requires external rotation

Similar to the greater trochanter of the hip and its proximity to the ilium, the outermost process of the shoulder, called the *greater tuberosity*, is located close to the *acromion* process of the scapula. The space under the acromion (see illustration) can become compressed, pinching soft tissue when the arm is abducted overhead. To avoid injury, the shoulder must externally rotate once the arm is abducted 90° from the shoulder. Failure to externally rotate can result in damage to the biceps tendon, the ligaments of the shoulder joint, the supraspinatus muscle or the acromio-clavicular joint.

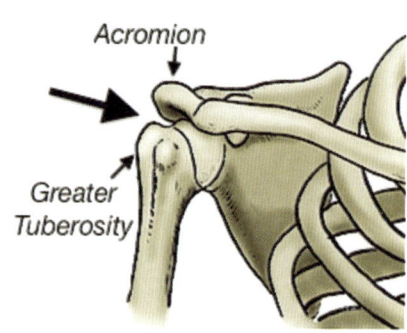

> The palms face downward until the arms are horizontal in order to take advantage of the ligament-releasing benefits of internal rotation. At 90°, the palms turn to face upward as the arms continue lifting overhead.

Shoulder dislocation

The most vulnerable position for the gleno-humeral joint is anterior and inferior, or downward and toward the breast. This section of the joint is poorly supported by ligaments and muscles and is, therefore, the weakest. The shoulder joint most often dislocates when the shoulder is rolled forward with the arm moving in an anterior-inferior direction.

The clavicle and its two joints

Commonly known as the collarbones, the two clavicles bridge the two scapulae (shoulder blades) with the *sternum* (breastbone). They provide anterior bracing of the shoulders and create the shoulder girdle. The two clavicles are the only long bones of the body that are horizontally positioned. They do not run straight across the front of the body but angle 60° forward to join the sternum. The clavicles move by rotating 30° at each end along a horizontal axis (picture hot dogs spinning on a commercial griller). The clavicles' participation in shoulder movement occurs primarily when circumduction is between 90 and 150°.[2]

The clavicles of humans have evolved to firmly brace the front of the shoulder girdle, while other mammals have only remnant-sized clavicles or none at all. Animals that are primarily runners benefit less from collarbones than climbers do. Cats, being both runners and climbers, have small clavicles embedded in their muscles, but they do not form a functional joint. This unique design gives cats the ability to squeeze through small spaces. Humans, however, have long, broad collarbones that keep the shoulders from collapsing forward. This may also be why we humans get into tight spots from which we seem unable to get out!

Not a fashion statement!

Recently touted as stylish, prominent collarbones are an indication of poor shoulder alignment. This loss of postural integrity causes the shoulder girdle to round forward, a position that predispose the biceps tendons to tearing and the rotator cuff muscles vulnerable to injury (details reviewed later in this chapter). The head and neck shift forward of the central axis, tightening the jaw and tensing the upper back muscles. This is not so chic a position!

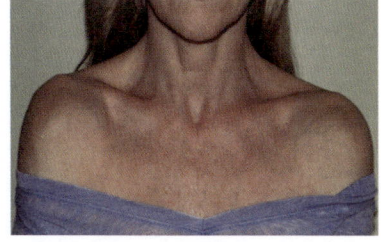

The acromio-clavicular joint

If you hang around a group of physically active people, it is not long before someone mentions an AC joint injury. The acromio-clavicular (AC) joint forms where the clavicle joins the acromion portion of the scapula at the outer shoulder. The AC joint pivots on its long axis when the arm raises overhead. The challenges of rapid movement, changes of position, and the necessity of maintaining alignment makes the AC joint an easy target for sports-related trauma. Ligament tears, joint separations, and fractures are the most common injuries to the AC joint. Often a large bump is noticed over this joint, a permanent deformity following an acromio-clavicular injury. In my personal experience of having suffered bilateral AC separations, these bumps are useful for keeping backpack straps from sliding off the shoulders!

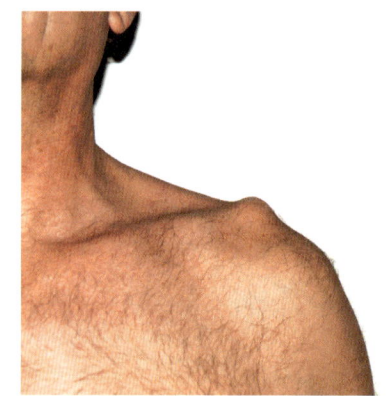

The Sterno-clavicular joint

The medial end of each clavicle affixes to the breastbone to form the *sterno-clavicular* joint. It also attaches to the first rib, held by thick ligaments and cushioned by an articular disc. This juncture is the only skeletal connection between the shoulder girdle and the torso. The entire weight and muscular power of the shoulders and arms are structurally supported at this location on each side of the breastbone.

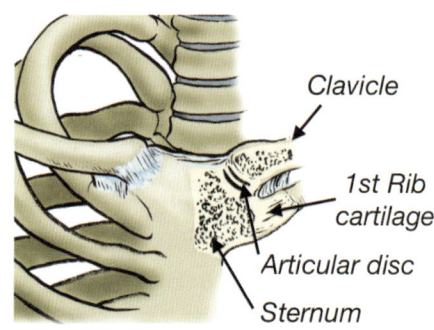

Chronic poor alignment of the shoulders can excessively strain the sterno-clavicular joints, causing them to become hypermobile and susceptible to injury. If the ligaments surrounding the joint capsules become overstretched, the joints become unstable and unable to brace the front of the shoulders properly against forces, such as those produced when jumping back into **Chatarunga Dandasana** (Four Limbed Staff Pose).

Mechanical stress on a hypermobile sterno-clavicular joint can cause the joint to become enlarged and swollen. This joint is also a common site for arthritis and bone infection.

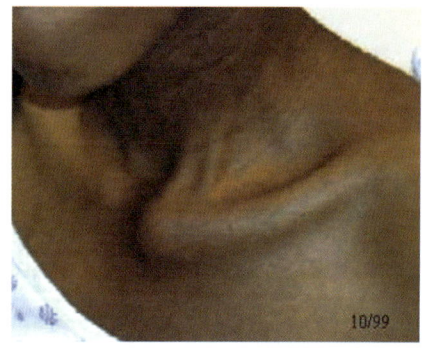

The scapulo-thoracic "joint"

A joint is defined as two or more bones directly united or connected through an intervening substance, such as cartilage.[3] Since none of the spinal vertebrae directly attach to the scapula, the scapulo-thoracic "joint" is technically not a joint. Physiologists, however, consider the scapula-thoracic articulation a "pseudo" joint because, mechanically, with its interconnected musculature, it functions as if it were a joint between the scapula and the thoracic spine.[3]

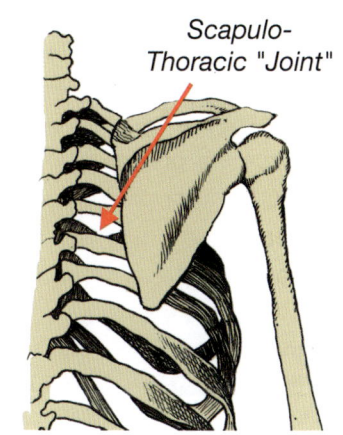
Scapulo-Thoracic "Joint"

Regardless of how it is categorized, the scapulo-thoracic articulation is extremely important to the mechanics of the shoulder. The principles of shoulder integrative alignment that will be presented in the following chapter focus specifically on the functionality of the scapulo-thoracic joint.

The scapula – fun facts

The shoulder blade, or scapula, "lives" on the back. Its upper medial edge is approximately 3 inches (5-6 cm) from the spine. At the bottom, this distance widens to nearly 7-8 inches. Vertically, the scapula spans the distance from the second to the seventh thoracic ribs. The *acromion* and the *coracoid* are two boney projections, or processes, that arise from the scapula. They extend over the gleno-humeral joint to provide ligament and muscular attachment.

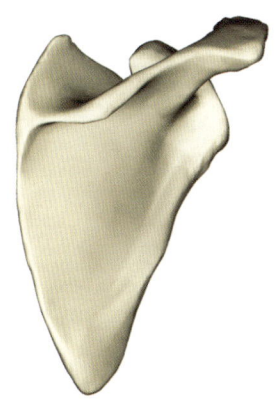

The scapula is contoured, having an inner surface curve with a radius of 30°. Additionally, the scapula does not sit squarely on the back in its neutral position, but angles 30° toward the front of the torso. The curved shape and angled orientation of the scapula on the back allows small movements of the scapula to amplify to large swings of the arm. Scapula movement is most active at 90-180° of circumduction.[4]

The glenoid fossa points its contoured surface outward like a radio-tracking dish, following the humeral head as the arm moves in space. It acts as a movable base that stabilizes the humeral head while it shifts into all its positions. Because the shoulder joint is relatively close to the body's core, small movements at the scapula become large movements when observed at the hand. Conversely, large movements of the arm can become excessive and misalign the shoulder.

Where go the palms, so go the shoulder blades

A common instruction offered by yoga teachers for shoulder alignment is to "put the shoulder blades into the back pants pockets." Another concept for shoulder alignment is that the shoulder blades move in the same direction as the palms of the hands. The heels of the hands correspond with the bottom tips of the shoulder blades. In practice, torque the heels of the palms toward the midline of the body to bring the shoulder blades closer toward the spine.

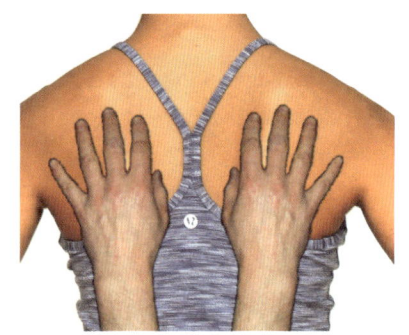

Keep your angel wings folded in!

Keep the scapulae on the back during asana. As long as we remain in human form, we keep our angel wings drawn in.

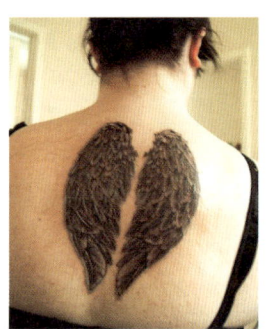

Specific joint and muscle involvement in circumduction

The term *circumduction* is used to describe shoulder movement because the shoulder overlaps multiple ranges and directions as it moves through its wide arc. Also, some movements do not conform to standard terminology. When the arms move from the side of the body to overhead, for the first 90° the arms are moving away from the body (*abduction*). Continuing past 90°, the arms are moving "toward" the midline of the body (*adduction*). When the arms are completely overhead, 180°, they are essentially in the same position after abduction/adduction as they would be if lifted overhead from flexion. Using the term circumduction reduces this confusion.

From **0-90°** of either shoulder flexion or abduction, movement occurs almost exclusively in the gleno-humeral joint. The supraspinatus and deltoid muscles, primarily, provide the action. At 90°, the upper ligaments of the joint capsule become taut, helping to support the arm.

Continuing from **90-150°,** the clavicle rotates at each end and the scapula begins to glide away from the spine. Additional muscles begin to contribute at this stage: the middle and upper trapezius and the serratus anterior. The rhomboids do not play a significant role in circumduction.

In the final **150-180°** of flexion or abduction, all previously-mentioned muscles are engaged with additional aid from the paraspinal muscles. When one arm is lifted, the scapula and spine shift toward the lifted arm side as the spinal muscles on the opposite side (contra-lateral) contract. If both arms are raised together, the muscles of both sides of the spine engage and the lumbar curve increases (lordosis).

Shoulder compensations

Limited shoulder mobility stiffens the upper spine and neck. The lumbar spine often compensates for this stiffness by deepening its curve. Over time, the curve may flatten if the lumbar spine ligaments weaken due to over-exertion.

If the thoracic spine is overly rounded (hyper-kyphosis), the shoulder blades are unable to fully retract toward the spine. The shoulder blades will become positioned chronically wide on the back and the front of the shoulders will round and drop forward, predisposing them to injury.

The serratus anterior

The *serratus anterior* arises as finger-like projections from the upper eight or nine ribs and inserts into the underside of the smooth, medial border of the scapula. When the arm swings forward, the serratus anterior muscle assists in bringing the shoulder forward. The serratus anterior has another important, albeit subtle, action that plays a central role in keeping the shoulders from rounding forward. A small section of the lower serratus anterior has the specific function of drawing the bottom tip of the shoulder blade forward, toward the back ribs. As will be discussed in the next chapter, this action provides a critical refinement in shoulder integrative alignment.

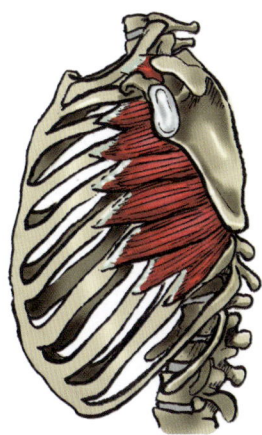

Serratus Anterior

Challenges of the serratus anterior

The good

The *rhomboid major* and the *teres major* create a cradle that secures the inferior tip of the scapula to the posterior rib cage. They assist the function of the serratus anterior in drawing the lower tip of the scapula tip forward.

The bad

Many students have a habit of tensing the middle *trapezius* to draw the shoulder blades onto the back. The trapezius muscle must not become overly tense or it will limit the actions of the rhomboids and the serratus anterior. It is more effective to *soften* the mid-trapezius and upper back muscles and simply allow the scapulae to gently slide closer. This approach allows the serratus anterior to be more engaged.

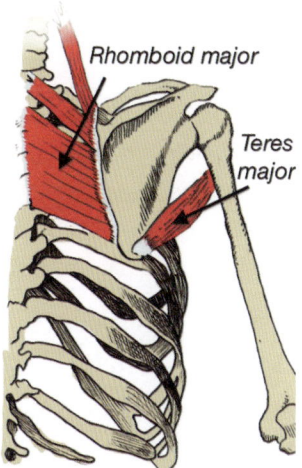

> Soften the mid-trapezius and upper back muscles and simply allow the scapulae to gently slide closer.
>
> Learn to move the arms and shoulders from the musculature below the armpits (axilla) instead of tightening and shrugging the shoulders.

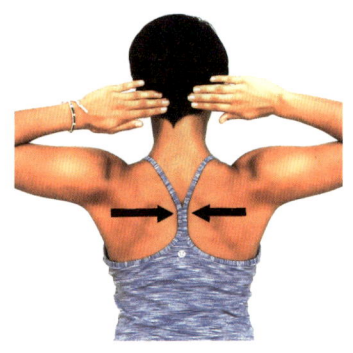

The ugly

The chest muscle, the *pectoralis minor*, has an antagonistic relationship with the serratus anterior. The pectoralis minor attaches to the front of the shoulder, pulling it down toward the chest. Its action opposes the serratus anterior. The muscles of the front body are approximately 30% stronger than those of the back. This is consistent with the relatively greater amount of front-body activity that humans perform. If the pectoralis minor overpowers the serratus anterior, the shoulders round forward and entrap the nerve and blood supply that course through the front of the neck and under the collarbones. This muscular imbalance can cause pain, weakness, numbness, or high blood pressure.

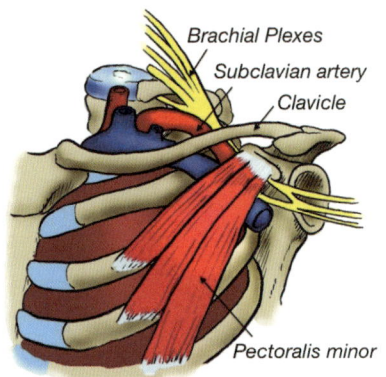

The serratus anterior receives its nerve supply from the *long thoracic nerve*, which originates from the roots of the cervical 5 to 7 spinal nerves. This nerve is subject to injury from stretch or compression trauma. Should the long thoracic nerve become damaged or paralyzed, the effect is observed in the shoulder blade "winging" off the back.[5]

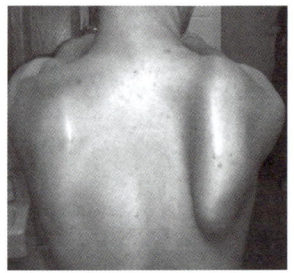

The Rotator Cuff

The *rotator cuff* consists of four short muscles that attach only between the scapula and the humerus. Their function is to move and to stabilize the gleno-humeral joint. The rotator cuff muscles are assisted by the large muscles of the upper torso. Conversely, the larger muscles are assisted by the rotator cuff muscles, which operate as "keys" to jumpstart movement that the large muscles are unable to initiate themselves.

The first letters of the four rotator cuff muscles spell out the useful mnemonic *SITS*.
- **S**upraspinatus
- **I**nfraspinatus
- **T**eres minor
- **S**ubscapularis

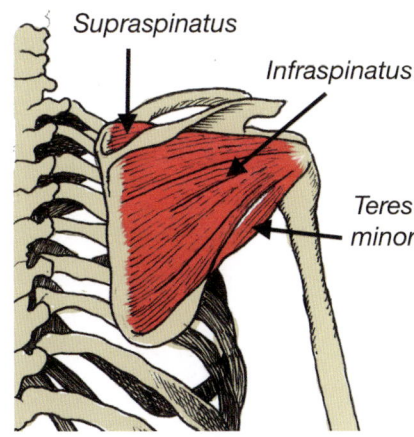
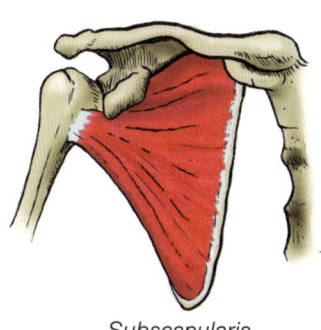

Subscapularis

Actions of the rotator cuff

External rotation: the *infraspinatus* and *teres minor* jointly externally rotate the shoulder. They also stabilize the humerus during abduction. The external rotators of the cuff are 30% weaker than their opposing internal rotators. They receive assistance from the trapezius and rhomboid muscles. The trapezius and rhomboid also adduct the shoulder but are not considered part of the rotator cuff. Shoulder shrugging engages the trapezius muscles and reduces its ability to assist in external rotation.

Internal rotation: the *subscapularis* attaches across the inner surface of the scapula. It stabilizes the shoulder, preventing it from slipping anteriorly. The subscapularis works with the pectoral muscles to internally rotate the humerus, especially when the arm is behind or at the side of the body.

Abduction: the *supraspinatus* spans across the top of the gleno-humeral joint. It initiates abduction when the arm is at rest along the side of the torso. The *deltoid*, the more powerful abductor of the shoulder, is unable to initiate abduction without assistance from the supraspinatus. The supraspinatus' involvement diminishes after abduction initiates and increases again when abduction is in the range of 90-180°. In its role as a stabilizer of the gleno-humeral joint, the supraspinatus prevents the head of the humerus from anterior-inferior dislocation, the shoulder's weakest point.

Rotator cuff injury

In 2006, the number of medical patients reporting shoulder and upper arm injuries was approximately 7.5 million. More than 4.1 million of these cases involved the rotator cuff.[6] The presence and the specific location of shoulder pain are diagnostic indicators of rotator cuff injury. Pain from rotator cuff injury is felt at the front of the shoulder. It can also be felt in the neck. Rotator cuff injury will limit shoulder motion, resulting from either an acute muscular tear or degenerative changes to the joint and tendons. Degenerative changes often result from over-use and repetitive injury, or loss of blood supply to the tendons of the rotator cuff muscles.

The most common rotator cuff injury is a tear of the supraspinatus. The cause is usually poor alignment or function of the deltoid muscle. If the deltoid muscle does not maintain its alignment (centered over the top of the shoulder), the supraspinatus, forced to carry a load normally handled by a well-aligned deltoid, becomes vulnerable. This scenario occurs when the shoulders round and drop forward. Rounded shoulders also compromise the posterior deltoid muscle, making it unable to stabilize the back of the shoulder. Strengthening the posterior (rear) deltoid can prevent rotator cuff injury and is often a key determinant for successful rotator cuff rehabilitation. *Push ups, Reverse Fly*, and *Bent-over Lateral Raise* are three gym exercises best suited to strengthening the posterior deltoid. In yoga practice, Plank Pose, **Chatarunga** and Reverse Plank can increase posterior deltoid strength.

Chatarunga Dandasana is a valuable asana for rotator cuff rehabilitation, although it is certainly not appropriate in the acute phases of injury. To be rehabilitative, Chatarunga requires precise alignment of the shoulders. Without correct alignment, Chatarunga becomes the cause of rotator cuff injury, not its cure.

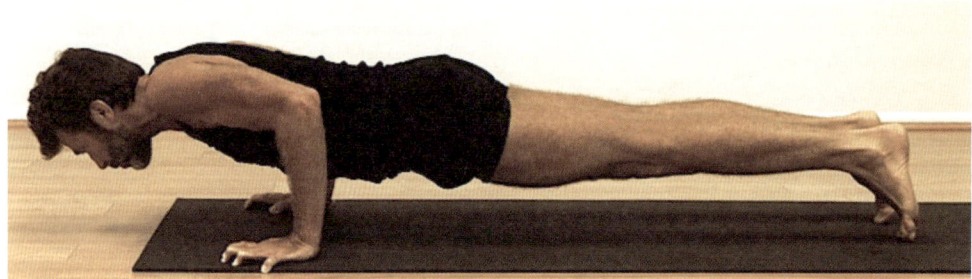

This chapter's exploration of shoulder anatomy sets the groundwork and is the rationale for the principles of *shoulder integrative alignment* that are presented in the next chapter.

31 Integrative Alignment of the Shoulders

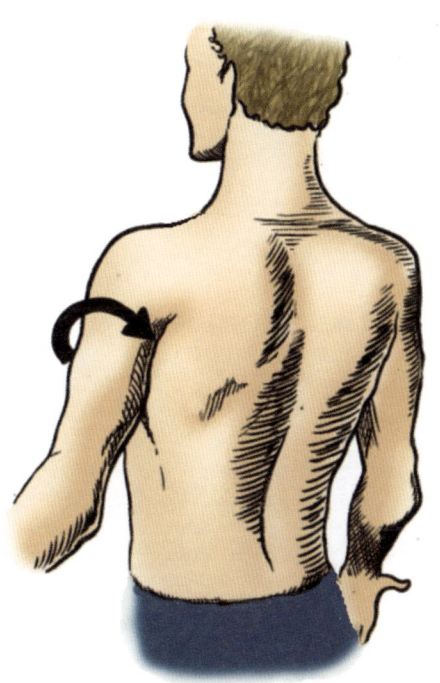

This chapter explores the step-by-step, integrative alignment principles of the shoulders and their relationship to the upper torso, arms, head and neck. These principles apply to every pose, whether standing on the feet or standing on the head. In forward bends and back bends alike, this set of instructions is used each and every time. Although the principles are precise and detailed, with practice they become easy to apply and second nature.

The physiological rules for the ligaments of the shoulders are the same as those that apply to the ligaments of other major joints of the body. For flexibility, move the joints in directions that loosen the ligaments. For stability, move the joints in directions that tighten ligaments.

Rules of engagement

When engaging any asana, use this three-step sequence every time:

1. Establish a stable and aligned foundation, from the ground up.
2. Move into the posture using the tools of flexibility:
   a. Loosen the joint ligaments
   b. Lengthen muscles from their bellies
3. Stabilize the posture by utilizing tools of strength:
   a. Tighten the joint ligament
   b. Contract the muscles from their bellies

Ligaments Loosen	Ligaments Tighten
•Flexion	•Extension
•Internal rotation	•External rotation
•Adduction	•Abduction

Postural pre-requisites for initiating shoulder integrative alignment

- Chest is positioned in front of the shoulders.
- Shoulder blades are hugged onto the back body.
- Lower rib cage is drawn back and does not jut forward.
- Ears are aligned over the shoulders.
- Arms are aligned with the shoulders. If the arms are straight, the middle finger is in line with the seam of the pants. If they are bent, the elbows are in line with the side body ribs.

Integrative alignment of the shoulder

The following sequence brings the shoulders into ideal alignment:

1. Lengthen the side body rib cage

- Deepen the armpits (axilla) from underneath without shrugging the shoulders. Keep the shoulders square and level.
- Scoop the bottom tip of the breastbone to secure the lower rib cage and keep it from jutting forward.
- Lengthen from "*Hips to Pits*" (according to Anusara yoga teacher Jaye Martin).

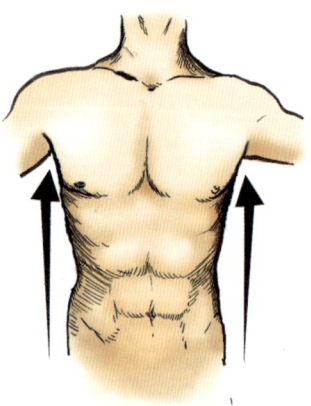

Side body lengthening brings the thoracic spine into extension, flattens the thoracic curve, and creates space in the joints that permits increased mobility.

2. Inflate the upper chest

- Expand the upper quadrants of the lungs with breath in all directions: 360° around the chest, below the armpits, and across the upper back.
- The expanded volume of the chest is maintained throughout both inhalation and exhalation.
- Increased chest volume creates an inflated barrier and prevents the shoulders from collapsing forward.

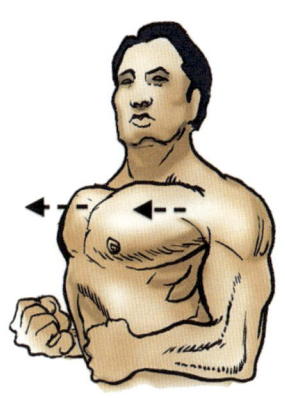

3. Head of arm bones internally rotate and draw back into the shoulder

- Pull the head of each humerus back into the shoulder joint simultaneously from its inner and outer aspects with equal speed and effort. Note that the *outer* shoulder has a tendency to move faster and farther than the *inner* (axillar) portion, a discrepancy that initiates external rotation and prevents the direction of movement from being purely posterior.
- To coordinate the movement of the arms with shoulder internal rotation, point the thumbs up, inward, or down.
- Move the arms using the musculature below the shoulders that forms the inner armpit and the side of the torso.
- Do not shrug the shoulders when drawing the arms back. This causes the upper trapezius and levator scapulae muscles to tense.

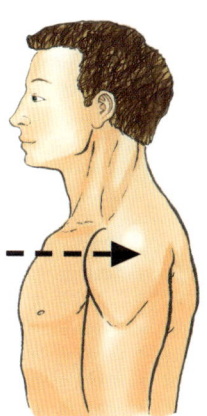

4. Lengthen collarbones and glide the shoulder blades toward the spine

- The clavicles and scapulae move at the same rate (1:1) but in opposite directions.
- Lengthen the clavicles laterally while drawing the scapulae medially toward the spine.

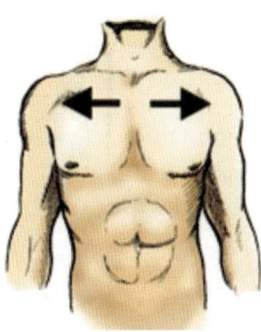 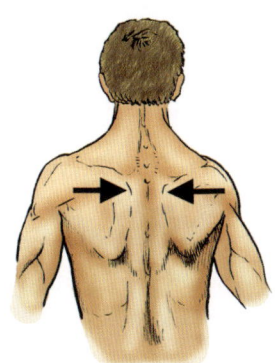

5. Externally rotate the humeral heads deep in the shoulder socket

- Keep the head of each humerus drawn deeply into the shoulder joint as it externally rotates.
- When humerus externally rotates, the triceps muscle always moves toward the midline of the body. When the arms are overhead, move the triceps toward the ear. When the arms are by the side of the body, move the triceps toward the side body ribs.
- External rotation of the shoulder tightens the ligaments and strengthens and stabilizes the joint.

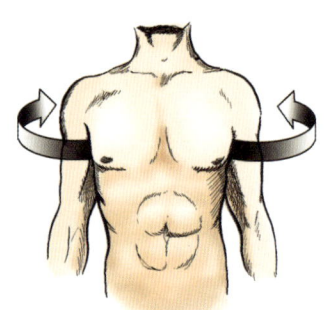

6. Lower tips of scapulae press forward onto the back

- Press the lower tips of the shoulders forward by engaging the serratus anterior muscles.
- The chest expands forward, as if the heart is leading the movement of the pose. A useful image taught in Anusara yoga is to press the shoulder blades forward "as if two hands are cradling the heart from behind".
- This final step brings refinement to shoulder integration and gives the serratus anterior sufficient mechanical advantage to resist the powerful forward and downward pull of the pectoralis minor muscles.

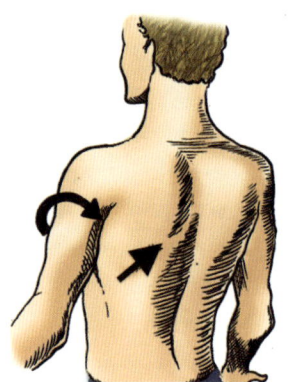

OK! This may seem like a lot to think about every time you move your shoulders. It is, however, what it takes to properly align the shoulders and integrate them with the thoracic spine, as well as to create the necessary foundation for the head and neck. Every asana engages each step of shoulder integration.

> The following checklist for shoulder alignment principles can be remembered or made into a mantra. Memorizing them is well worth the effort.
>
> - Lengthen side body rib cage
> - Inflate the upper chest
> - Internally rotate and draw head of arm bones back
> - Lengthen collarbones and glide shoulder blades toward the spine
> - Externally rotate arm bones deep in their sockets
> - Press the lower tips of the scapulae onto the back

The following asana demonstrate how to apply the shoulder alignment principles.

Vasisthasana — Side Plank Pose

In Side Plank Pose, keep the arms in a "T" position while supporting the torso. Lengthen the clavicles and glide the shoulder blades onto the back. Once in the full posture, externally rotate the humeral heads and press the tips of the shoulder blades forward.

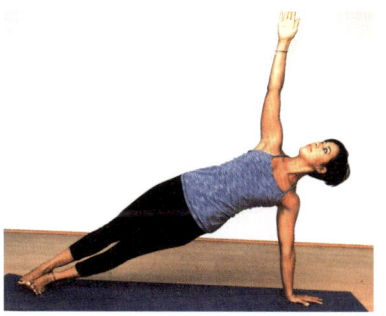

Side Plank Pose has more in common with Downward Facing Dog than Plank Pose and would be better called Side-Facing Downward Dog. If the transition into Side Plank is from Plank Pose, lift firmly from the hips, stacking one over the other. The lower arm is not directly vertical under the shoulder. That position would place the force of the pose on the shoulder's weakest point, anterior and inferior. Instead, the arm is forward, as it would be in Downward Facing Dog. This position of the arm retains the integrity of the "T" formation between the lower arm and the shoulder.

Gomukhasana — Cow Face Pose

A tendency in **Gomukhasana** is to roll the shoulders forward when attempting to bring the arms behind the back. To prevent this, begin the pose by inflating the chest and lengthening the collarbones, keeping the shoulders back as much as possible. Internally rotate the shoulders and draw the head of the arm bones back. Once the hands are clasped or the stretch of the arms has reached its limit, externally rotate the shoulder joints. The final effort of the posture is to draw the lower tips of the shoulder blades forward onto the back ribs. Avoid jutting the lower rib cage forward.

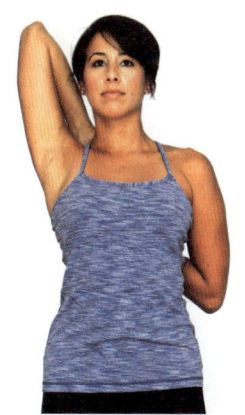

Seated Spinal Twist

Students often roll or drop their shoulders forward when attempting to bind the hands or grasp the knee. Instead, square and lengthen the collarbones. Expand the chest forward while firmly keeping the head of the humerus bones back.

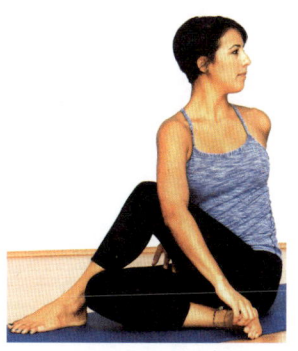

Shown as incorrect

Bhujangasana assist   Cobra assist

There are many methods to assist a Cobra Pose. In the one illustrated, a strap is placed around the back of the student, crossing through the center of the scapulae. The assistant, seated in front of the student, holds the ends of the strap and uses his feet to firmly support and press back the humeral heads and encourage the collarbones to lengthen. The student expands her chest forward to complete the pose.

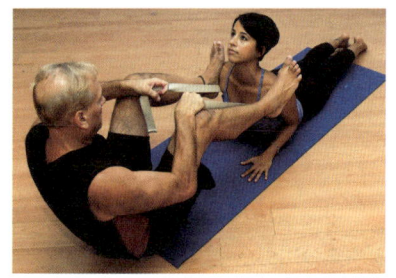

Chatarunga Dandasana   Four Limbs Staff Pose

Chatarunga Dandasana may seem challenging for yoga students who assume that great arm strength is required to suspend the torso in a straight position. Although strength does play a role, the pose is accomplished primarily by distributing more of the body weight forward (toward the head) over the fulcrum created by the forearms and hands. Shoulder integration is required to create a strong pose and not to injure the shoulders. Hold the elbows firmly to the side body ribs and draw the humeral heads deep into the shoulder sockets. Lengthen the collarbones and draw the shoulder blades firmly onto the back body. Additional alignment instructions for the arms will be presented in Chapter 32.

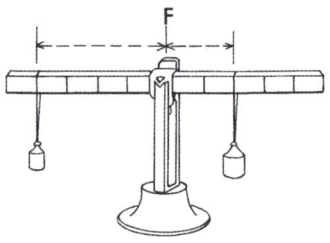

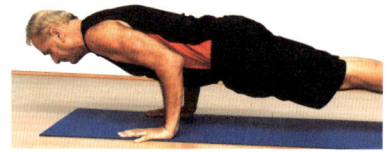

The most common misalignment in Chatarunga is for the elbows to spread apart and lose contact with the side body. This forces the shoulders to roll forward and drop toward the floor. The splayed elbow position pushes the humeral heads in the anterior-inferior direction, where the shoulders are most unstable. If Chatarunga is practiced repetitively in this fashion, the shoulder's tendons and ligaments become overstretched and weakened, predisposing the shoulder joints to dislocation.

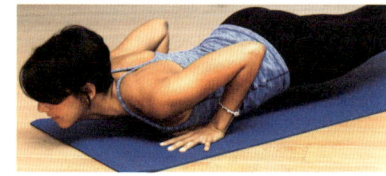

Shown as incorrect

32 The Upper Extremities

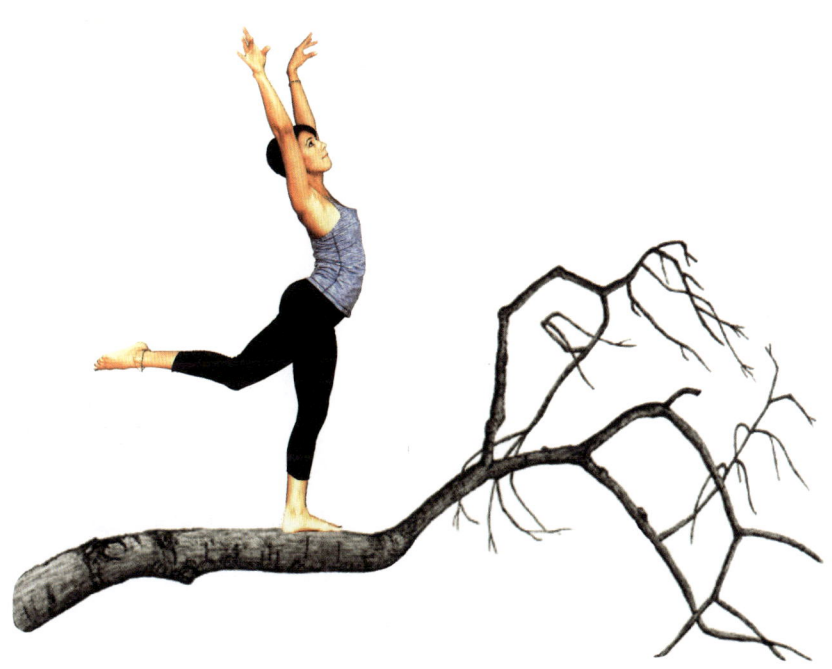

Out on a limb

Whether performing an arm-balancing pose or simply standing in Tadasana, the arms maintain a structural relationship with the shoulders. The upper extremities are considered an extension of the shoulders and the principles of shoulder integrative alignment are established before the arms are engaged.

There are numerous muscles that attach from the shoulders to the arms. The two muscles most associated with the arms are the biceps and the triceps. The *biceps brachii* (from the Latin *biceps,* meaning *two heads*, and *brachii,* meaning *arm*) flexes the elbow. The *triceps brachii* extends it. The biceps has two heads (muscle bundles), and the triceps, three heads.

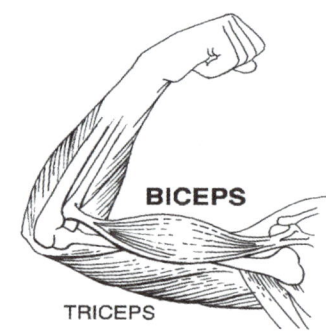

Pre-requisites for upper extremity principles

Apply these general principles, some already introduced in Chapter 5, before engaging the nuances of arm alignment:

Move from the core, using the shortest levers

Lift the arm, using muscles that are as close to the shoulder as possible. This action enlists the strong upper torso muscles to raise the arms. When lifting the arms from the side body, yogis often unconsciously use and overstrain the forearm muscles and hands, even though there is no mechanical way to lift the arms from these outer body parts.

Bones draw to the midline, muscles extend out

When yoga teachers tell students to "reach out the arms," they are instructing students to move from their extremities, not their core. Instead, draw the arm bones into the shoulder joint and toward the core while the muscles extend outward. This approach ensures core muscle involvement and prevents strain on the muscle tendons.

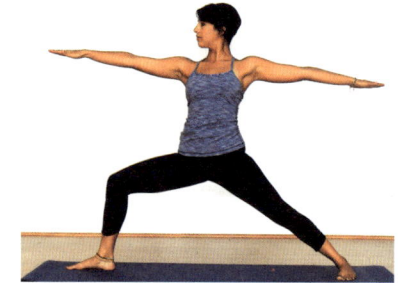

When extending the arms in Warrior Two Pose, students often forcefully contract their forearm muscles, rather than working from their core. Preferably, use the middle deltoid, supraspinatus, and latissimus dorsi muscles to support the arms. Draw the arm bones into the shoulders; then extend the arm muscles outward.

Triceps muscle rotates toward the midline

When the arms are at the side of the torso, as in **Chaturanga Dandasana**, roll the back of each arm (triceps) medially, toward the side body ribs. When the arms are overhead, as in **Urdvha Hastasana**, rotate the triceps muscles forward towards the ears.

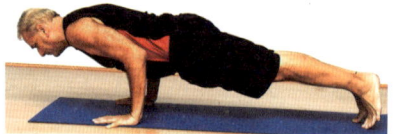

Chaturanga Dandasana

Use the triceps muscle to extend the elbow

It is common for the elbows to inadvertently bend in poses where the arms are held overhead. If students' arms are not straight in poses that call for straight arms, they should more fully engage the triceps muscle. "Draw the outer elbow toward the armpit" is a helpful verbal cue for triceps extension.[1]

Straightening the arms often requires added effort. This is because the triceps muscle is most efficient when the arms are flexed and the elbows are bent 20-30°. This is the position of power and readiness, what is needed, for example, to swing an axe. Muscles at rest do not lengthen beyond their most efficient position without additional effort.

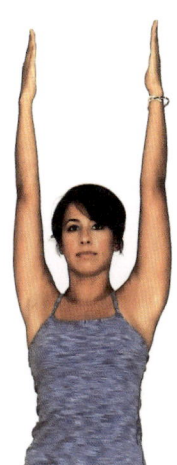

Samasthiti – equal tension and balance

Maintain subtle, energetic balance in length and tension between the entire *radial* (thumb) and *ulnar* (small finger) surfaces of the arm. When the arms are weight bearing, as they are in Downward Facing Dog, the floor provides a firm foundation from which equal and balanced energy can be established. When the arms float freely, as in **Urdvha Hastasana**, the quality of Samasthiti must be brought to the pose though actual muscular action. Samasthiti in the arms helps bring Samasthiti to the rest of the body. It greatly improves the integrative alignment of the chest, upper back, and shoulders.

Try This:

Stand in Urdvha Hastasana. Notice whether the energetic and muscular tension along each side of each arm is the same or is different. Once that is determined, lengthen through the ulnar (small finger) side of the arms. This causes the front of the body to lengthen as well. Next, lengthen the radial (thumb) side of the arms. This causes the back to round and the chest to sink. Most yoga students need to energetically lengthen through the ulnar side of their arms more than the radial side.

Lengthen through the ulnar side of the arms to draw the triceps muscles toward the midline, to open the chest and to establish Samasthiti in upper extremities.

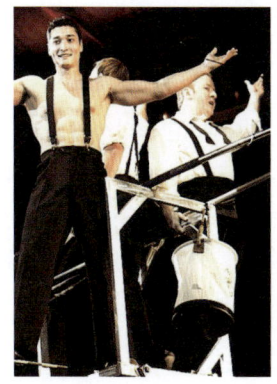

Ta da!

The elbow

Mobility of the elbow is vital to the overall function of the arm and to the specific action of moving the hand to the mouth. The elbow consists of three bones joined together into a simple hinge joint. The humerus (upper arm) joins and articulates with the *radius* and *ulna* of the forearm. Because elbow motion is integrated with the overall mobility of the arm and shoulder, the elbow joint appears to be capable of moving in multiple directions. Extensive crisscrossed ligaments, however, bind the radius to the ulna and prevent any movement of the elbow joint other than *flexion* and *extension*.

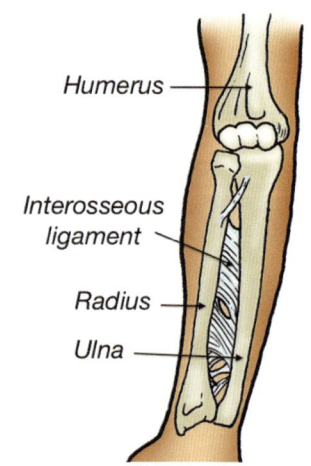

The primary forearm bone involved with elbow motion is the ulna. It forms an intricate hinge joint with the humerus. The radius, being minimally involved in elbow movement, is free to rotate the forearm and wrist, regardless of the position of the arm or the degree of elbow flexion or extension.

Elbow flexion

Elbow flexion is measured from a straight-arm position (zero degree point) as it bends toward the shoulder, reaching its full range at 140° to 160°.

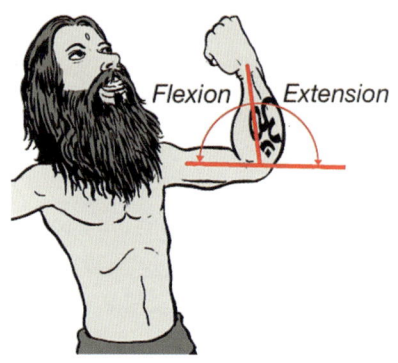

Elbow extension

Technically, the elbow joint does not extend and is only capable of flexion. In other words, no natural movement extends the elbow beyond the position of the arm being straight. Movement that goes beyond straight is considered *hyperextension* and not extension. When the elbow straightens from a flexed position, commonly referred to as *extension*. Physiologists specifically call this movement "relative" extension. The same considerations are presented with the design of the knee joint.

To prevent the elbow from hyperextending, there is a large boney hook on the posterior part of the ulna, called the *olecranon process*, which locks into the back of the humerus as the elbow straightens.

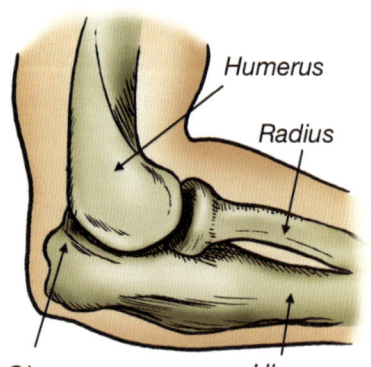

Hyperextension of the elbow

Some flexible yoga students habitually hyperextend their elbows, moving them beyond the straight-arm position. This is usually the result of overly flexible ligaments allowing the joints to exceed a mechanically desirable range. If hyperextension occurs habitually, the ligaments become weakened, causing muscle tendon strain and increasing the likelihood of degenerative damage to the elbow.

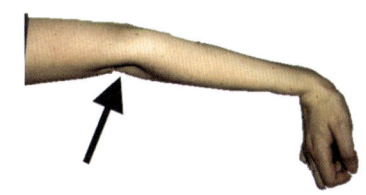

Use the following steps to remedy hyperextension in arm balancing poses:

- Micro-bend the elbows.
- Squeeze the elbows from side-to-side (radius-to-ulna) using their accessory muscles.
- Turn the hands slightly inward.
- Counter-rotate the arms (instructions to follow on next page) to stabilize the normalized elbow position.

The "eyes" of the elbows

The inner elbow creases are sometimes called the *eyes* of the elbows. In Downward Facing Dog and other arm balancing poses, the elbows' eyes face inward, pointing toward the clock positions of ten to two o'clock.

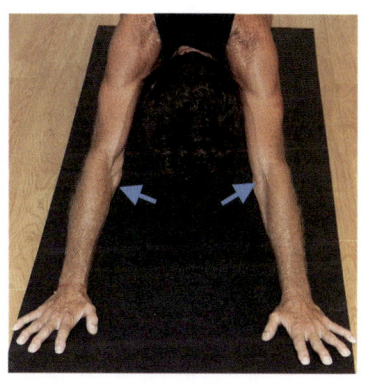

Students who hyperextend their elbows should face the eyes of the elbows directly toward each other, looking straight across, "eye-to-eye". The greater the degree of hyperextension, the more direct the elbow creases should face each other.

The forearm

As stated, the radius plays only a minor role in elbow motion. It is, however, the primary rotator of the forearm and wrist. The ulna does not participate in wrist rotation, but essentially remains stationary as the radius arcs around it. The forearm can move into *pronation* (palm facing down) and *supination* (palm facing up).

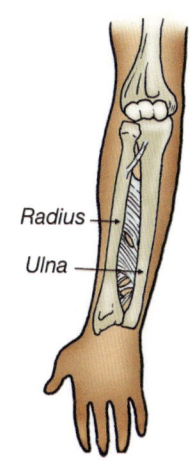

The full range of forearm rotation is 180°. In yoga and in daily activities, the forearm may seem to have a far greater range. Many students can rotate the forearm in what looks like a full circle of nearly 360°. The additional range, however, comes from movement of the shoulder.

Upper extremity alignment

As with the legs, there are alignment principles for the arms that provide flexibility, stability, and are therapeutic for rehabilitating injuries. Because the arms can find neutral in many positions, describing their orientation in terms of what is the front and what is the back can be challenging.

Lift the forearms

The ventral forearm (palm-side) and wrist move posterior. In Downward Facing Dog, lift the underside of the forearms and wrists to prevent injury and align the arms. Piano students and computer geeks already know the value of this instruction.

Middle fingers in line with the seam of pants

- Individuals may have a different ratio of the lengths of the upper and lower arm bones. With the arms at the side in **Tadasana**, however, correct alignment for most students is the same: the middle fingers line up with the outer seam of the pants.

- If the back (dorsum) of the hand faces forward, it indicates that the shoulders are rolled forward.

- Tension should be equal on the thumb and small finger side of arms. If the thumb side of the arm is longer, the front of the body has become shortened and tight. **Urdvha Hastasana** (Upward Hands Pose) is a good pose for observing these differences.

These subtle hand positions are good indicators of shoulder integrative alignment.

Arm counter-rotation provides stability

For the greatest support and stabilization of the arms, rotate the forearm radially (in the direction of the thumb) while externally rotating the upper arm (triceps toward the midline). The effect is a "towel-twisting" action that locks the elbow without hyperextension and protects the joints and soft tissues from injury. The musculature of the entire arm is more efficient and powerful when this action is engaged.

> **Technically Speaking**
>
> The ventral surface of the body is the front or abdominal side. With the forearm, ventral is the palm side since the palms face forward in the anatomically neutral posture. The dorsum is the back of the body (think of dorsal fin) and the back of the hand.

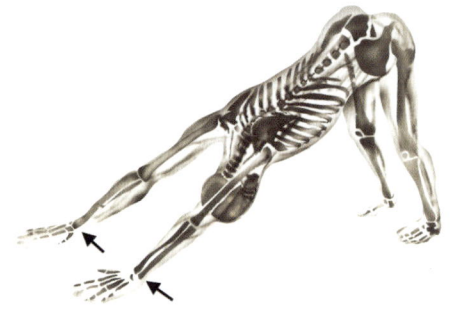

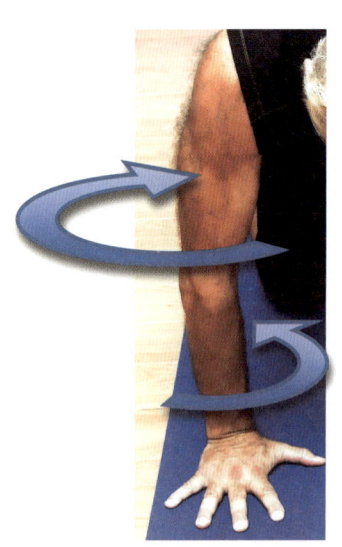

Arm alignment with the side body ribs

When aligning the legs, the hips are vertical over the ankles and the knees "find their place". The same holds true for the arms. The elbows are not forced into a straight-line alignment between the shoulders and hands, but instead, come into position effortlessly after the center of the wrists align vertically with the shoulders.

In postures where the arm is bent, the "end" of the extremity is not the hand but the elbow. Whether in **Siddhasana** (Seated Pose) or in the more strenuous **Chaturanga Dandasana**, the elbows are in line with the shoulder and with the side-body rib cage. When shoulder *integrative alignment* is engaged, the elbows come into position without additional effort. Aligning the elbows with the side body ribs is critical for safely performing Chaturanga Dandasana. In the pose, the forearms are vertical, aligned at 90° angles to the upper arm. If the elbows divert from the side body, the integrity of shoulder alignment is lost.

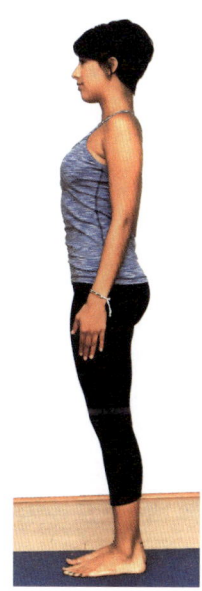

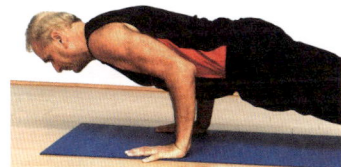

Chaturanga Dandasana

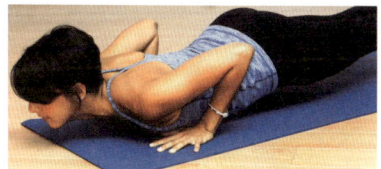

Shown as incorrect

How wide apart are the arms in arm-balancing poses?

In Headstand, Downward Facing Dog Pose, and all other two-handed balancing poses, the center of the wrists align vertically with the outer edge of the shoulders.

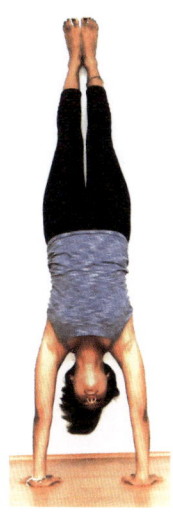

Carrying Angle

Back in medieval times, the peasants who could carry the largest water buckets or bundles of wood were more highly desired, or so the story goes. The further away the forearm deviated from the side of the body, the bigger the bucket that could be carried; hence the name, *carrying angle*. A larger angle is more common for women than men.

Anatomically, degree of angle is determined by the direction of a small impression located at the hinge of the elbow called the *trochlear groove*. A larger angle brings the forearm further away from the body. Larger carrying angles presents challenges in arm balancing poses.

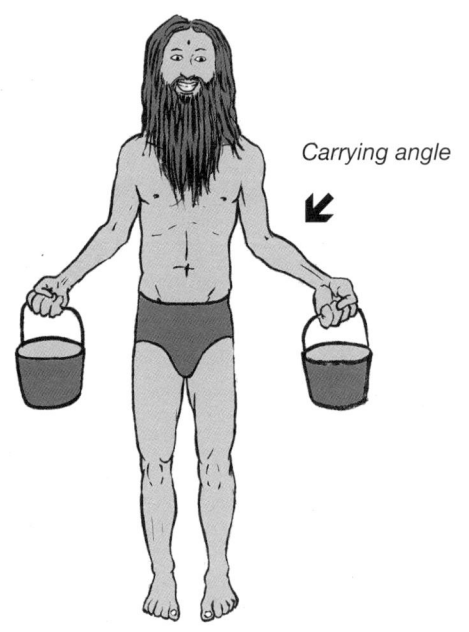

Carrying angle

Carrying on with the carrying angle

When the hands are placed on the mat, an excessive carrying angle causes misalignments throughout the upper extremities. An excessive carrying angle causes the hands to turn inward, the elbows point out and the shoulders roll forward.

To compensate for a large carrying angle, place the hands wider than usual on the mat. Turn the hands outward, toward the small finger side (ulnar deviation).

Elbow hyperextension often accompanies a large carrying angle. If this is the case, still keep the hands wider apart to compensate for the carrying angle. Then, modify for hyperextension by pointing the hands slightly inward and have the elbow creases face directly toward each other.

In the next chapter, the anatomy of the wrist and hand and the alignment of these structures will be explored. Their alignment continues to follow the seamless flow and interdependence of movement that occurs through the rest of the upper extremities and shoulders.

33 The Wrists and Hands

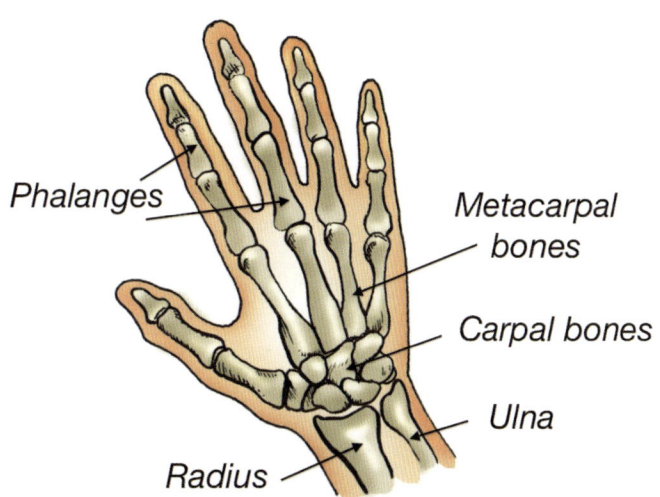

The hands are the extraordinary end users for the combined actions performed by the upper extremities. The hand's ability to hold, seize, and grasp is called *prehension*. It has reached a level of sophistication that has single-handedly elevated the human experience far above the rest of our animal brethren. Not only is the hand a masterful, mechanical apparatus, but also, through touch and feel, the hand provides vast amounts of sensory information to the brain and nervous system.[1]

The anatomy of the wrists and hands is comparable to that of their counterparts of the lower extremities, the ankles and feet. Although there are clear differences between the two regions, alignment strategies are similar. The wrists and hands are being reviewed together in this chapter because their functionality is completely interconnected.

The bones that comprise the wrist are called *carpal bones*, and the bones that form the palm are *metacarpals*. These correspond in the feet to tarsal bones and metatarsals, respectively. The bones of the fingers and toes are called *phalanges*. In the hand, the first phalange, what we call the thumb, is positioned on the heel of the hand instead of in line with the other phalanges, as on the feet.

The carpal bones of the wrist are a tightly-fitted group of eight, irregularly-shaped bones that arrange in two distinct lines: a *distal row*, consisting of bones close to the hand that articulate with the metacarpals; and a *proximal row*, bones that adjoin the radius and ulna.

Mechanically, the two rows perform slightly different actions. The distal row takes a greater role in wrist extension while the proximal row's role is more pronounced in flexion.

- Distal row: extension
- Proximal row: flexion

This information, which may seem somewhat obscure, becomes a useful tool when trying to pinpoint the cause of wrist pain and devise yoga therapy to resolve it.

Wrist and hand relationship

The centerline of the hand passes through the phalanges of the third finger and the third metacarpal. It runs perpendicular to the wrist crease, with which it forms an inverted "T".

In arm-balancing asana, such as Downward Facing Dog, align the wrist creases parallel to the front of the yoga mat and put less emphasis on the position of the centerline of the hands.

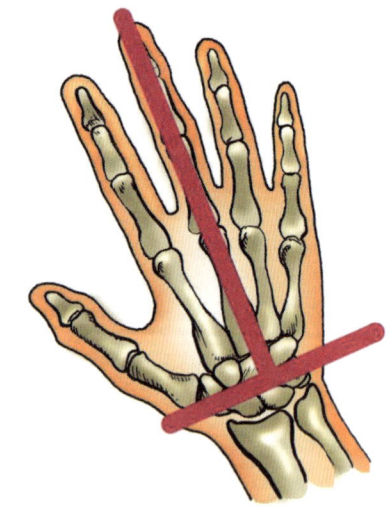

Anatomical terminology for the hands

- Ventral or palmar - refers to the palm of the hand
- Dorsal - refers to the back of the hand
- Supination - the palm turning upward
- Pronation - the palm turning downward

Wrist wrap

A fibrous band of connective tissue wraps around the wrist. It is called the *transverse carpal ligament*; also referred to as the *flexor retinaculum*. On the palmar side, the band overlaps a major nerve supply to the hand, the *median nerve*. It anchors the flexor tendons of the ventral forearm close to the forearm bones and wrist. The transverse carpal ligament tightly wraps around the carpal bones, preventing them from spreading apart.

Many of the muscles that provide movement of the hand originate in the forearm. They are either long muscles originating near the elbow, or short muscles that arise mid-forearm, closer to the wrist. Small interosseous muscles (the muscles between the finger bones) provide the more finely tuned, detailed movements of the hands.

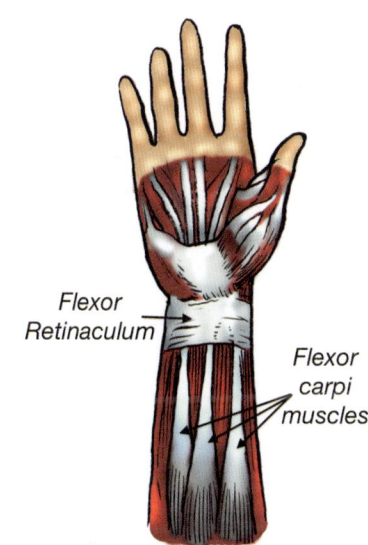

Arch of the palm

Comparing the inner and outer heels of the hand, it is easily observed that the muscle and flesh on the heel of the thumb (*thenar*) is more pronounced than the heel on the small finger side (*hypothenar*).

The space formed between the two heels is referred to as the *arch of the palm*. This arch can best be viewed by placing the hands in Namaste´ turned upside down. When all four heels come together, the space created at the center of the wrists is approximately the size of a kidney bean.

When the hands are weight-bearing, press both heels evenly into the ground and maintain the arch. Since the hypothenar heel is smaller and less developed than the thenar heel, additional pressure may be needed on this outer heel to create balance across the palm. Pressure on the outer heel of the hand stabilizes the shoulders by activating shoulder external rotation.

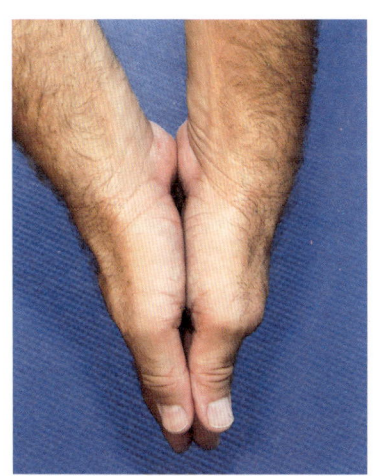

The *transverse* (metacarpo-phalangeal) arch, formed by the knuckles, also supports the palm by toning and vaulting the palmar fascia and musculature in a fashion similar to the transverse arch of the feet. Apply pressure evenly to the bottom of each knuckle of the arch.

A handprint exerting correct pressure resembles an upside down horseshoe.

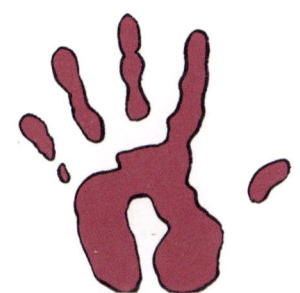

Weight bearing alignment of the hand

As with the feet, there is an ideal sequence for pressing the hands into the floor in order to best engage the arches:

- Index finger knuckle (metacarpal-phalangeal joint -1)
- Heel of thumb (thenar heel -2)
- Outer knuckle (metacarpal-phalangeal joint -3)
- Outer heel of the hand (hypothenar heel -4)

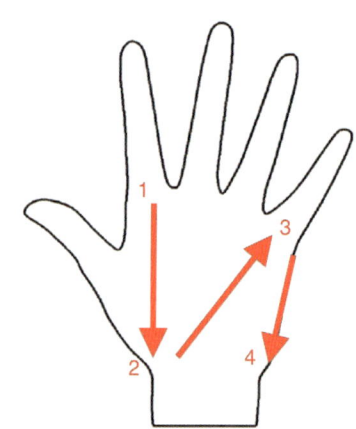

Additional refinements in hand placement

The precision of hand placement is important, especially for the rehabilitation of the wrist or hand. After the four points of the hands are grounded, the following instructions provide additional refinements in the alignment of the hands:

- Press the remaining knuckles down, spreading and distributing weight evenly across the transverse arch.
- The pad of each fingertip (distal phalange) presses fully to the floor.
- The nail bed of each finger (thumb excluded) is flat and level with equal pressure placed on both the inner and outer sides of each finger.
- The fingers do not spread apart, but instead extend straight out from the knuckles.
- The joints within each finger, the *inter-phalangeal* joints, are lifted, making the fingers appear claw-like.

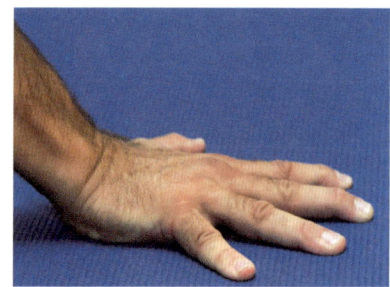

Keep the foundation stable

Once a foundation is established in the hands, it remains stable, well grounded, and unaltered. The palm remains vaulted and muscularly engaged; the hand being supported by its heels and transverse arch. The fingers act as "outriggers" that can apply subtle pressure from the finger pads to re-establish a stable foundation as the body shifts.

Spider-fingers

The wrist position that produces maximum strength and efficiency is 40° in extension and 15° in ulna deviation (flexed toward the ulna). This configuration is referred to as *spider-fingers*. With the wrist in this position, the arches are well formed, the fingers curved, and body weight distributed evenly across each finger pad. For most types of injuries to the wrist and hands, *spider-fingers* is an excellent therapy.

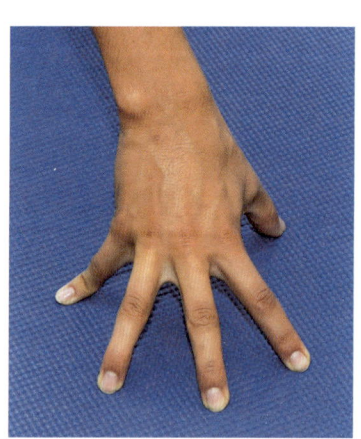

Flexion of the wrist

Wrist (palmar) flexion is not a position that can support significant weight. Rather, it is used in gripping and clasping. Palmar flexion is often seen in traditional Indian dance and hand Mudra practice. Flex the wrist by drawing in the transverse carpal ligament. This deepens the wrist crease and increases muscle tone in the arches of the palm. Pianists and computer keyboard workers will recognize this vaulting of the wrist as necessary for performing well and avoiding injury.

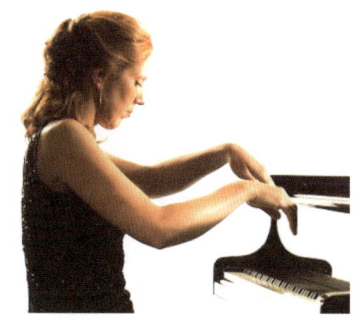

Wrist extension – less than you think

Wrist extension, called *dorsi-flexion*, is the bending back of the hand. In arm-balancing postures such as Handstand or **Urdhva Dhanurasana** (Upward Bow Pose), it may appear that the wrists need to extend 90° or beyond to carry the full weight of the asana. Anatomically, however, the wrist's actual range of motion is 85°, both for flexion and extension. This range is further reduced when the wrist either pronates or supinates.[2] In spite of the apparent ease with which some yoga students take their wrists beyond anatomical limits, especially in extension, it is not safe or healthy for the wrists.

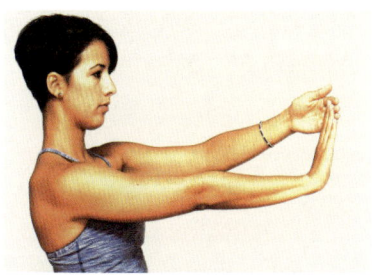

Hyperextension overstretches and weakens the ligaments of the wrist. It causes the carpal bones to widen and potentially collapse the *carpal tunnel*, crushing the median nerve. The tendons of the forearm muscles are also held firmly to the wrist by these same ligaments. If the ligaments become loose, the forearm tendons lift away from the wrist, causing increased strain and tendonitis. Hyperextension also often causes the arches of the palm to collapse and reduces the intrinsic strength of the hands. Wrist hyperextension, however, is very easy to commit during yoga practice. In fact, students unaware of the anatomical design of the wrists often try to force the wrists to extend to a full right angle (90°). For flexible students, hyperextension is easy and therefore may feel natural, making these students unaware of the damage they are doing to their wrists.

Asana should avoid exploiting the loose structural design of the wrists and practice Asteya (non-stealing). When carefully observing even the most advanced arm-balancing poses, one can see that it is not necessary for the wrists to be at a full right angle (90°).

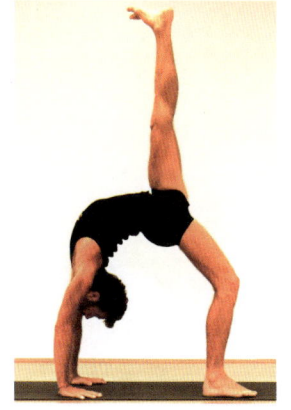

Urdhva Dhanurasana (Upward Bow Pose) places substantial force on the wrists. It challenges yoga students with highly mobile wrists to resist extending them beyond the normal limit. It is common for students to complain of wrist pain immediately after performing this pose. Although the Upward Bow Pose requires the hands to rest flat on the floor, the wrists can still maintain an angle of extension that is close to 85°. The greater the chest expands forward and the shoulder blades press from the back, the less strain will be transferred to the wrists. Utilizing the shoulder alignment principles, in fact, provides the extra degrees needed for the wrists to create a flat foundation in the pose without the wrists having to exceed 85° of extension.

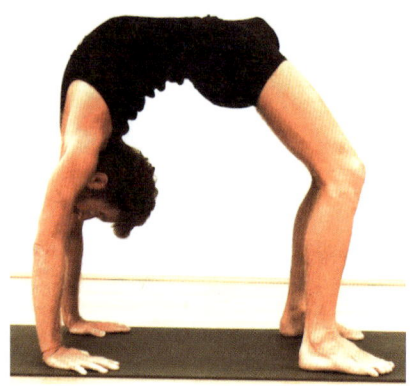

> **Reducing strain on the wrists**
> - Hug the transverse carpal ligament firmly to the wrist. The same muscular action increases the vaulting of the arches of the palm and strengthens *spider-fingers*.
> - Keep wrist range of motion to less than 85°.
> - Bring the shoulders into full integrative alignment by drawing the humeral heads fully into the shoulders and the shoulder blades onto the back.

Carpal Tunnel Syndrome

A frequent injury to the wrist is *Carpal Tunnel Syndrome* (CTS). Reported complaints range from 5% in the general population to nearly 50% in occupations that require repetitive movement, firm grasping, or exposure to constant vibration.[3,4] Yoga practice can be challenging and possibly aggravating for students who have this injury.

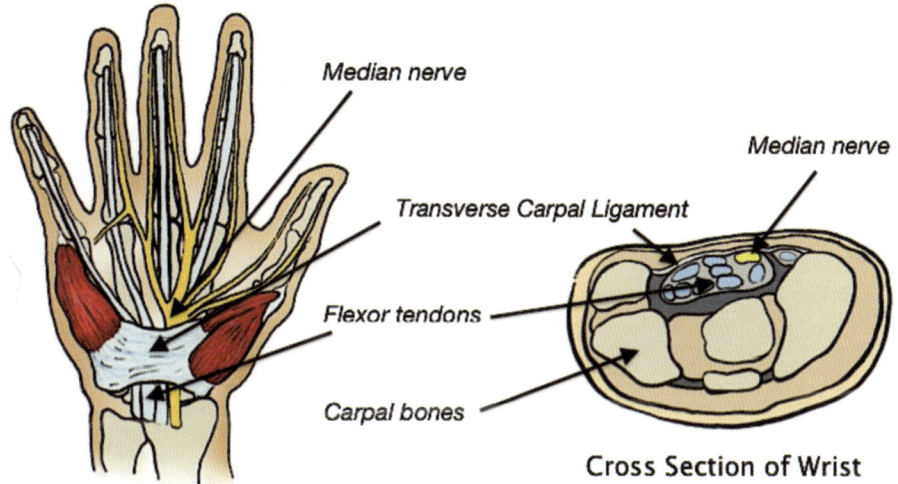

Cross Section of Wrist

Carpal tunnel syndrome often occurs when the transverse carpal ligament becomes traumatized and overstretched. The weakened ligament causes the carpal bones to shift from their tightly aligned configuration and spread apart. This collapses the tunnel between the bones on the inner wrist and entraps the median nerve. Inflammation often engorges the limited space and further compresses the nerve. Complaints of pain, numbness, or weakness in the hand and fingers are common. If Carpal Tunnel Syndrome is suspected, there are some general diagnostic signs of the condition. CTS symptoms increase if the wrist is held firmly in flexion for more than a minute of time. Tapping on the inner wrist can produce sharp or tingling pain. It is important to neurologically test the function of the median nerve to accurately determine CTS. Even with medical testing, however, CTS is easily misdiagnosed. Carpal Tunnel Syndrome is an overused label for many other painful conditions of wrist and hand.

In addition to securing the carpal bones, the transverse carpal ligament also secures the forearm tendons, which can become inflamed, adhered, or damaged. In some instances, the cause of apparent CTS is actually *tendonitis*. Other localized conditions confused with CTS are bone fractures of the wrist and arthritis of the thumb. With these other conditions, there is usually no significant nerve compression or positive findings in neurological testing. Additional causes of CTS-like symptoms originate in the central nervous system and brain. These conditions are rare and it is best to first consider issues localized in the wrist.

If carpal tunnel syndrome is present, yoga students often find postures such as Downward Facing Dog and the Handstand painful to perform. The alignment principles presented earlier in this chapter - sequencing of hand placement, guarding against wrist hyperextension, and maintaining the palmar arches - are useful for limiting trauma or rehabilitating the wrists if damage has already occurred. In poses where it is possible, engaging *spider-fingers* is very therapeutic. As in all situations, the overall asana must be correctly aligned. If a position that greatly reduces or eliminates the symptoms cannot be found, asana should be stopped.

The following two postures are therapeutic for Carpal Tunnel Syndrome, tendonitis, and wrist strengthening, in general.

Sphinx Pose

Sphinx Pose is a relatively easy posture that rehabilitates the wrists and is good for the upper extremities in general. Activate, integrate and correctly align the hands, wrists, shoulders, and upper spine. Press the hands down into all four corners. This causes the wrist creases to lift, which, as noted, is the best position for strengthening injured ligaments and tendons. Sphinx Pose is an excellent posture to use as yoga therapy when full arm-balances are not possible or if the severity of injury or pain is great.

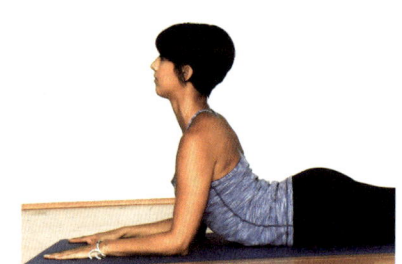

"Popeye™ arms" therapy

This yoga therapy pose helps relieve strain and discomfort in the wrists and the flexor tendons. It is especially relieving after performing asana such as **Urdhva Dhanurasana** (Upward Bow Pose).

Bring the arms straight out to the sides. Bend the elbows to 90° and fully flex the wrists. Straighten the elbows and arms again, keeping the wrists in flexion the entire time.

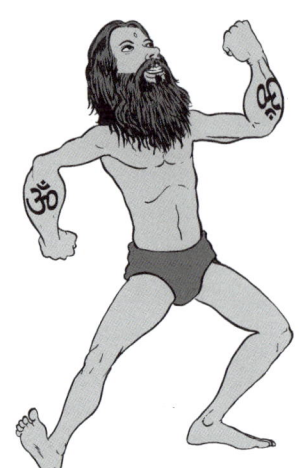

> Pain and injury are our two greatest teachers.
> If we listen carefully to the advice they give us, yoga will help us heal.

34 The Head and Neck

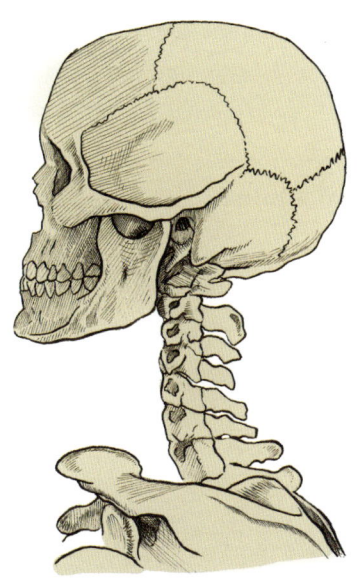

For most of us, the reflection looking back each morning from the bathroom mirror represents our identity. What we see - the head and neck - is the most expressive and interactive region of our body. The body below is something from which we feel more disassociated, perhaps only a framework for displaying clothes. Along with the hands, our head and neck are the way we collaborate with the world.

Yoga practice is an opportunity for the rest of the body to become animated, conscious, and articulate. Keeping the head and neck from dominating our movements requires awareness and applying the principles of integrative alignment designed for the body below. Of course the head and neck have their own alignment principles that must be engaged so they too can function seamlessly with the body as a whole.

A balancing act

Like a bowling ball balanced on a stick, the average adult head weighs 9-11 pounds, propped up on a stack of seven cervical vertebrae that each weigh in at 2-4 ounces each. These seven vertebrae form an anteriorly convex curve (lordosis) that helps provide stability. The shoulders provide the primary foundation for the head and neck. When the head, neck and shoulders are in alignment, the weight of the head can be safely supported.

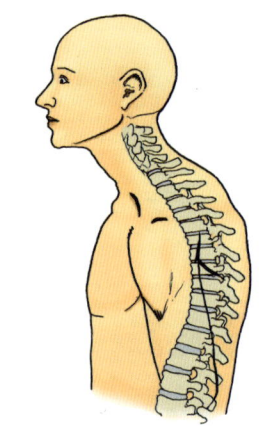

Incorrect, forward-positioned head

The cervical spine

The cervical spine comprises seven small vertebrae. The obliquely facing facet joints of these vertebrae are ideally oriented for the multi-directional movements of the neck. The lower five cervical vertebrae have the same structure as the rest of the spinal vertebrae while the top two, the *atlas* and *axis*, are specialized in both design and function.

Ranges of motion in the cervical spine:	
• Flexion	40°
• Extension	75°
• Lateral flexion	35-45° bilaterally
• Rotation	45-50° bilaterally

Atlas, the first cervical vertebra (C1)

Just as the mythological god Atlas braces the earth upon his upper back and shoulder, the *atlas* vertebra supports the base of the skull on its upper surface. The atlas is the only vertebra that does not have an anterior body. Instead, it is a ring of bone with two lateral masses affixed on opposing anterior and posterior arcs of the ring.

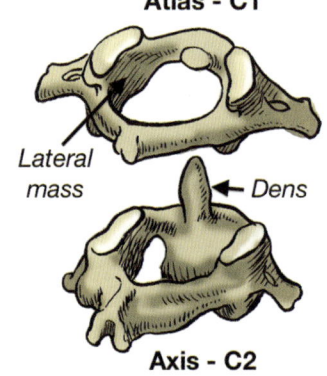

The Axis (C2)

The second cervical vertebra, the axis, is the neck's swivel point, where most rotation occurs. A large, anterior, tooth-like process called the *odontoid process*, or the *dens* (Latin for *tooth*), acts as a pivot point on which the atlas rotates. The brain stem, the oldest and most vital portion of the nervous system, descends from the skull to the C2 vertebra. Improper movement or misalignment of C1 and C2 can interfere with brain stem signals and impair the basic body functions that they control, including those of the heart and lungs.

The anterior compartment of the neck

The majority of nerves and blood vessels that serve the head and upper extremities pass through the anterior lower region of the neck, a region referred to as the *anterior compartment*. Shoulder integrative alignment principles are essential for keeping the anterior compartment from collapsing and compressing these delicate structures. Broadening the chest and lengthening the collarbones keep the anterior compartment open.

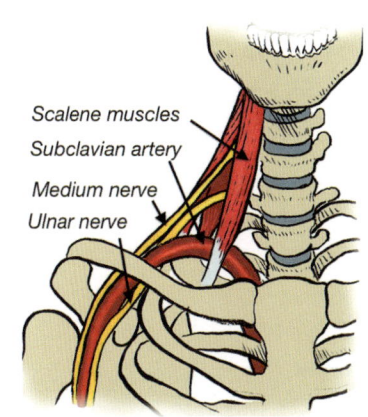

Can you see the collarbones?

As presented in Chapter 30, a deep, visible recess above protruded collarbones is a sign that the shoulders have rounded forward and lost their integrative alignment. This misalignment collapses the anterior compartment and can cause damage to the blood vessels and nerves, particularly when the arms and shoulders are moving at the far end of their ranges.[1]

Foundation for the head and neck

The shoulders and upper thoracic spine create the foundation for the head and neck. The muscles that support and move the head and neck anchor to the shoulders and upper back. All strategies for aligning the head and neck, therefore, begin by setting this foundation using the principles of *shoulder integrative alignment*.

Head and neck posture

- Align the head and neck with the central axis of the body.
- Align the center of the ear canal with the center point of the middle deltoid muscle. The middle deltoid muscle forms a cap over the outer shoulder joint. The jaw joint (tempromandibular joint or TMJ) abuts the ear canal and also aligns over the shoulders.
- Align the posterior fontanel of the skull vertically over the inner ear canals, completing the vertical alignment through the body's central axis.

> A healthy cervical curve positions the ears directly over the shoulders

Head games

Teachers often lead students into postures using instructions such as, "turn your head", or "look left or right", encouraging initiation of the postures from the perspective of the head. A more precise asana instruction would be to move from the neck and let the head follow. An even more precise instruction would be to begin movement by turning from the upper chest.

Managing the cervical curve

The depth of the cervical curve significantly affects mobility and stability in the cervical spine. A deep curve brings stability but limits mobility. Lengthening the cervical spine creates mobility, but compromises stability. This principle is especially important in Headstand Pose.

> For most yoga students, the ideal cervical curve is one that, when lying in **Savasana,** would comfortably round over a *small-sized lemon*.

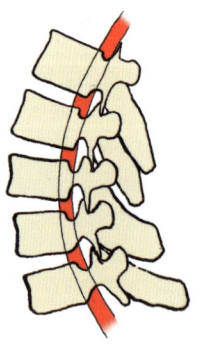 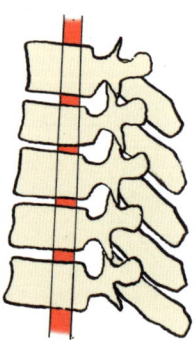

Normal lordotic curve   *Flattened curve*

Excessive extension of the neck compresses the cervical spine and can cause injury to the vertebral discs. In **Matsyasana** (Fish Pose), create the pose by opening the chest and drawing the shoulders onto the back. Keep the throat drawn back to protect the neck from hyperextending.

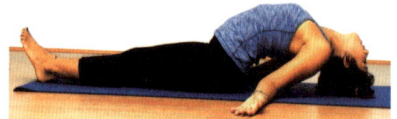

Matsyasana variation

Shoulder Stand, Plow Pose, Bridge Pose

In these asana, none of the vertebrae of the neck or any portion of the spine touches the floor. The pose rests on the back of the skull, the shoulder blades, and the back of the arms. The small lemon-sized cervical curve is maintained and does not flatten. To avoid compressing the cervical spine when coming out of these poses, lengthen the neck but do not flatten it to the floor.

The pencil test:
A pencil should be able to slide under the neck and be retrieved from between the shoulder blades if the spine is properly lifted from the floor in any of these asana. The spinous process of the 7th cervical vertebra, being oversized and prominent, serves as a convenient marker. If space can be maintained below C7, the neck is in a good position. Bruises or calluses are sometimes visible on the skin that covers C7 for yoga students who do not keep the spine properly lifted.

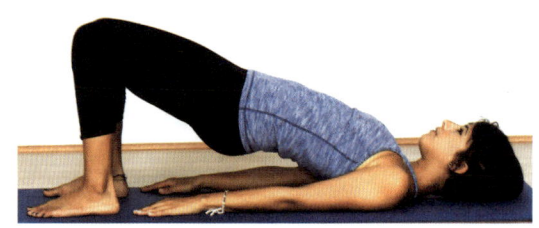

Cervical spine instability

Whiplash injuries occur when the weight of the head thrashes forward and backward rapidly. Whiplash injuries can alter the curve in the neck, straightening or even reversing it. A trauma-induced straight or reversed curve makes supporting the weight of the head extremely difficult. In the initial stages of recovery when the weak and inflamed muscles cannot support the head, an immobilizing, orthopedic collar may be needed.

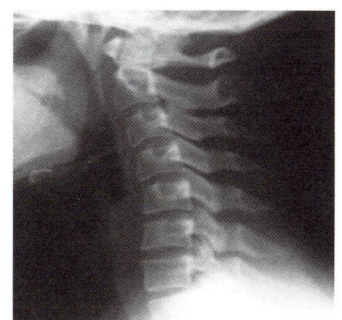
Whiplash

Whiplash is not the only cause of flattened cervical curves. Head-down working positions and poor postural habits, particularly those acquired while the spine was developing, can result in the formation of a flattened curve. In the early phases of a flattened curve, the spine is often hypermobile and unstable. If the correct curve is not established within a number of years, degenerative changes in the spine occur and mobility then becomes limited, an attempt by the body to rectify an unstable state.

Hypermobility

Hypermobility in the neck not only results from direct injury and poor postural habits. It also occurs as a compensation for limited mobility, either in other cervical vertebrae, the thoracic spine, or the shoulders. Limited mobility in the thoracic region is problematic for the neck. A small degree of thoracic joint fixation or the habit of not fully engaging the upper thoracic spine can cause compensatory hypermobility in the cervical spine. The lumbar spine is similarly subject to compensatory hypermobility in response to thoracic-spine immobility.

Is Headstand safe?

In the ongoing debate about the safety of yoga, detractors who believe asana are inherently dangerous, a virtual snake pit of trauma, usually make **Sirsasana** (Headstand) the central point of their argument. To them, Headstand is simply unsafe and end of story. Far on the other side of the argument are those who believe that yoga is divinely inspired and that every asana unconditionally creates health and eternal wisdom. The question of safety in Headstand Pose is important to yoga teachers, students, and health professionals alike. To be clear, there is no answer that is incontrovertibly right, but the question of Headstand safety can be explored in a way that will help individuals make wise personal choices.

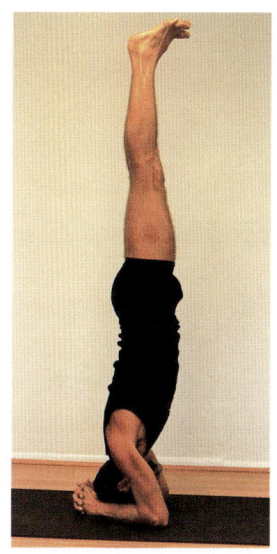

Inversions, in general, have many benefits for the health of the body. Headstand Pose in particular has great value. Inversion postures reverse gravitational stress and its downward drag on the skin and other connective tissues of the body.

Blood circulation in the legs is under constant demand to pump against gravity. Inversions temporarily reduce pressure on the veins, giving the valves and smooth muscles respite from the pressure.

Inversions improve lymphatic drainage. The *lymphatic system* is a secondary circulatory system to the cardio-vascular system. Lymph is a watery fluid created from blood that is located within body tissue. Lymph is important for circulating the white blood cells of the immune system and for carrying away metabolic waste products from the cells. Lymph re-enters the blood system at two points located under the clavicles in the upper chest. Since there is no built in lymphatic pump, inversions can assist in re-circulating the lymph, especially if edema (tissue swelling) is present.

Inversion postures improve balance. While inverting, yogis engage muscles from a different orientation and work from new centers of gravity. For example, when standing, the feet naturally pronate (flatten) and the inner heels drop to the floor. When inverted, the feet are non-weight bearing and the inner heels supinate (sickle). In inversion postures, yoga students can learn to press through the inner heels, an important action for safe knee function.

Headstands increase bone density. Loading weight through the bones of the skull and spine stimulates bone density. In many indigenous cultures, people routinely carry half their body weight on the top of their head. Incidence of bone density loss (osteoporosis) and spinal fractures are very low in these populations, even in locations where nutrition is poor. Compared to epidemic levels of bone loss in Western societies, this finding strongly supports the benefits of axially loading the spine and skull. In cultures where loading weight onto the head is not common practice, Headstand may be the best option.

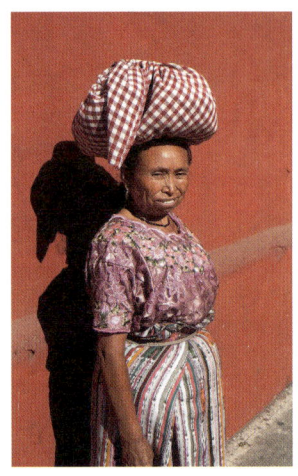

Alignment

Women walking with heavy bundles on their head in indigenous cultures have nearly flawless posture regardless of age. No doubt they learn early in life that precise alignment is necessary to safely carry their loads. Maintaining an "S" curve throughout the entire spine is critical for safely loading the head, neck, and spine. Although one is upside down, Headstand provides the same benefit. With balanced curves and precise shoulder alignment, the spine can best balance the weight of the body. Headstand is essentially a reversed Tadasana (Mountain Pose) and uses all of the alignment principles of Tadasana to equally distribute the weight of the body.

Where is the head placed for Sirsasana One?

A curved spine can support ten times the weight of a straight spine. Too much curve, however, will result in spinal compression. Finding the *sweet spot* for correct head placement is essential in keeping Headstand safe and therapeutic.

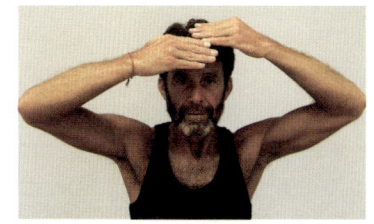

The best method to determine the sweet spot is for the student to place the top of their head against a wall in **Ardha Uttanasana** while an assistant observes the point of contact that best established the cervical and lumbar curves.

If assistance for Headstand is not possible, a reliable spot for head placement is approximately twelve finger-widths from the tip of the nose. If the cervical curve is flatter than normal, then the point of contact for the head is closer to the forehead by one or two finger-widths. Moving the point on the head forward causes the cervical curve to deepen by shifting the center of gravity forward. This adjusted position can rehabilitate a flattened cervical curve and help develop a more desired arc. Conversely, if the cervical curve is already too deep, the contact point on the head moves an extra finger-width or two back toward the center of the skull.

The rest of the foundation in **Sirsasana One** comes from arm placement. The three points of contact - the skull and the two elbows - form three corners of an equilateral triangle. The ulnar edge of each forearm presses firmly into the mat, acting as long extensions of the elbows. The wrists remain perpendicular to the floor and the palms firmly cup and support the skull.

Considerations for the Headstand

For yoga students with a healthy cervical spine, Headstand and its variations are beneficial and belong in a personal practice. Receiving instruction and assistance while learning these poses is invaluable. There are a few conditions, however, that make most inversions contra-indicated.

- Glaucoma, retinal detachment, or any condition where intraocular pressure is increased.
- Uncontrolled high blood pressure.
- Low blood pressure. This can cause a student to faint and fall out of the pose, which could lead to potential injury.
- Any condition where the vertebral or cerebral artery blood flow is compromised, such as advanced atherosclerosis.
- Spinal disc prolapse or advanced degenerative disc disease.
- Spinal arthritis that has produced significant degeneration or severe bone loss.
- Acute inner ear or sinus infections.
- Menstruation. Some traditions of yoga caution headstand practice during menstruation or pregnancy. Medicals professionals have yet to determine the basis for this prohibition.

Musculature of the neck

The head's center of gravity is slightly forward of the body's central axis. This can be experienced when falling asleep while sitting and "nodding off". When the neck muscles release, the head drops to the chest. To compensate for this naturally anterior position of the head, the muscles of the upper back and neck, particularly the trapezius muscles, develop to be stronger than their anterior counterparts. This pattern of muscle development predisposes the neck muscles to residual tension, possibly triggering vestigial memories from our evolutionary past where the trapezius muscles raised the hairs on the back.

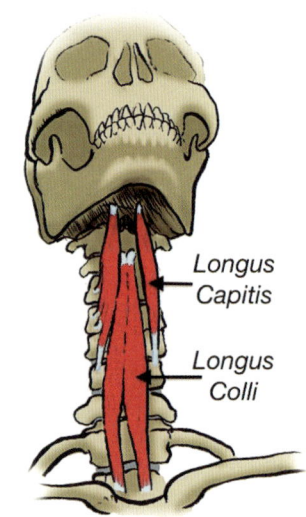

The muscles that maintain the cervical curve are the sterno-cleido-mastoid (SCM), scalenes, rectus capitus, and longus colli.

The *longus colli* is the primary muscle that straightens the neck from a curved position. It also stabilizes the cervical curve, helping to maintain its neutral position. Engaging the longus colli protects the neck from hyperextension and compression. To engage the longus colli, simply draw the throat back. The longus colli and many of the muscles of the neck are engaged by aligning a small, horseshoe-shaped bone suspended within the muscles of the anterior neck called the *hyoid bone*.

The hyoid bone

The *hyoid bone* is often unknown to yoga students. It is located in the center of the throat and is the only structural bone in the human body that is non-articular, meaning it does not attach directly to any other bones.

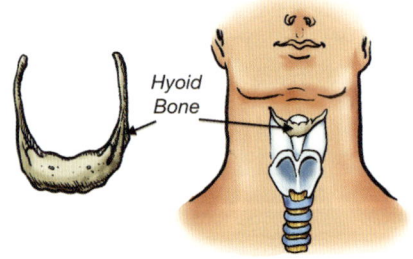

The hyoid bone anchors muscular attachments from the tongue to the larynx (voice box) and is involved, therefore, with the intricate movements of the tongue. The position of the hyoid bone influences the swallowing mechanism and the function of the tempromandibular joint (TMJ). Misalignment of the hyoid can adversely affect the digestive system.

Hyoid alignment – the smiling throat of Buddha

When directing students to move their heads in a posture, teachers often tell students to lift or tuck their chin. This can inadvertently compress or tighten the tempromandibular joints. Alignment of the head is best achieved by moving the head not from the chin but from the neck, and, more specifically, from the hyoid bone.

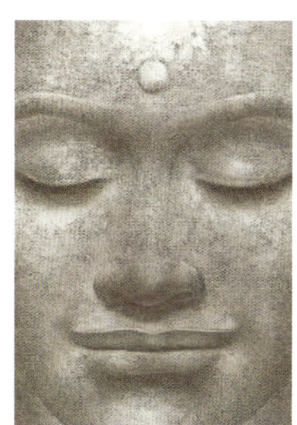

The hyoid bone is aligned by the same muscular action that creates a soft, subtle smile, one that mimics the smile we see depicted on images of Buddha and on the Mona Lisa. Hyoid bone alignment has been referred to as *the smiling throat.* Draw the hyoid bone back and gently lift the corners of the bone up and back toward a point behind the lower ears. This action creates a small, soft smile. Big smiles of the mouth tend to engage muscles of the face and jaw and less from those of the throat. Sufferers of TMJ syndrome will benefit from practicing with a small Buddha smile.

How to move the neck

- Begin all movements of the neck by drawing the throat back. Lift the hyoid bone back and up with the *smiling throat*. This action flattens the cervical curve and increases flexibility in the cervical spine.

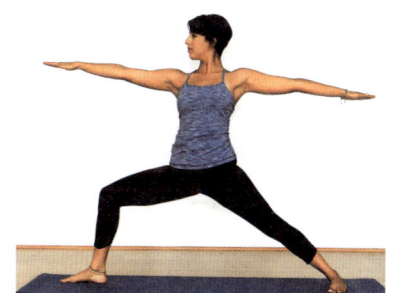

- To rotate the neck, turn from the lower ears, the level where Frankenstein's electrodes were located. This action engages the C2 (axis) vertebra.

- To flex or extend the neck, tilt from the upper ears. This action glides the occiput on the C1 vertebra (atlas).

- In **Warrior Two**, to rotate the head toward the front hand, draw the throat back and rotate from below the ear, C2.

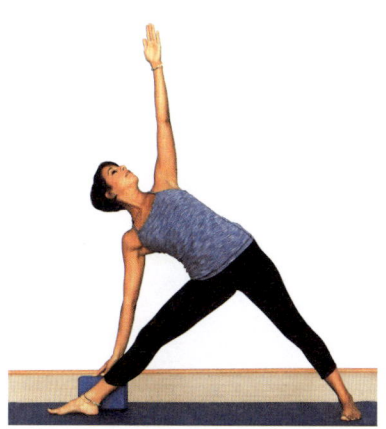

- In **Triangle Pose**, use the steps listed above for moving the neck: draw back the throat and rotate from the lower ear. An additional step can make rotation easier by opening the facet joints. After the throat is drawn back, tilt the lower ear of the pose down toward the lower shoulder before rotating the head toward the raised hand.

> **Neck movement tips**
> Draw the throat back. Turn from below ears. Flex and extend from above ears.

How to align the head

- With minimal effort, *float* the head on the neck, centered between the shoulders.
- Lift the head from the body's central axis, drawing up from the roof of the mouth (soft palate) through the back of the skull (posterior fontanel).
- Keep the eyes horizontal, deep and soft in their sockets. Eyelids remain in line with each other.
- Horizontally, align the roof of mouth (soft palate) with the ear canals.
- With a subtle "nod" that does not disturb the alignment of the roof of the mouth, lift the posterior ridge of the occiput (back of skull), as if a hand were gently lifting the hair at the nape of the neck.[2]

Therapeutic movements of the neck

The neck has nearly fifty individual vertebral movements. Techniques can be used to separately move each vertebra and determine if their mobility is normal, immobile, or hypermobile. Students can use this information to modify their neck movements and restore balance to the cervical spine. To accomplish this, we use a procedure that moves the head in a stair-step or "turtle-neck" fashion. It can be performed by oneself or with assistance.

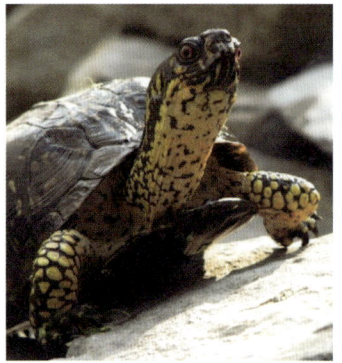

The procedure:

- Starting at the lowest vertebra of the neck, slowly move the head forward, segment-by-segment, avoiding extraneous nodding motions. This action has a "stair-climbing" feel.

- At each step between the vertebrae, move the head in a side-to-side, figure-eight motion. Figure-eight movements shear across each vertebral facet surface in all directions of motion. Keep the face moving forward as it glides without adding extraneous tipping, rotation or nodding movements.

- Move the head slowly and meticulously to access each subtle motion.

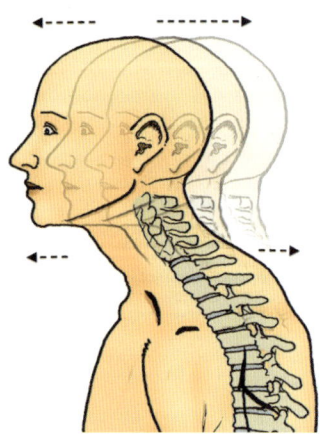

- Be aware of any vertebrae that feel "stuck" where movement is unable to smoothly step to the next segment. If a stuck section is found, continue to go back over that section, repeating the figure-eight movement until the missing joint motions become fluidly joined with the rest.

- Notice any segments that tend to "jump" over a step without engaging. In this situation, remain at that spot and slowly figure-eight until some isolated movement can be felt. The sensation is best described as "catching an edge". With patience and precision, this procedure can be very effective.

- If this procedure is performed with an assistant, the student lies supine and remains completely passive. The assistant gently stair-steps the head, keeping the face flat to the ceiling. The assistant performs the same procedure of figure-eight rocking as described for the self-administered procedure.

Easy on the eyes

As mentioned earlier, some students habitually move their eyes before engaging any other body part. This behavior constrains the upper thoracic spine and keeps it from fully participating in the pose. A useful instruction is to think of the eyes as being located on the upper, inner chest and to "look" first from those eyes and let the head and neck simply "go along for the ride".

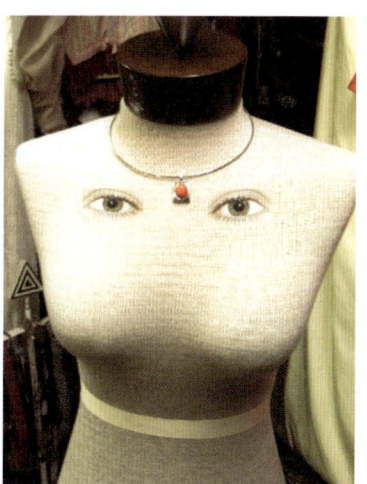

In some yoga traditions, students are taught to keep their eyes deep in the sockets, maintaining a soft passive gaze. This encourages students to take in the world, instead of forcing themselves onto it. This introspective point of view is not only a valuable metaphor for how to approach life but also prevents the eyes from dominating the initial movements of asana.

Using an eye pillow for Savasana

The eyes are delicate organs. They are filled with fluid, and changes of pressure within eyeballs can increase stress on the retinas and lenses. In the presence of any eye disease that increases ocular fluid pressure, such as glaucoma, it is important to be cautious when placing direct pressure on the eyes. Pressure on the eyeballs can also stimulate the 5th and 10th cranial nerves to lower cardiac pulse rate. This phenomenon, called *oculocardiac reflex*, is calming to the body. An eye pillow can stimulate this response and is appropriate if no pre-existing eye pressure conditions are present.

That's it! You made it! Congratulations!

If you started from the beginning of the book and ended up here, you made it through material amassed over thirty years of study and condensed into this one text. There were many details presented so I hope you have been compassionate with yourself and trusting in the fact that most learning comes by doing. In a surprisingly short amount of time, most of this material will seem second nature.

My hope is that you will continue on your studies and application of alignment to asana practice with ceaseless and rigorous dedication. When in doubt about a particular detail concerning alignment, come back to the book as a reference to make it more clear and refined. Better yet, go back to page one and begin a second reading!

My intention in writing this book has been to share information that will help you pursue your yoga practice as a life-long experience that will provide you with better health and increased wellbeing. The information in this book will support you on that journey.

Namasté

Steven Weiss, MS, DC, RYT

Footnotes and References

Chapter 1
1. "Yoga in America" Market Study." *Yoga Journal*, Feb. 26, 2008.
2. "Yoga is Fastest Growing Sport in America", *Bloomberg TV*, 8/23/2010.
3. Public lecture at Omega Institute, Rhinebeck, NY. Ram Dass explains the Hindu concept that the most we can ever know of God is no more than the broad direction that the finger points. Beyond what we can see, the rest is mystery. July, 1993.
4. *Pranayama*: breath control practice that moves life force through the tissues of the body
5. Paraphrased excerpt of B.K.S. Iyengar from film, "Enlighten Up", Kate Churchill, Balcony Releasing, 2008.
6. Paraphrased excerpt of B.K.S. Iyengar from film, "Enlighten Up", Kate Churchill, Balcony Releasing, 2008.
7. "Common yoga injuries…How to Avoid Them", Herndon, James, MD, Revolution Health, 2012.

Chapter 2
1. "How Yoga Can Wreck Your Body!", Broad, William, NY Times Sunday magazine, Sheila Glaser, 2012.
2. Candace Pert, PhD, Workshop at Omega Institute, Rhinebeck, NY,1995.

Chapter 3
1. Freeman, Richard, The Mirror of Yoga, Shambhala Publications, 2010, pg. 3.

Chapter 4
1. "Highlander", Film director Russell Mulcahy, 1986.

Chapter 5
1. The concept of a universal alignment blueprint is attributed to John Friend, presented during his international national workshops from 2009-2012. More details on the blueprint are presented in Chapter 10.
2. John Friend, founder of Anusara Yoga, Universal Principles of Alignment, live at Covens Center, Miami, FL, 2010.
3. "Goldilocks and the Three Bears" was first published in 1837 by British author, Robert Southey.
4. Suzie Hurley, "Divine Play of Anusara", Garden of the Heart Yoga Center, Sarasota, FL, July, 2011.
5. The periphery of the body moves faster than at the core. This concept is frequently presented in Anusara yoga classes and workshops.
6. Concept presented by B.K.S. Iyengar. John Friend formulated a similar set of principles using the terms "Muscular energy and Organic energy".

Chapter 6
1. "Form Follows Function", Attributed to American architect Louis Sullivan,1896- Wikipedia online.
2. Robin, Mel, <u>A Physiological Handbook for Teachers of Yogasana</u>, Fenestra Books, 2002.

Chapter 7
1. Robin, Mel, <u>A Physiological Handbook for Teachers of Yogasana</u>, Fenestra Books, 2002, pg. 273.
2. Eighty to ninety percent of the body's connective tissue consists of these four main types. There are numerous variations in these classifications and the percentages vary.
3. Robin, Mel, <u>A Physiological Handbook for Teachers of Yogasana</u>, Fenestra Books, 2002, pg. 275.
4. Robin, Mel, <u>A Physiological Handbook for Teachers of Yogasana</u>, Fenestra Books, 2002, pg. 173-274.
5. Robin, Mel, <u>A Physiological Handbook for Teachers of Yogasana</u>, Fenestra Books, 2002. pg. 274.
6. Robin, Mel, <u>A Physiological Handbook for Teachers of Yogasana</u>, Fenestra Books, 2002, pg. 27.

Chapter 9
1. Teach PE.com, Anatomy, structure, skeletal muscle, #17.
2. Synerstretch: For Total Body Flexibility, Health for Life, 1984.
3. Robin, Mel, <u>A Physiological Handbook for Teachers of Yogasana</u>, Fenestra Books, 2002.
4. Robin, Mel, <u>A Physiological Handbook for Teachers of Yogasana</u>, Fenestra Books, 2002.
5. Norkin & Levangie, <u>Joint Structure and Function: A Comprehensive Analysis,</u>1992.
6. Carvalho et al, <u>Journal of Strength and Conditioning Research</u>, "Acute Effects Of A Warm-Up Including Active, Passive, And Dynamic Stretching On Vertical Jump Performance", 11/5/2011.
7. webmd.com/fitness-exercise/news/20110217
8. Morton et al, <u>Journal of Strength and Conditioning Research</u>, "Resistance training vs. static stretching: effects on flexibility and strength", 12/25/2011.
9. exrx.net/WeightTraining/Tidbits (internet reference).
10. Crago, P. E., Houk, J. C., and Rymer, W. Z., (1975). Influence of motor unit recruitment on tendon organ discharge. *Neuroscience Abstracts,* 1: 280.
11. Signorile, Joseph, PhD, *Bending the Aging Curve,* Human Kinetics, 2011.
12. Bass, Clarence, Carol, "Ripped", Ripped Enterprises, 2011.

Chapter 10
1. When cartilage receives blood supply, hydroxyapatite crystals form and turn it into bone. This is the mechanism for infant-to-adult development of the long bones. The jaw, clavicle, and flat bones (skull, sternum, ribs, scapula and pelvis) form directly from periosteum and do not use this system.
2. Heinegård, Dick, "Molecular Events in Cartilage Formation and Remodeling", <u>Arthritis Research</u>, Supplement A , 2001.
3. NIH Osteoporosis and Related Bone Diseases National Resource Center, "Bed Rest and Immobilization: Risk Factors for Bone Loss", 1/2012.
4. Levy et al, "Associations of Fluoride Intake with Children's Bone Measures at Age 11", <u>Community Dentistry and Oral Epidemiology</u>, 2009. Vol. 37, pg. 416-426.
5. Becker, Robert, Selden, Gary, <u>The Body Electric: Electromagnetism and the Foundation of Life,</u> William Morrow,1985.

Chapter 11

1. John Friend, Yoga Therapeutics Workshop, Miami, FL, March, 2009.
2. Christopher Baxter, "Mula and Meditation" workshop, Mandala Yoga, Sarasota, FL, 12/2011.
3. Anusara Yoga uses a system of "loops and spirals" in its depiction of the Universal Principles of Alignment. Much of the inspiration for the Alignment Grid is drawn from that model. B.K.S. Iyengar is purported to have formulated similar concepts to loops and spirals in the 1970's (Joan White). Iyengar's work, however, was considerably expanded and codified by John Friend.
4. Friend, John, Anusara Teaching Training Manual, Anusara Press, 2008.

Chapter 12

1. Education. Yahoo .com, "The Femur", Gray's Anatomy of the Human Body, 2009.
2. Sesej, Nahhas et al, "The Influence of Age at menarche on Cross-sectional Geometry of Bone in Young Adulthood", Science Direct.com, Bone, Vol 51, Issue 1, Pg.s 38-45, 2012.
3. Baxter, Christopher, "The ADC's of Core", Sarasota, FL, 1/2012.
4. Schafer, DC, R.C., Clinical Biomechanics- Musculoskeletal Actions and Reactions, Baltimore: Williams & Wilkins, 1983.
5. Woodley, Kennedy, "Anatomy in Practice: the Sacrotuberous Ligament", New Zealand Journal of Physiotherapy, Vol. 33,3, 11/2005.
6. Cole, Roger, Ph.D, "Protect the Sacroiliac Joints in Forward Bends, Twists, and Wide-Legged Poses", Yoga Journal (On-line teachers/1027).
7. Cole, Roger, Ph.D, "Protect the Sacroiliac Joints in Forward Bends, Twists, and Wide-Legged Poses", Yoga Journal (On-line teachers/1027).
8. Sacro Occipital Reasearch Society International, (Internet- our technique defined).
9. DeJarnette, Major,DC , Sacro Occipital Technique, Nebraska City, NE, 1984, pg.s Preface, 66, 95.
10. John Friend, Yoga Therapeutics Workshop, Miami, FL, March, 2009.

Chapter 13

1. This aspect of hip release is fully inspired by Anusara's *Inner Spiral*.
2. Forward tailbone scoop is fully inspired by Anusara's *Scoop the Tailbone*.
3. Schafer, DC, R.C., Clinical Biomechanics- Musculoskeletal Actions and Reactions, Baltimore: Williams & Wilkins, 1983. There are more sophisticated variations of this test used in chiropractic and orthopedic settings where eight separate points of reference are observed.
4. DeJarnette, Major,DC , Sacro Occipital Technique, Nebraska City, NE, 1984, pg.s Preface, 66, 95.
5. DeJarnette, Major,DC , Sacro Occipital Technique, Nebraska City, NE, 1984, pg.s Preface, 66, 95.

Chapter 14

1. Yoga teacher and researcher Doug Keller orientates this action from the front hips points, what are called the *anterior superior iliac spines* (ASIS). In inward hip release, the ASIS move closer together.
2. The specific location in the upper inner thighs from which the *roll in* and *spread apart* actions initiate is the lesser trochanter, a small boney prominence that juts out from the upper, medial surface of the femur bones. It is the attachment point for the iliopsoas and psoas major muscles.
3. The psoas major, along with its companion hip flexor muscles, attaches to the lesser trochanter located on the upper medial thigh. More about the psoas major muscle and its importance to structural alignment is presented in chapter 26.
4. Offering another approach, yoga teacher and author Richard Freeman describes the action of *forward tailbone scoop* as lifting the second sacral segment towards the navel. Doug Keller follows his own methodology for creating an action similar to *forward tailbone scoop* by advising students to *spread* the two ASIS away from the midline.

Chapter 15
1. The bottom tip of the breastbone forms a tail-like structure called the xiphoid process. In CPR classes, the xiphoid process is identified as the place to avoid when performing chest percussion as it can break off and puncture the liver underneath.
2. A detailed review of the anatomy and structural mechanics of the rib cage and the thoracic spine is presented in Chapter 28.

Chapter 16
1. A simple reflection of a phrase offered by Anusara yoga teacher Sianna Sherman in workshop, Feb 2007 Sarasota, FL.

Chapter 17
1. The major hip ligament is the "Y" ligament, which consists of three parts: iliofemoral, pubofermoral, and ischiofermoral. The ligamentum teres, another femoral ligament, attaches to the femur head, offers minor additional support, and, from the ligament's hollow core, brings arterial supply to femur head.
2. A minor ligament, the iliotrochanteric, responds with the opposite action.

Chapter 18
1. Calais-Germain, Blandine. Anatomy of Movement, Eastland Press, 1993.
2. This stretch resembles Gaenslen's test, an orthopedic examination procedure that evaluates the stability of the sacroiliac joints. Forward tailbone scoop protects the sacroiliac joints from sprain while stretching the iliopsoas and extending the hip.
3. Morton et al, Journal of Strength and Conditioning Research, "Resistance training vs. static stretching: effects on flexibility and strength", 12/25/2011.

Chapter 19
1. *Shins in-Thighs apart* is a term commonly used in Anusara Yoga.
2. Numerous muscles are involved in *Thighs apart*: the gluteus maximus and medius, tensa fascia lata, and the adductor group.
3. Kapangji, I.A., The Physiology of the Joints, Volumes 1-3. NY: Church Livingston, 1982.
4. Draganich-LF; Jaeger-RJ; Kralj-AR Department of Surgery, University of Chicago
5. Baratta et al, "Muscular coactivation. The role of the antagonist musculature in maintaining knee stability", American Journal of Sports Medicine, 1988, pgs. 113-122.

Chapter 20
1. en.wikipedia.org/wiki/Ham
2. Dictionary.com
3. Woodley, Kennedy, "Anatomy in Practice: the Sacrotuberous Ligament", New Zealand Journal of Physiotherapy, Vol. 33,3, 11/2005.
4. John Friend, Anusara therapeutics workshop, Miami, 2007.

Chapter 21
1. The TFL "locks" the knee in full extension and laterally rotates it when in flexion.
2. American Academy of orthopedic surgeons, (internet- OrthoInfo), 2007.
3. Additional support and alignment is provided by the patella via the menisco-patellar ligament
4. Numerous smaller ligaments attach to the knee, its menisci and the patella and can be a common source of pain. In cases where knee pain cannot be isolated to the cruciates or the collaterals, these smaller tissues merit evaluation.

5. Lateral muscles: iliotibial band, biceps femoris (primarily the long head). Medial muscles: gracilis, sartorius, semimembranosus, semitendinosus. bi-lateral muscles: quadriceps (these fibers attach to both collateral ligaments).
6. The angle used to measure tibial torsion is that created by a line drawn from the knee to the back outside ankle with the leg in neutral position, neither flexed nor bent, and the femur centered over the knee.
7. Bursas are small pads between tendons that serve as spacers and prevent tendons from rubbing against each other and causing irritation.
8. Tuckerman et al, "Outcomes of meniscal repair: minimum of 2-year follow-up", Bull Hospital of Joint Diseases, NYU-Hospital for Joint Diseases Department of Orthopaedic Surgery.

Chapter 22
1. Kapangji, I.A., The Physiology of the Joints, Volume Two, NY: Church Livingston, 1982, pgs. 136-150.
2. Anusara Yoga instructors refer to this action as the *calf loop*.
3. Kapangji, I.A., The Physiology of the Joints, Volume Two, NY: Church Livingston, 1982, pgs. 136-150.
4. Deltoid refers to a type of quadrilateral shape, similar in shape to a *leaf*. In the body, there exists the deltoid muscle of the shoulder, the deltoid of the hip (the joined portion of the gluteus maximus and the TFL) and the deltoid ligament of the ankle.
5. American Academy of Orthopaedic Surgeons; American Orthopaedic Foot and Ankle Society, ©1995-2012.

Chapter 24
1. Kapangji, I.A., The Physiology of the Joints, Volume 3. NY: Church Livingston, 1982, pg. 20. According to the Dlema Index, resistance to axial compression on a column is directly proportional to the square of the number of curvatures plus one.
2. Shamji, Mohammed, Phd, "Surprising Find May Yield New Avenue of Treatment for Painful Herniated Discs", Duke Medicine News and Communications, DukeHealth.org, 6/2010.
3. Kapangji, I.A., The Physiology of the Joints, Volume Three, NY: Church Livingston, 1982, pg.. 108.
4. Sato et al, "In Vivo Intradiscal Pressure Measurement in Healthy Individuals and in Patients With Ongoing Back Problems", Spine, Volume 24, number 23, 1999, pg.s. 2468-2474. Breath retention may help initiate the Valsalva effect but should not continue while postures are being performed. Breath retention is best utilized while in sitting or lying postures, the usual positions for pranayama.
5. Kapangji, I.A., The Physiology of the Joints, Volume Two, NY: Church Livingston, 1982, pg. 170-185.
6. Being able to evaluate all 336 subtle, segmental movements may seem like an overwhelming task, however it is a skill, readily learned, and the day-to-day practice of a chiropractor.

Chapter 25
1. "Chartbook on Trends in the Health of Americans 2006, Special Feature: Pain", National Centers for Health Statistics.
2. Vallfors B. "Acute, Subacute and Chronic Low Back Pain: Clinical Symptoms, Absenteeism and Working Environment". Scan J Rehab Med Suppl 1985,11: 1-98.
3. Kapangji, I.A., The Physiology of the Joints, Vol. Three, NY: Church Livingston, 1982, pg. 126.

Chapter 27
1. Koch, Liz "The psoas is NOT a hip flexor", Pilates Digest (internet source), 9/8/2009.

Chapter 28
1. Kapangji, I.A., The Physiology of the Joints, Volume 3, NY: Church Livingston, 1982, pg 132.

Chapter 29

1. Kapangji, I.A., The Physiology of the Joints, Vol 3, NY: Church Livingston, 1982, pg. 146-161.
2. Kapangji, I.A., The Physiology of the Joints, Volume 3, NY: Church Livingston, 1982, pg. 148.
3. Kapangji, I.A., The Physiology of the Joints, Volume 3, NY: Church Livingston, 1982, pg. 150.
4. Kolar et al, "Stabilizing function of the diaphragm: dynamic MRI and synchronized spirometric assessment", Journal of Applied Physiology, 109:1064-1071, 2010.
5. Douillard, John, DC, PhD, "The Invincible Athlete", Workshop, Westport CT, 1991.
6. Douillard, John, DC, PhD, "The Invincible Athlete", Workshop, Westport CT, 1991.
7. Raman, MD, Krishna, A Matter of Health, Integration of Yoga and Western Medicine for Prevention and Cure. Madras, India: Eastwest Books, 1998.
8. Ornish, Dean, MD, Program for Reversing Heart Disease, Mass Paperback Books, 1996.
9. Freeman, Richard, Omega Institute Workshop - Astanga Flow, 1998. Richard Freeman describes hatha yoga as the general term for the physical forms of yoga. "Ha" means sun and "tha" means moon. Hatha joins together and interpenetrates these two opposite patterns, awakening the kundalini (energy serpent) of the body.
10. Freeman, Richard, Yoga Breathing, Shambala Press, 2002.
11. A pelvic floor exercise named after Arnold Kegel, MD thought to improve prolapse and muscular weakness in various genital, urinary and uterine conditions. Engaging Mula bandha may help in cases of prostatitis or incontinence.
12. The floor of the pelvis (perinium) contains the vestigial musculature of tail wagging. Engaging Mula bandha and may trigger a phantom energy, perhaps stirring up archetypal body "memories" for the yogi.

Chapter 30

1. Kapangji, I.A., The Physiology of the Joints, Vol 1, NY: Church Livingston, 1982, pg. 60-65
2. Kapangji, I.A., The Physiology of the Joints, Vol 1, NY: Church Livingston, 1982, pg. 44-52.
3. Kapangji, I.A., The Physiology of the Joints, Vol 1, NY: Church Livingston, 1982, pg. 38-42
4. Kapangji, I.A., The Physiology of the Joints, Vol 1, NY: Church Livingston, 1982, pg. 38-42
5. Duncan et al, "Incidence, Recovery, and Management of Serratus Anterior Muscle Palsy after Axillary Node Dissection", Physical Therapy, Vol 63 /Number 8, August 1983, pgs. 1243-7.
6. American Academy of Orthopaedic Surgeons, 2006 Common Shoulder Injuries, topic A00327

Chapter 32

1. White, Joan, Iyengar Yoga workshop, Omega Institute for Holistic Studies, Rhinebeck, NY, July 2009.

Chapter 33

1. Kapangji, I.A., The Physiology of the Joints, Volume 1, NY: Church Livingston, 1982, pg. 164.
2. Kapangji, I.A., The Physiology of the Joints, Volume 2, NY: Church Livingston, 1982, pg. 134.
3. deKrom MC, Kester AD, Knipschild PG, "Risk factors for carpal tunnel syndrome". American Journal of Epidemiology. Dec 1990; 132(6) 1102-10. Medscape Research.
4. Miller, BK, "Carpal tunnel syndrome: a frequently misdiagnosed common hand problem", Nurse Practitioner. ASU, Tempe College of Nursing, 1993 Dec:18(12):52-6.

Chapter 34

1. John Friend, Anusara Therapeutics workshop, Tuscon, AZ 2007.
2. Anusara yoga teachers refer to this action as *skull loop*.

Additional source material:

Draganich-LF; Jaeger-RJ; Kralj-AR Department of Surgery, University of Chicago

Dimon, Jr., Theodore, Anatomy of the Moving Body. Berkeley, CA: North Atlantic Books, 2001.

Earle, Roger, Baechle, Thomas, NSCA's Essentials of Personal training, National Strength and Conditioning Commission, Human Kinetics, 2004.

Earle, Roger, Baechle, Thomas, Essentials of Strength Training and Conditioning Human Kinetics, 2000.

ExRx.net. "Weight Training Glossary". (Online) http://www.exrx.net/WeightTraining/Glossary.html#anchor1279833.

Freeman, Richard, The Mirror of Yoga, Shambhala Publications, 2010.

Friend, John, Anusara Yoga-Therapy Training Manual, Tucson, AZ, 1007.

Friend, John, Anusara Therapeutic and Alignment trainings, personal notes, 2004-2008.

Iyengar, BKS, Tree of Yoga Shambhala Pubilcations, Boston 1988.

Iyengar, B.K.S., Light on Yoga- British Edition. London: Thorsons, 2001.

Iyengar, B.K.S., Light on Life. USA: Rodale Press, 2005.

Keller, Doug, Anusara Yoga, Hatha Yoga in the Anusara Style. VA: DoYoga Productions, 2001.

Keller, Doug, Yoga as Therapy. VA: DoYoga Productions, 2004.

Schafer, DC, R.C., Clinical Biomechanics- Musculoskeletal Actions and Reactions, Baltimore: Williams & Wilkins, 1983.

The Body Worker. "Anatomy and Kinesiology". (Online) http://www.thebodyworker.com/muscleslegchart.htm.

University of Washington. "Musculoskeletal Atlas". (Online) http://depts.washington.edu/ventures/UW_Technology.

Wells, Katharine, Luttgens, Kathryn, Kinesiology- Scientific Basis of Human Motion. Philadelphia: W.B. Saunders Company, 1976.

http://education.yahoo.com/reference/gray/subjects/subject/57

http://education.yahoo.com/reference/gray/subjects/subject/59

Photographic Acknowledgements

Preface	Cart at Mae Taeng, Thomas Kriese, 2010, Wikimedia Commons
Introduction	Hindu Om Symbol, 2008, Wikimedia Commons
Chapter 1	B.K.S. Iyengar, Mutt Lunker, 2008, Wikimedia Commons
Chapter 2	Siddhasana, Mirzolot2, Yoga, art and science, Wikimedia Commons
Chapter 3	Fire- P3200034, Jgisbert, MorgueFile
Chapter 4	Larus Canus , Nyman, Bengt, Stockholm, 2010, Wikimedia Commons
Chapter 5	Iceberg Baffin Island, Ansgar Walk, 2000, Wikimedia Commons
Chapter 5	Interior door hinge, Infrogmation, New Orleans, 2011, Wikimedia Common
Chapter 5	Leyland Station with train, Ben Brooksbank, 1963, Wikimedia Commons
Chapter 6	Sports fishing, US National Oceanic and Atmospheric Administration
Chapter 7	Yeti, Pandy Corina, 2007, Wikimedia Commons
Chapter 7	Bodybuilder girl, Gamer1606, 2007, Wikimedia Commons
Chapter 9	Overspagat, 2006, Wikimedia Commons
Chapter 11	Lock Nr.9 - Moskva River, A. Savin, 2011, Wikimedia Commons
Chapter 12	Gears DCS_3537, K. Connors, morgueFile
Chapter 14	Hello Kitty PEZ dispenser, Deborah Austin, 2009, Wikimedia Commons
Chapter 18	Body builder-Kevin Sperling, MCS Seaman, Eric Cutright, USN, 2007
Chapter 19	Gold Diggers of 1933, Warner Brothers "42nd Street", Wikimedia Common
Chapter 21	Two-part iron hinge, Audrius Meskauskas, 2006, Wikimedia Commons
Chapter 21	Joni Mitchell, Paul C Babin, Whoknoze, 1974, Wikimedia Commons
Chapter 22	Left ankle sprain, Hildgrim, 2006, Wikimedia Commons
Chapter 24	Scoliosis patient in Cheneau brace, Weiss, HR, 2007, Wikimedia Common
Chapter 24	Scoliosis Cobb Skoliose Info Forum, Germany, 2005, Wikimedia Common
Chapter 24	Scoliosis, Weiss, Goodall, BioMed Central, Ltd, 2008, Wikimedia Common

Chapter 25	Baby playing with feet, Anita Peppers, morgueFile
Chapter 26	Big Butts, Alias 0591- Netherlands, 2009, Wikimedia Commons
Chapter 26	IMG_7278 springs, morgueFile
Chapter 29	Exhausted runner, Mary K Baird, 2007, morgueFile
Chapter 29	Throat, Creative Commons Attribution-Share, Wikimedia Commons
Chapter 29	Heart, Idhayam, 2005, Wikimedia Commons
Chapter 29	Parrot cartoon-1872, Lear, Edward, Wikimedia Commons
Chapter 29	Hindi-Yoga darshan parmarthik trust, 2011, Wikimedia Commons
Chapter 29	Siddhasana, Mirzolot2, Yoga, art and science, Wikimedia Commons
Chapter 30	Right Scapula, Body Pts 3D Anatomography, 2012, Wikimedia Commons
Chapter 30	Tabattoo II, Lauren Liston, 2012, Wikimedia Commons
Chapter 31	Fulcrum, P., S. Foresman, #2010061110041093 Wikipedia Foundation
Chapter 32	Biceps Pearson S. Foresman, #2010061110041093, Wikipedia Foundation
Chapter 32	Ta-da! Dombrowski, Quinn, Russavia, 2011, Wikimedia Commons
Chapter 33	Sarah Beth Briggs (piano), Clive Barda, OTRS #2011070810011038, 2010
Chapter 34	Buddha, Kittyela_P1000528_h, morgueFile
Chapter 34	Turtle IMG_2142, morgueFile
Chapter 34	mf118, Jeotocski, 2007, morgueFile
Chapter 34	Auge (Eye)- 1983, Leviathan, Wikimedia Commons- 2009.

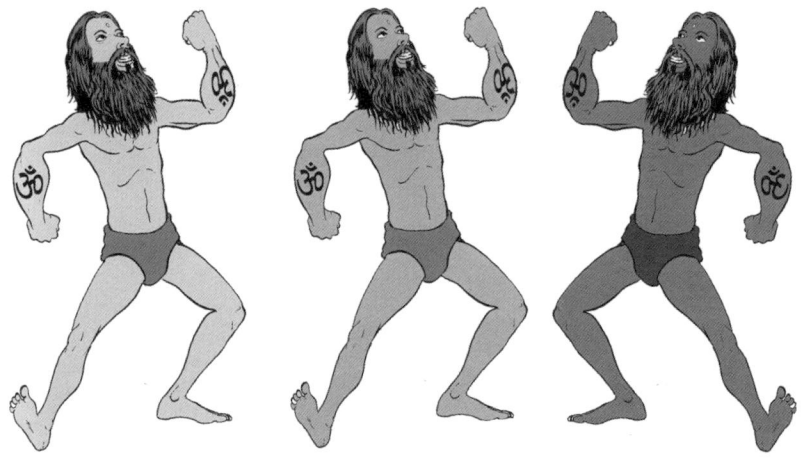

Acknowledgements

I am grateful to the many people whose expertise and support has been invaluable to the creation of "The Injury-Free Yoga Practice".

I wish first to acknowledge the teachers that I have studied with directly, who have guided my practice and professional development over thirty-years. Some inspired my personal growth and yoga practice, while others shared information that influenced the direction of this book. The most notable are Joan White, Kofi Busia, Glenn Black, Betsey Downing, Jaye Martin, John Friend, Doug Keller, and Christopher Baxter. I am particularly grateful to Jaye Martin, who has been my weekly instructor for the past twelve years. I treasure his exceptional ability to impart his knowledge of alignment in a clear, accessible fashion. Jaye also appears as a model for many of the photographs in this book, especially on the cover.

Special appreciation to BKS Iyengar and John Friend for their inspiring teachings and groundbreaking approaches to alignment-based asana.

A special thank you to the Omega Institute for Holistic Studies in Rhinebeck, New York. Being on staff for seventeen years as a wellness practitioner and yoga teaching faculty introduced me to many great teachers and provided a unique opportunity to explore my craft.

Thanks to Christin Neisler, who gracefully modeled for many of the photographs.

Many thanks go to Walter Fritz for his photography and photo enhancements. Thanks to Cheryl Chaffee at Garden of the Heat Yoga for use of her studio space.

I appreciate Ben Schikowitz for the skillful and creative illustrations featured in this book. Ben's abilities and willingness to work under a tight deadline was much appreciated. I am honored to have his work centrally featured in *The Injury-Free Yoga Practice.*

I have deep appreciation for Esther Veltheim, who has been a constant support throughout the development of the book. Esther provided editing, proofreading, photography and equipment, referrals and a steady stream of creative suggestions. Much gratitude is given to Esther in the creation of this book. Thanks also to the International BodyTalk Association for their support.

To Debra Gitterman, the primary editor and all around wordsmith, for her patience and professionalism and for being a voice of reason in leading us through the arduous editing process.

To Ronni Geist for the style and formatting set up, her editing skills and advice. To Cliff Berry for his cover design and formatting assistance. To Carol Weiss, for graphic design and photographic assistance. To my son, Joshua Nodiff, for his photo studio work and helping to make sense out of Word for Mac!

To William Wohlsifer, Esq. for his legal advice and friendship.

Thank you, all!

About the author:

Steven Weiss has 32 years experience as a holistic chiropractor and nutritionist. Dr. Weiss teaches anatomy, alignment principles, yoga therapeutics and nutrition for yoga teacher trainings around the United States and Asia. He spent seventeen years as resident faculty at the Omega Institute for Holistic Studies in Rhinebeck, New York. Steven's teaching is a unique, hands-on approach that incorporates skills from his background. Dr. Weiss also serves as a chiropractic college post-graduate instructor and member of the International Association of Yoga Therapists. More information can be found at AlignByDesignYoga.com on the web or at FaceBook.

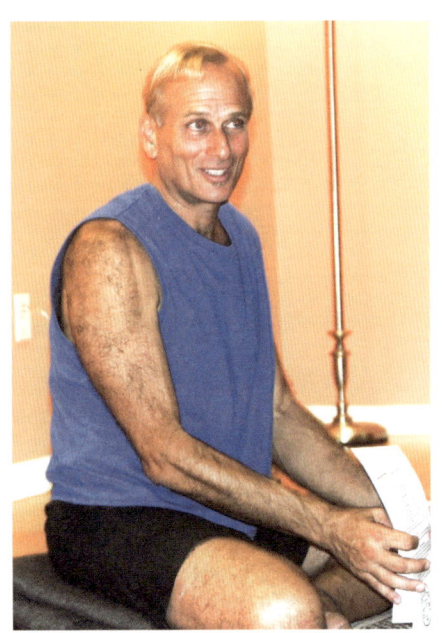

About the Illustrator:

Ben Schikowitz a self-taught artist, drummer and massage therapist. He comes from Prince Edward Island, Canada. Ben has worked at the Omega Institute for Holistic studies in Rhinebeck, New York for many years, supervising the campus art studio and teaching classes. While there, Ben had the great fortune to study Bodytuning® and Yoga with Glenn Black. Ben studied art with visionary greats such as Alex and Alllyson Grey, Robert Venosa and Martina Hoffman, and Laurence Caruana. Ben currently lives in Chapel Hill NC where he practices art and massage. Ben can be contacted through FaceBook at Benjamin John Schikowitz.

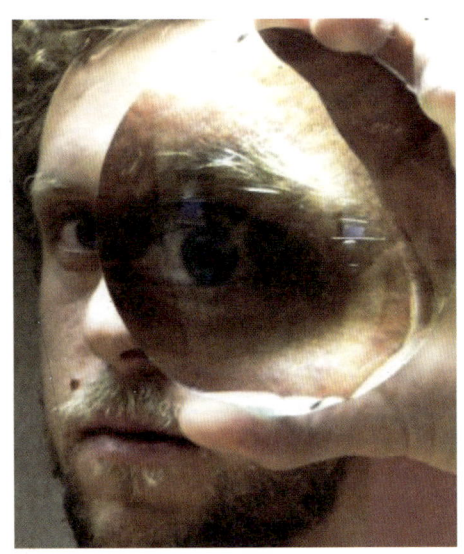